Diffuse Lung Disease

Editor

JEFFREY P. KANNE

RADIOLOGIC CLINICS
OF NORTH AMERICA

www.radiologic.theclinics.com

Consulting Editor
FRANK H. MILLER

November 2016 • Volume 54 • Number 6

ELSEVIER

1600 John F. Kennedy Boulevard • Suite 1800 • Philadelphia, Pennsylvania, 19103-2899

http://www.theclinics.com

RADIOLOGIC CLINICS OF NORTH AMERICA Volume 54, Number 6
November 2016 ISSN 0033-8389, ISBN 13: 978-0-323-47693-5

Editor: John Vassallo (j.vassallo@elsevier.com)
Developmental Editor: Donald Mumford

Radiologic Clinics of North America (ISSN 0033-8389) is published bimonthly by Elsevier Inc., 360 Park Avenue South, New York, NY 10010-1710. Months of issue are January, March, May, July, September, and November. Periodicals postage paid at New York, NY and additional mailing offices. Subscription prices are USD 460 per year for US individuals, USD 784 per year for US institutions, USD 100 per year for US students and residents, USD 535 per year for Canadian individuals, USD 1002 per year for Canadian institutions, USD 660 per year for international individuals, USD 1002 per year for international institutions, and USD 315 per year for Canadian and international students/residents. To receive student and resident rate, orders must be accompanied by name of affiliated institution, date of term and the signature of program/residency coordinator on institution letterhead. Orders will be billed at individual rate until proof of status is received. Foreign air speed delivery is included in all *Clinics* subscription prices. All prices are subject to change without notice. **POSTMASTER:** Send address changes to *Radiologic Clinics of North America*, Elsevier Health Sciences Division, Subscription Customer Service, 3251 Riverport Lane, Maryland Heights, MO63043. **Customer Service: Telephone: 1-800-654-2452** (U.S. and Canada); **1-314-447-8871** (outside U.S. and Canada). **Fax: 1-314-447-8029. E-mail: journalscustomerservice-usa@ elsevier.com (for print support); journalsonlinesupport-usa@elsevier.com (for online support)**.

Reprints. For copies of 100 or more of articles in this publication, please contact the Commercial Reprints Department, Elsevier Inc., 360 Park Avenue South, New York, New York 10010-1710. Tel.: +1-212-633-3874; Fax: +1-212-633-3820; E-mail: reprints@elsevier.com.

Radiologic Clinics of North America also published in Greek Paschalidis Medical Publications, Athens, Greece.

Radiologic Clinics of North America is covered in *MEDLINE/PubMed (Index Medicus), EMBASE/Excerpta Medica, Current Contents/Life Sciences, Current Contents/Clinical Medicine, RSNA Index to Imaging Literature, BIOSIS, Science Citation Index,* and *ISI/BIOMED.*

Contributors

CONSULTING EDITOR

FRANK H. MILLER, MD
Chief, Body Imaging Section and Fellowship
Program; Medical Director of MRI; Professor,
Department of Radiology, Northwestern
University Feinberg School of Medicine,
Chicago, Illinois

EDITOR

JEFFREY P. KANNE, MD
Professor and Chief of Thoracic Imaging, Vice
Chair of Quality and Safety, Department of
Radiology, University of Wisconsin School of
Medicine and Public Health, Madison,
Wisconsin

AUTHORS

AYODEJI ADEGUNSOYE, MD
Department of Pathology, The University of
Chicago, Chicago, Illinois

JITESH AHUJA, MD
Acting Instructor, Department of Radiology,
University of Washington, Seattle, Washington

DEEPIKA ARORA, MD
Division of Rhematology, Multicare Health
System, Tacoma, Washington

JOSEPH AZOK, MD
Section of Thoracic Imaging, Imaging Institute,
Cleveland Clinic, Cleveland, Ohio

ABIGAIL V. BERNIKER, MD
Cardiothoracic Clinical Fellow, Department of
Radiology and Biomedical Imaging, University
of California, San Francisco, San Francisco,
California

BRETT W. CARTER, MD
Department of Diagnostic Radiology,
University of Texas MD Anderson Cancer
Center, Houston, Texas

ALICIA M. CASEY, MD
Co-Director of Interstitial Lung Disease
Program, Pulmonary Division, Department
of Medicine, Boston Children's Hospital,
Harvard Medical School, Boston,
Massachusetts

JAY CHAMPLIN, MD
Department of Radiology, University of
Washington, Seattle, Washington

JONATHAN H. CHUNG, MD
Department of Radiology, The University of
Chicago, Chicago, Illinois

PHUONG-ANH T. DUONG, MD
Department of Radiology and Imaging
Sciences, Emory University Hospital, Emory
University School of Medicine, Atlanta,
Georgia

RACHAEL EDWARDS, MD
Department of Radiology, University of
Washington, Seattle, Washington

BRETT M. ELICKER, MD
Associate Professor of Clinical Radiology;
Chief, Cardiac and Pulmonary Imaging
Section, Department of Radiology and
Biomedical Imaging, University of California,
San Francisco, San Francisco, California

CAROL FARVER, MD
Department of Pathology, Cleveland Clinic,
Cleveland, Ohio

MARTHA P. FISHMAN, MD
Co-Director of Interstitial Lung Disease
Program, Pulmonary Division, Assistant
Professor, Department of Medicine, Boston
Children's Hospital, Harvard Medical School,
Boston, Massachusetts

CHRISTOPHER J. FRANÇOIS, MD
Associate Professor, Department of Radiology,
University of Wisconsin, Madison, Madison,
Wisconsin

JAMES A. FRANK, MD
Professor of Medicine, Division of Pulmonary,
Critical Care, Allergy and Sleep, San Francisco
VA Medical Center, San Francisco, California

TERI J. FRANKS, MD
Senior Pulmonary and Mediastinal Pathologist,
Department of Defense, Defense Health
Agency, Joint Pathology Center, Silver Spring,
Maryland

JEFFREY R. GALVIN, MD
Professor of Radiology and Internal Medicine,
Department of Diagnostic Radiology and
Nuclear Medicine, University of Maryland
School of Medicine, Baltimore, Maryland; Chief
of Thoracic Imaging, Department of Thoracic
Radiology, American Institute for Radiologic
Pathology, Silver Spring, Maryland

SUBHA GHOSH, MD
Section of Thoracic Imaging, Imaging Institute,
Cleveland Clinic, Cleveland, Ohio

MATTHEW D. GILMAN, MD
Department of Radiology, Massachusetts
General Hospital, Boston, Massachusetts

J. DAVID GODWIN, MD
Professor, Department of Radiology, University
of Washington, Seattle, Washington

TRAVIS S. HENRY, MD
Assistant Professor of Clinical Radiology,
Cardiac and Pulmonary Imaging Section;
Director, Cardiothoracic Imaging Fellowship;
Department of Radiology and Biomedical
Imaging, University of California, San
Francisco, San Francisco, California

ALIYA HUSAIN, MD
Department of Pathology, The University of
Chicago, Chicago, Illinois

KIRK T. JONES, MD
Professor, Department of Pathology, University
of California, San Francisco, San Francisco,
California

JEFFREY P. KANNE, MD
Professor and Chief of Thoracic Imaging, Vice
Chair of Quality and Safety, Department of
Radiology, University of Wisconsin School of
Medicine and Public Health, Madison,
Wisconsin

SETH KLIGERMAN, MD
Associate Professor of Radiology, Department
of Diagnostic Radiology and Nuclear Medicine,
University of Maryland School of Medicine,
Baltimore, Maryland

JOANNA E. KUSMIREK, MD
Department of Radiology, Virginia
Commonwealth University, Richmond,
Virginia

EDWARD Y. LEE, MD, MPH
Chief, Division of Thoracic Imaging; Associate
Professor, Department of Radiology, Boston
Children's Hospital, Harvard Medical School,
Boston, Massachusetts

JASON LEMPEL, MD
Section of Thoracic Imaging, Imaging Institute,
Cleveland Clinic, Cleveland, Ohio

BRENT P. LITTLE, MD
Department of Radiology and Imaging
Sciences, Emory University Hospital, Emory
University School of Medicine, Atlanta, Georgia

ANDREA L. MAGEE, MD
Department of Radiology, The University of
Chicago, Chicago, Illinois

SHAMSELDEEN MAHMOUD, MD
Section of Thoracic Imaging, Imaging Institute, Cleveland Clinic, Cleveland, Ohio

MARIA DANIELA MARTIN, MD
Department of Radiology, University of Wisconsin, Madison, Wisconsin

STEVEN M. MONTNER, MD
Department of Radiology, The University of Chicago, Chicago, Illinois

DAVID M. NAEGER, MD
Associate Professor of Clinical Radiology, Department of Radiology and Biomedical Imaging, University of California, San Francisco, San Francisco, California

SUDHAKAR PIPAVATH, MBBS
Department of Radiology, University of Washington, Seattle, Washington

MELISSA PRICE, MD
Department of Radiology, Massachusetts General Hospital, Boston, Massachusetts

RAHUL D. RENAPURKAR, MD
Sections of Thoracic Imaging and Cardiovascular Imaging, Imaging Institute, Cleveland Clinic, Cleveland, Ohio

BRADLEY S. SABLOFF, MD
Department of Diagnostic Radiology, University of Texas MD Anderson Cancer Center, Houston, Texas

MARK L. SCHIEBLER, MD
Professor, Department of Radiology, University of Wisconsin, Madison, Madison, Wisconsin

PAUL G. THACKER, MD
Associate Professor of Radiology and Pediatrics, Department of Radiology and Radiological Science, Medical University of South Carolina, Charleston, South Carolina

MYLENE T. TRUONG, MD
Department of Diagnostic Radiology, University of Texas MD Anderson Cancer Center, Houston, Texas

SARA O. VARGAS, MD
Staff Pathologist; Associate Professor; Department of Pathology, Boston Children's Hospital, Harvard Medical School, Boston, Massachusetts

REKHA VIJ, MD
Department of Pulmonology and Critical Care, The University of Chicago, Chicago, Illinois

CAROL C. WU, MD
Department of Diagnostic Radiology, University of Texas MD Anderson Cancer Center, Houston, Texas

SHAMSEL DEEN MAHMOUD, MD
Center of Clinical Imaging, Imaging Institute, Cleveland Clinic, Cleveland, Ohio

MARIA DANIELA MARTIN, MD
Department of Radiology, University of Wisconsin, Madison, Wisconsin

STEVEN M. MONTNER, MD
Department of Radiology, The University of Chicago, Chicago, Illinois

DAVID M. NAEGER, MD
Associate Professor of Clinical Radiology, Department of Radiology and Biomedical Imaging, University of California, San Francisco, San Francisco, California

SUDHAKAR PIPAVATH, MBBS
Department of Radiology, University of Washington, Seattle, Washington

Massachusetts General Hospital, Boston, Massachusetts

RAHUL D. RENAPURKAR, MD
Sections of Thoracic Imaging and Cardiovascular Imaging, Imaging Institute, Cleveland Clinic, Cleveland, Ohio

BRADLEY S. SABLOFF, MD
Department of Diagnostic Radiology, University of Texas MD Anderson Cancer Center, Houston, Texas

MARK L. SCHIEBLER, MD
Professor, Department of Radiology, University of Wisconsin, Madison, Wisconsin

PAUL G. THACKER, MD
Associate Professor of Radiology and Pediatrics, Department of Radiology and Radiological Science, Medical University of South Carolina, Charleston, South Carolina

MYLENE T. TRUONG, MD
Department of Diagnostic Radiology, University of Texas MD Anderson Cancer Center, Houston, Texas

SARA O. VARGAS, MD
Pathologist, Associate Professor, Department of Pathology, Boston Children's Hospital, Harvard Medical School, Boston, Massachusetts

REXHA VU, MD
Department of Pulmonology and Critical Care, The University of Chicago, Chicago, Illinois

CAROL C. WU, MD
Department of Diagnostic Radiology, University of Texas MD Anderson Cancer Center, Houston, Texas

Contents

Idiopathic interstitial pneumonias are a heterogeneous group of diffuse lung diseases characterized by distinct clinicopathologic entities with the usual interstitial pneumonia (UIP) being the most common. The pattern of UIP can be seen in idiopathic pulmonary fibrosis (IPF) as well as in secondary causes, most commonly in connective tissue diseases. IPF is usually progressive and associated with a very poor prognosis, and newer therapies pose a risk of serious complications; therefore, diagnostic certainty is crucial. This article reviews the radiologic findings in UIP with clinical correlation and histopathologic features along with its significance for prognosis and monitoring of patients.

Connective tissue diseases (CTDs) are a heterogeneous group of conditions characterized by circulating autoantibodies and autoimmune-mediated organ damage. Common CTDs with lung manifestations are rheumatoid arthritis, scleroderma or systemic sclerosis, Sjögren syndrome, polymyositis/dermatomyositis, systemic lupus erythematosis, mixed connective tissue disease, and undifferentiated connective tissue disease. The most common histopathologic patterns of CTD-related interstitial lung disease are nonspecific interstitial pneumonia, usual interstitial pneumonia, organizing pneumonia, and lymphoid interstitial pneumonia. Drug treatment of CTDs can cause complications, including opportunistic infection.

The management of hypersensitivity pneumonitis (HP) depends on early identification of the disease process, which is complicated by its nonspecific clinical presentation in addition to variable and diverse laboratory and radiologic findings. HP is the result of exposure and sensitization to myriad aerosolized antigens. HP develops in the minority of antigenic exposures, and conversely has been documented in patients with no identifiable exposure, complicating the diagnostic algorithm significantly. Prompt diagnosis and early intervention are critical in slowing the progression of irreversible parenchymal damage, and additionally in preserving the quality of life of affected patients.

The direct toxicity of cigarette smoke and the body's subsequent response to this lung injury leads to a wide array of pathologic manifestations and disease states that lead to both reversible and irreversible injury to the large airways, small airways, alveolar walls, and alveolar spaces. These include emphysema, bronchitis, bronchiolitis, acute eosinophilic pneumonia, pulmonary Langerhans cell histiocytosis, respiratory bronchiolitis, desquamative interstitial pneumonia, and pulmonary fibrosis. Although these various forms of injury have different pathologic and imaging manifestations, they are all part of the spectrum of smoking-related diffuse parenchymal lung disease.

Childhood interstitial lung disease represents a rare and heterogeneous group of diseases that can result in significant morbidity and mortality, some leading to death during infancy. CT is the imaging test of choice. Although many CT findings are nonspecific and a definitive diagnosis usually cannot be reached by CT alone, the interpreting radiologist is instrumental in defining disease extent and refining the diagnosis. Chest CTs are of key importance in guiding site selection for lung biopsy and for following disease progression and response to treatment. Thus, from the radiologist's perspective, ensuring maximal quality of CT imaging and interpretation is paramount.

Occupational lung diseases span a variety of pulmonary disorders caused by inhalation of dusts or chemical antigens in a vocational setting. Included in these are the classic mineral pneumoconioses of silicosis, coal worker's pneumoconiosis, and asbestos-related diseases as well as many immune-mediated and airway-centric diseases, and new and emerging disorders. Although some of these have characteristic imaging appearances, a multidisciplinary approach with focus on occupational exposure history is essential to proper diagnosis.

 Video content accompanies this article at http://www.radiologic.theclinics.com.

Pulmonary vasculitis is a relatively uncommon disorder, usually manifesting as part of systemic vasculitis. Imaging, specifically computed tomography, is often performed in the initial diagnostic workup. Although the findings in vasculitis can be nonspecific, they can provide important clues in the diagnosis, and guide the clinical team toward the right diagnosis. Radiologists must have knowledge of common and uncommon imaging findings in various vasculitides. Also, radiologists should be able to integrate the clinical presentation and laboratory test findings together with imaging features, so as to provide a meaningful differential diagnosis.

Acute lung injury (ALI) is the clinical syndrome associated with histopathologic diffuse alveolar damage. It is a common cause of acute respiratory symptoms and admission to the intensive care unit. Diagnosis of ALI is typically based on clinical and radiographic criteria; however, because these criteria can be nonspecific, diagnostic uncertainty is common. A multidisciplinary approach that synthesizes clinical, imaging, and pathologic data can ensure an accurate diagnosis. Radiologists must be aware of the radiographic and computed tomographic findings of ALI and its mimics. This article discusses the multidisciplinary diagnosis of ALI from the perspective of the imager.

Multimodality, noninvasive imaging is increasingly used in the identification and management of pulmonary hypertension (PH). Chest radiography, ventilation-perfusion scintigraphy, and Doppler echocardiography are frequently the initial studies used to evaluate patients suspected of having PH. However, their ability to evaluate the right ventricle (RV) and pulmonary vasculature is limited. Computed tomography (CT) and magnetic resonance (MR) imaging are increasingly used to identify causes of PH and assess the effect of PH on RV function. This article describes the noninvasive imaging techniques and findings, particularly CT and MR imaging, used in the diagnosis and management of suspected or known PH.

Eosinophilic lung diseases encompass a broad range of conditions wherein patients present with pulmonary opacities and eosinophilia of the serum, pulmonary tissue, or bronchoalveolar lavage fluid. Many of these entities can be idiopathic or are secondary to parasitic infection, exposure to drugs, toxins, or radiation. These diseases exhibit a wide range of imaging findings, including consolidation, ground-glass opacities, nodules, and masses. Diagnoses often require bronchoalveolar lavage and/or biopsy to confirm respiratory eosinophilia and to exclude other entities, such as infection or malignancy. Treatment entails administration of corticosteroids, removal of inciting agents, and treatment of underlying infection.

Small airways diseases, or bronchiolitis, encompasses many conditions that result in bronchiolar inflammation and/or fibrosis. Bronchioles are distal airways within secondary pulmonary lobules that are only visible on imaging when abnormal. High-resolution computed tomography plays an important role in diagnosing small airways diseases. The predominant direct high-resolution computed tomography sign of bronchiolitis includes centrilobular nodules, whereas air trapping is the main indirect finding. This article reviews bronchiolar anatomy, discusses the differential diagnosis for cellular and constrictive bronchiolitis with a focus on key imaging features, and discusses how to distinguish important mimics.

Imaging of the large airways is key to the diagnosis and management of a wide variety of congenital, infectious, malignant, and inflammatory diseases. Involvement can be focal, regional, or diffuse, and abnormalities can take the form of masses, thickening, narrowing, enlargement, or a combination of patterns. Recognition of the typical morphologies, locations, and distributions of large airways disease is central to an accurate imaging differential diagnosis.

PROGRAM OBJECTIVE

The objective of the *Radiologic Clinics of North America* is to keep practicing radiologists and radiology residents up to date with current clinical practice in radiology by providing timely articles reviewing the state of the art in patient care.

TARGET AUDIENCE

Practicing radiologists, radiology residents, and other health care professionals who provide patient care utilizing radiologic findings.

LEARNING OBJECTIVES

Upon completion of this activity, participants will be able to:

1. Review imaging techniques for both small and large airway diseases.
2. Discuss updates in imaging, evaluation, and prognosis of interstitial lung disease of infants.
3. Recognize imaging techniques for diffuse lung diseases such as idiopathic pulmonary fibrosis, pulmonary hypertension, and occupational lung disease, among others.

ACCREDITATION

The Elsevier Office of Continuing Medical Education (EOCME) is accredited by the Accreditation Council for Continuing Medical Education (ACCME) to provide continuing medical education for physicians.

The EOCME designates this enduring material for a maximum of 15 *AMA PRA Category 1 Credit*(s) ™. Physicians should claim only the credit commensurate with the extent of their participation in the activity.

All other health care professionals requesting continuing education credit for this enduring material will be issued a certificate of participation.

DISCLOSURE OF CONFLICTS OF INTEREST

The EOCME assesses conflict of interest with its instructors, faculty, planners, and other individuals who are in a position to control the content of CME activities. All relevant conflicts of interest that are identified are thoroughly vetted by EOCME for fair balance, scientific objectivity, and patient care recommendations. EOCME is committed to providing its learners with CME activities that promote improvements or quality in healthcare and not a specific proprietary business or a commercial interest.

The planning committee, staff, authors and editors listed below have identified no financial relationships or relationships to products or devices they or their spouse/life partner have with commercial interest related to the content of this CME activity:

Ayodeji Adegunsoye, MD; Jitesh Ahuja, MD; Deepika Arora, MD; Joseph Azok, MD; Abigail V. Berniker, MD; Brett W. Carter, MD; Alicia M. Casey, MD; Jay Champlin, MD; Jonathan H. Chung, MD; Phuong-Anh T. Duong, MD; Rachael Edwards, MD; Brett M. Elicker, MD; Carol Farver, MD; Martha P. Fishman, MD; Anjali Fortna; Christopher J. François, MD; James A. Frank, MD; Teri J. Franks, MD; Jeffrey R. Galvin, MD; Subha Ghosh, MD; Matthew D. Gilman, MD; J. David Godwin, MD; Travis S. Henry, MD; Aliya Husain, MD; Kirk T. Jones, MD; Seth Kligerman, MD; Joanna E. Kusmirek, MD; Edward Y. Lee, MD, MPH; Jason Lempel, MD; Brent P. Little, MD; Andrea L. Magee, MD; Shamseldeen Mahmoud, MD; Maria Daniela Martin, MD; Frank H. Miller; Steven M. Montner, MD; David M. Naeger, MD; Melissa Price, MD; Rahul D. Renapurkar, MD; Bradley S. Sabloff, MD; Erin Scheckenbach; Mark L. Schiebler, MD; Karthik Subramaniam; Paul G. Thacker, MD; Mylene T. Truong, MD; Sara O. Vargas, MD; John Vassallo; Rekha Vij, MD; Carol C. Wu.

The planning committee, staff, authors and editors listed below have identified financial relationships or relationships to products or devices they or their spouse/life partner have with commercial interest related to the content of this CME activity:

Jeffrey P. Kanne, MD is a consultant/advisor for PAREXEL International Corporation and Genentech, A Member of the Roche Group.

Sudhakar Pipavath, MBBS is a consultant/advisor for Boehringer Ingelheim GmbH and Imbio.

UNAPPROVED/OFF-LABEL USE DISCLOSURE

The EOCME requires CME faculty to disclose to the participants:

1. When products or procedures being discussed are off-label, unlabelled, experimental, and/or investigational (not US Food and Drug Administration [FDA] approved); and
2. Any limitations on the information presented, such as data that are preliminary or that represent ongoing research, interim analyses, and/or unsupported opinions. Faculty may discuss information about pharmaceutical agents that is outside of FDA-approved labelling. This information is intended solely for CME and is not intended to promote off-label use of these medications. If you have any questions, contact the medical affairs department of the manufacturer for the most recent prescribing information.

TO ENROLL

To enroll in the *Radiologic Clinics of North America* Continuing Medical Education program, call customer service at 1-800-654-2452 or sign up online at http://www.theclinics.com/home/cme. The CME program is available to subscribers for an additional annual fee of USD 315.

METHOD OF PARTICIPATION

In order to claim credit, participants must complete the following:
1. Complete enrolment as indicated above.
2. Read the activity.
3. Complete the CME Test and Evaluation. Participants must achieve a score of 70% on the test. All CME Tests and Evaluations must be completed online.

CME INQUIRIES/SPECIAL NEEDS

For all CME inquiries or special needs, please contact elsevierCME@elsevier.com.

RADIOLOGIC CLINICS OF NORTH AMERICA

THE CLINICS ARE AVAILABLE ONLINE!
Access your subscription at:
www.theclinics.com

RADIOLOGIC CLINICS OF NORTH AMERICA

Preface
Diffuse White Stuff in the Lungs: Challenges and Advances

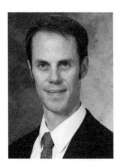

Jeffrey P. Kanne, MD
Editor

Diffuse lung disease is a challenging area of medicine for clinicians, radiologists, and pathologists. Many diffuse lung diseases are uncommon or rare, and expertise in diagnosis and treatment is limited. High-resolution computed tomography (HRCT) plays a central role in the diagnosis and management of patients with known or suspected diffuse lung disease. In some cases, HRCT findings in conjunction with clinical evaluation are sufficient to establish a high-confidence diagnosis. In others, surgical biopsy may be required as part of the evaluation. For some patients, a diagnosis is not reached until multidisciplinary review of clinical, radiologic, and pathologic data leads to a consensus, and for some patients, the consensus diagnosis may ultimately be an unclassifiable diffuse lung disease.

Recognizing characteristic HRCT appearances of certain diffuse lung diseases can greatly influence the practice of our clinical colleagues in disciplines such as pulmonology and rheumatology and affect the outcomes of our mutual patients. In some cases, accurately described and interpreted HRCT scans can obviate surgical lung biopsy. Furthermore, the radiologist may be the first to suggest the presence of a systemic illness, such as collagen vascular disease or sarcoidosis, in patients presenting with vague or nonspecific respiratory signs and symptoms. New advances in the treatment of idiopathic pulmonary fibrosis have led to increasing requests for radiologists to accurately classify the pattern of pulmonary fibrosis.

This issue of *Radiologic Clinics of North America* focuses on imaging of diffuse lung disease with a particular focus on HRCT. Each article provides a wealth of knowledge for readers regarding the spectrum of diffuse lung disease ranging from pulmonary fibrosis to occupational lung disease. The authors include up-to-date information on these constantly evolving topics and provide high-quality illustrations to help radiologists and non-radiologists alike in their clinical practices.

It is my hope that readers will build on their existing knowledge, adopt current terminology, and integrate well-established information in addition to useful tips put forth by the authors in order to provide better care to their patients. I extend my gratitude to the authors for their high-quality, thoughtful articles, which will serve our readers well.

Jeffrey P. Kanne, MD
Department of Radiology
University of Wisconsin School
of Medicine and Public Health
600 Highland Avenue
MC 3252
Madison, WI 53792-3252, USA

E-mail address:
kanne@wisc.edu

Radiol Clin N Am 54 (2016) xv
http://dx.doi.org/10.1016/j.rcl.2016.08.010
0033-8389/16/© 2016 Published by Elsevier Inc.

radiologic.theclinics.com

Imaging of Idiopathic Pulmonary Fibrosis

Joanna E. Kusmirek, MD[a],*, Maria Daniela Martin, MD[b], Jeffrey P. Kanne, MD[b]

KEYWORDS

- Idiopathic interstitial pneumonia • Idiopathic pulmonary fibrosis • Usual interstitial pneumonia
- HRCT

KEY POINTS

- High-resolution computed tomography (HRCT) findings are crucial in the multidisciplinary diagnosis of idiopathic pulmonary fibrosis (IPF).
- If the HRCT pattern is consistent with usual interstitial pneumonia (UIP) and the clinical presentation is concordant, lung biopsy is not indicated.
- Most patients with a UIP pattern on HRCT have IPF, but the pattern can also occur with connective tissue disease, asbestos exposure, and drug toxicity, so thorough clinical evaluation is necessary.
- Mimics of UIP on HRCT include nonspecific interstitial pneumonia, fibrotic hypersensitivity pneumonitis, fibrosing sarcoid, asbestosis, and drug reaction.
- HRCT carries prognostic value in IPF and plays an important role in longitudinal monitoring as well as detection of complications such as infection, acute exacerbation, and cancer.

INTRODUCTION

Idiopathic interstitial pneumonias (IIPs) include a group of diffuse parenchymal lung diseases with variety of clinicopathologic presentations. The recent classification by the American Thoracic Society (ATS)/European Respiratory Society (ERS) from 2013,[1] divides IIPs into (Box 1): (1) chronic fibrosing IIPs, including idiopathic pulmonary fibrosis (IPF) and idiopathic nonspecific interstitial pneumonia (NSIP); (2) smoking-related IIPs, including respiratory bronchiolitis–associated interstitial lung disease (RB-ILD) and desquamative interstitial pneumonia (DIP); (3) acute or subacute IIPs, including cryptogenic organizing pneumonia (COP) and acute interstitial pneumonia; and (4) rare IIPs, including lymphoid interstitial pneumonia and idiopathic pleuroparenchymal fibroelastosis.

The ATS/ERS 2013 update on IIPs also proposed a classification based on disease behavior because the IIPs represent a heterogeneous group of diseases with different prognoses[1] (Table 1).

IPF is the most common of the IIPs and is a chronic, progressive, fibrosing lung disease of unknown cause characterized by the histopathologic pattern of usual interstitial pneumonia (UIP).[2]

The prognosis is poor in most cases, with median survival ranging from 2.5 to 3.5 years.[3–5] However, progression and prognosis can be variable, and although most patients experience rapid progression, some patients remain fairly stable.[6–8] The prevalence of IPF is estimated to range from 14 to 42.7 per 100,000 in the United States, and from 1.25 to 23.4 per 100,000 in Europe; it is higher among men than women. The annual incidence is estimated at be 6.8 to 16.3 per 100,000 in the United States and 0.22 to 7.94 per 100,000 in Europe.[9–11]

Cigarette smoking is strongly associated with IPF, with up to two-thirds of patients with IPF being

Disclosures: Consultant for Parexel International, Genentech (J.P. Kanne).
[a] Department of Radiology, Virginia Commonwealth University, 1250 East Marshall Street, Richmond, VA 23298, USA; [b] Department of Radiology, University of Wisconsin, 600 Highland Avenue, Madison, WI 53792-3252, USA
* Corresponding author.
E-mail address: joanna.kusmirek@vcuhealth.org

Radiol Clin N Am 54 (2016) 997–1014
http://dx.doi.org/10.1016/j.rcl.2016.05.004
0033-8389/16/$ – see front matter © 2016 Elsevier Inc. All rights reserved.

radiologic.theclinics.com

Box 1
Classification of IIPs according to the official ATS/ERS (2013)

Chronic fibrosing IIPs

Idiopathic pulmonary fibrosis

Idiopathic nonspecific interstitial pneumonia

Smoking-related IIPs

Respiratory bronchiolitis–associated interstitial lung disease

Desquamative interstitial pneumonia

Acute or subacute IIPs

Cryptogenic organizing pneumonia

Acute interstitial pneumonia

Rare IIPs

Idiopathic lymphoid interstitial pneumonia

Idiopathic pleuroparenchymal fibroelastosis

Data from Travis WD, Costabel U, Hansell DM, et al. An official American Thoracic Society/European Respiratory Society statement: update of the international multidisciplinary classification of the idiopathic interstitial pneumonias. Am J Respir Crit Care Med 2013;188(6):733–48.

current or former smokers. No evidence of direct causation has been established; however, the highest risk of developing IPF exists for patients who have most recently quit.[12] Smoking also adversely affects survival in IPF.[13]

Table 1
Classification of IIP based on disease behavior according to the American Thoracic Society/European Respiratory Society 2013 update.

Reversible and self-limited disease	Many cases of RB-ILD
Reversible disease with risk of progression	Cellular NSIP and some fibrotic NSIP, DIP, COP
Stable with residual disease	Some fibrotic NSIP
Progressive irreversible disease with potential for stabilization	Some fibrotic NSIP
Progressive irreversible disease despite therapy	IPF, some fibrotic NSIP

Data from Travis WD, Costabel U, Hansell DM, et al. An official American Thoracic Society/European Respiratory Society statement: update of the international multidisciplinary classification of the idiopathic interstitial pneumonias. Am J Respir Crit Care Med 2013;188(6):733–48.

CLINICAL PRESENTATION

IPF should be considered in the differential diagnosis of unexplained chronic exertional dyspnea, dry cough, or both in adults, especially older patients, because the typical age of presentation is the sixth and seventh decades of life.[2] Physical examination may reveal inspiratory crackles and digital clubbing. Pulmonary function tests typically show low lung volumes with restrictive physiology and reduced carbon monoxide diffusion capacity in the lung (DLco). There are several issues that should be addressed by clinicians while evaluating patients for IPF, as listed in **Table 2**.

Gastroesophageal reflux disease (GERD) and aspiration occur frequently in patients with IPF[15,16] and are often asymptomatic.[17] Survival and functional advantage are seen in those treated for GERD as opposed to those who are not.[18] It is debated whether or not GERD contributes to the development of IPF or is an effect (possibly by altered mechanics).[17] GERD was also proposed as a causative/contributing factor to the development of acute exacerbations in IPF.[19]

IMAGING TECHNIQUE/PROTOCOLS

Pulmonary fibrosis on chest radiography most commonly manifests as reticulation and linear opacities[20] along with decreased lung volumes (**Fig. 1**). Linear opacities are nonspecific and can be seen in other conditions, including emphysema, pulmonary Langerhans cell histiocytosis, and lymphangioleiomyomatosis; however, lung volumes are preserved or increased with these diseases. When pulmonary fibrosis is suspected clinically or on chest radiographs, high-resolution computed tomography (HRCT) of the chest should be obtained (**Table 3**). Because of advances in computed tomography (CT) technology, the distinction between conventional CT and HRCT have become blurred. Current multidetector CT scanners acquire volumetric data compatible with HRCT images and allow multiplanar reformats,[21] which greatly help in evaluation, especially in assessment of honeycombing (**Fig. 2**). Volumetric CT acquisition with multidetector CT is generally preferred to noncontiguous imaging, despite slightly higher radiation exposure.[22–24] The effective radiation dose from chest CT is usually less than 5 mSv,[23] with doses of approximately 2 mSv or less readily achievable on current scanners. In the lungs, the natural high contrast between air and tissue allows low-dose HRCT imaging. Using low-dose technique and newer reconstruction algorithms, particularly iterative reconstruction (IR), can reduce the dose by up to

Table 2
Differential diagnosis/clinical correlation in suspected IPF

Clinical Question if Known/Suspected IIP	Significance	Action
History of CTD or any systemic symptoms suggestive of such	This completely alters therapy and may change prognosis in patients with UIP pattern on HRCT[14]	Check autoimmune panel
Hypersensitivity pneumonitis	Often mimics IPF; high level of certainty is required because newer therapies for IPF carry significant risk of complications and high costs	Thorough interrogation for any possible exposure and correlation with symptoms timing; may consider BAL in selected cases. The utility of sensitivity panels is questionable[2]
Asbestos, other dust, or chemical exposure	To exclude asbestos-related lung disease or other extrinsic lung injury	Correlation with possible exposure (eg, asbestos, silica, coal)
Drug exposure	To exclude drug-induced lung injury	Stop the offending medication, follow up with HRCT
Sarcoidosis	To exclude possibility of fibrosing sarcoidosis	Assessment for other systemic symptoms and additional findings
Smoking history and exposure	To exclude smoking-related lung disease or assess for coexistent injury (combined emphysema fibrosis)	Correlation with history, referral to smoking cessation program
Gastroesophageal reflux	May cause silent aspiration and progression of fibrosis	24-h pH monitoring and pH-impedance testing. Treatment even if asymptomatic
Family history	Familial fibrosis accounts for 5%–10% of cases	Early identification of affected family members

Abbreviations: BAL, bronchoalveolar lavage; CTD, connective tissue disease; HRCT, high-resolution computed tomography.

50% without loss of imaging quality.[25–29] Note that IR techniques are vendor specific and some of them carry inherent problems such as over-smoothing and long reconstruction time.[26] Prone images may help distinguish mild pulmonary fibrosis from mild dependent atelectasis (**Fig. 3**). Expiratory images are useful in differential diagnosis, because they can aid in detection of lobular

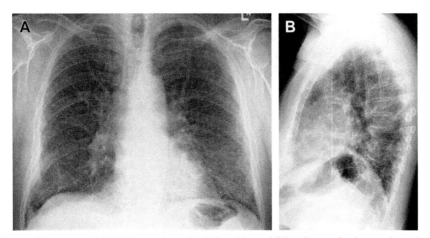

Fig. 1. A 79-year-old woman with IPF. Posteroanterior (*A*) and lateral (*B*) radiographs show volume loss and reticular opacities in the lungs bases. The findings are nonspecific, and high-resolution computed tomography (HRCT) is the examination of choice to characterize diffuse lung disease.

Table 3
Suggested parameters for CT evaluation of IIP

HRCT	Evaluation of IIP	Additional Remarks
Contrast	None	
Respiratory phase	Suspended full inspiration to total lung capacity (single breath hold 4–6 s)	Expiratory images should be considered in the initial evaluation of patients suspected of having IIP
Positioning	Supine	Prone if suspected or known asbestosis (carina through diaphragm) or suspected atelectasis
Slice thickness	1.0–1.25	
Slice Interval	0.625–1.25 mm	
Dose	Use ALARA standards	
mAs	Recommend using AEC to target effective dose <4 mSv AEC	80 mAs or less is sufficient for most patients, except for those who are very obese
Kilovoltage Peak (kV)	100–140	100 for small adults and 140 for large adults
Reconstructions	Soft tissue High spatial frequency Coronal and sagittal reformations Axial MIPs (optional)	

Abbreviations: AEC, automatic exposure control; ALARA, as low as reasonably achievable; MIP, maximum intensity projection.
Data from Refs.[21,30,31]

air trapping, a finding that is more associated with hypersensitivity pneumonitis (HP) and connective tissue disease (CTD) than IPF.

COMPUTED TOMOGRAPHY IMAGING FINDINGS

The primary role of HRCT is to distinguish chronic fibrosing lung diseases with a UIP pattern from those with non-UIP pattern and to suggest an alternative diagnosis when possible.[32] In the appropriate clinical setting, the presence of a definite UIP pattern on HRCT is sufficient to establish a diagnosis of IPF without performing a surgical lung biopsy because the likelihood of histopathologic UIP being present exceeds 95%. The characteristic HRCT features of UIP are:

1. Subpleural and basilar distribution
2. Reticulation
3. Honeycombing
4. Ground-glass opacity absent or less extensive than reticulation
5. Traction bronchiectasis (common but not a requirement)
6. Architectural distortion and volume loss

Distribution

Up to 30% of patients with histopathologic UIP can have upper lobe predominant pulmonary

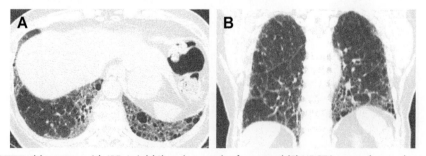

Fig. 2. A 79-year-old woman with IPF. Axial (A) and coronal reformatted (B) HRCT images show volume loss, architectural distortion, subpleural and basal predominant reticulation, traction bronchiectasis, and mild honeycombing.

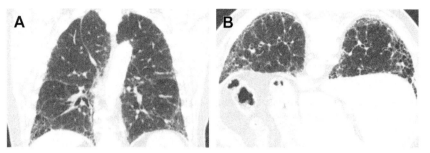

Fig. 3. An 81-year-old man with IPF. Coronal reformatted HRCT image (*A*) shows subpleural and basal predominant reticulation and honeycombing. Prone image (*B*) shows peripheral reticulation and honeycombing.

fibrosis, which strongly suggests chronic HP (**Fig. 4**).[33] In contrast, more than 90% of patients with IPF have a subpleural predominant distribution of fibrosis; central predominance is highly suggestive of an alternative fibrotic lung disease. As the disease progresses, it often seems to creep up the periphery of the lung.

Reticulation

Reticular abnormality refers to a fine network of lines, most commonly associated with architectural distortion.[33] According to Hunninghake,[34] the presence of subpleural lines in the upper lobes is also suggestive of a UIP pattern when other findings are present. Gruden and colleagues[35] suggest that upper lobe reticulation is essential to establish a radiologic diagnosis of UIP pattern, but this is not a requirement in the current ATS guidelines.[2]

Honeycombing

Honeycombing is the most specific finding of a UIP pattern on HRCT and is present in most patients with histopathologic UIP.[36,37] In a study by Flaherty and colleagues,[38] honeycombing on HRCT indicated the presence of UIP with a sensitivity of 90% and specificity of 86%. It is defined as "clustered cystic air spaces, typically of comparable diameters on the order of 3–10 mm but

occasionally as large as 2.5 cm."[39] What constitutes honeycombing on HRCT is unclear; possibly dilated small airways, but its presence is a sign of advanced fibrosis and is associated with a worse prognosis (see **Figs. 2** and **3**).[37,40] At present, the presence of honeycombing is required in order to establish a definite UIP pattern on CT.[2] However, the assessment of honeycombing on HRCT is subjective and can be challenging. There is significant interobserver disagreement among radiologists from across the world, including expert radiologists.[40,41] The most common cause of disagreement is the presence of mimics of honeycombing, especially traction bronchiectasis and bronchiolectasis and paraseptal emphysema.

Ground-Glass Opacity

Ground-glass opacity in areas of reticulation is thought to represent pulmonary fibrosis at less than the resolution of HRCT. Ground-glass opacities away from areas of fibrosis (reticulation, traction bronchiectasis, or bronchiolectasis) are thought to represent active inflammation or some other process.[42–44]

Other

Mediastinal and hilar lymph node enlargement are present on HRCT in up to 70% to 86% of patients with a UIP pattern (typically <15 mm).[45–47]

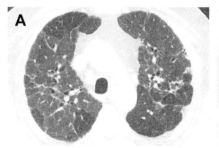
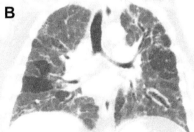

Fig. 4. A 65-year-old man with chronic (fibrotic) HP. Axial (*A*) and coronal reformatted (*B*) HRCT images show mosaic attenuation with patchy ground-glass opacity and lobular areas of decreased attenuation. Peribronchial fibrosis is present with mild traction bronchiectasis and an upper lobe predominance.

Asymmetric distribution of the findings is common, occurring in up to 25% of cases.[35,48]

DIAGNOSTIC CRITERIA AND CORRELATION WITH PATHOLOGY

Based on jointly published multidisciplinary guidelines for the diagnosis and management of IPF (ATS, ERS, Japanese Respiratory Society, and Latin American Thoracic Association, 2011),[2] there are 3 categories of UIP diagnosis by HRCT: definite UIP pattern, possible UIP pattern, and inconsistent with UIP pattern (Table 4). A definite UIP pattern consists of basilar and subpleural predominant reticulation, honeycombing with or without traction bronchiectasis, and absence of features suggesting another diagnosis. Patients with UIP pattern and concordant clinical presentation do not require lung biopsy. Possible UIP pattern on HRCT includes all of the imaging findings of definite UIP pattern except for honeycombing (Fig. 5). The category of patterns inconsistent with UIP is selected if any 1 of the following imaging findings are present: upper or midlung predominance, peribronchovascular predominance, ground-glass opacity that is more extensive than reticulation, profuse micronodules (bilateral, predominantly upper lobes), discrete cysts (multiple, bilateral, away from areas of honeycombing), diffuse mosaic attenuation or air trapping (involving 3 or more lobes and bilateral), and consolidation. Patients with possible UIP and inconsistent with UIP require further evaluation and may need lung biopsy. Many patients with HRCT findings of a possible UIP pattern have a histologic diagnosis of UIP on lung biopsy.[49–51] IPF can be diagnosed by clinical and radiologic criteria in about two-thirds of cases.[50] Morbidity and mortality associated with lung biopsies in patients with fibrosis is high (3%–4% in most studies).[52] The most important factor contributing to 30-day mortality after the procedure is an acute exacerbation of IPF, a phenomenon that is characterized by diffuse alveolar damage (DAD) superimposed on UIP.[53] It would be beneficial to improve the selection criteria and limit the number of biopsies, which was addressed in a recent study by Chung and colleagues[51] of 201 patients with a possible UIP HRCT diagnosis. The subjects were divided into 2 groups: probable UIP (all the typical UIP findings except honeycombing) versus indeterminate UIP (findings not sufficiently characteristic to be classified as definite, probable, or inconsistent with UIP). There was a statistically significant difference between the proportions of UIP diagnosis on histology in these 2 subgroups, with 82.4% of the subjects with probable UIP on HRCT having a probable or definite UIP diagnosis

Table 4
Three categories of UIP diagnosis by HRCT

Pattern	HRCT Findings	Likely Diagnosis	Further Management
Definite UIP	Basilar and subpleural predominant reticulation Honeycombing with or without traction bronchiectasis	IPF, asbestosis, collagen vascular disease, familial fibrosis, chronic HP, or drug-related pulmonary fibrosis	If no evidence of collagen vascular disease and other mentioned entities, the diagnosis of IPF can be established and therapy introduced
Possible UIP	As above except for honeycombing	As above	Requires further evaluation and possibly surgical lung biopsy
Inconsistent with UIP	Upper or midlung predominance, peribronchovascular predominance, ground-glass opacity more extensive than reticulation, profuse micronodules, discrete cysts (away from areas of honeycombing), diffuse mosaic attenuation or air trapping, consolidation	Suggests a diagnosis other than UIP	Requires further evaluation and possibly surgical lung biopsy

Data from Raghu G, Collard HR, Egan JJ, et al. An official ATS/ERS/JRS/ALAT statement: idiopathic pulmonary fibrosis: evidence-based guidelines for diagnosis and management. Am J Respir Crit Care Med 2011;183(6):788–824.

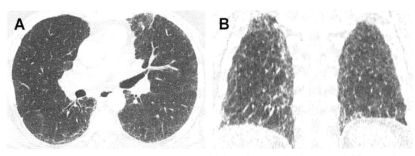

Fig. 5. A 54-year-old man with possible UIP pattern. Axial (*A*) and coronal reformatted (*B*) HRCT images show subpleural and basal predominant reticulation without honeycombing.

on histology as opposed to 54.2% of subjects with indeterminate UIP. This finding suggests that selected patients with possible UIP diagnosis on HRCT, after multidisciplinary discussion, could avoid lung biopsy.

Gruden and colleagues[54] proposed that UIP can be diagnosed in the absence of honeycombing based on certain findings (reticulation with lobular distortion, nonsegmental distribution with lower lobe predominance and upper lobe involvement, traction bronchiectasis, and heterogeneity without inconsistent features).

A confident diagnosis of UIP based on HRCT is correct in 80% to 95% of cases using pathology as a reference.[36,55–57] In a series described by Hunninghake and colleagues,[49] the sensitivity, specificity, accuracy, and positive predictive value of the diagnosis of IPF were 77%, 72%, 75%, and 85%, respectively. In a study described by Rhagu and colleagues,[50] the sensitivity and specificity of the radiologic diagnosis of IPF were 78.5% and 90%, respectively. Other investigators report similar numbers. In a study by Silva and colleagues,[58] the correct diagnosis was made in 84% cases of UIP. Despite the high accuracy of HRCT for the diagnosis of UIP, a substantial number of patients who ultimately are diagnosed with IPF do not have HRCT findings that allow a confident diagnosis of UIP. The interobserver agreement for the CT diagnosis of UIP/IPF is moderate to excellent[59–61]; however, distinguishing NSIP from UIP can be challenging, especially with fibrotic or advanced NSIP. The probability of UIP diagnosis on pathology increases with age. Patients 65 to 70 years old and older are very likely to have pathologic diagnosis of UIP even if the HRCT pattern is not typical.[62]

DIFFERENTIAL DIAGNOSIS
Nonspecific Interstitial Pneumonia

NSIP accounts for most of the disagreements among observers for the IIPs.[55] HRCT findings that favor NSIP rather than UIP include the presence of ground-glass opacity, which is found in most cases (Table 5). Subpleural sparing is highly suggestive of NSIP,[63–65] being present in 64% of patients with NSIP, in 11% with chronic HP, and in 4% with IPF (Fig. 6).

Fine reticulation and traction bronchiectasis may be present in NSIP, but honeycombing is typically absent.[65,66] However, both the histologic and radiologic appearances of NSIP are heterogeneous.[67,68] In a study by Hartman and colleagues,[67] honeycombing was present in 30% of the study patients. Some patients with IPF have HRCT findings similar to those of NSIP, and biopsy may be necessary to distinguish these entities.[34] It has also been recognized that some patients with HRCT findings consistent with NSIP have a UIP histologic diagnosis. In a series described by Flaherty and colleagues,[55] most patients with typical HRCT findings of NSIP had a histologic diagnosis of UIP at surgical lung biopsy (26 of 44; 59%), specifically 17 of 25 patients with probable NSIP and 9 of 19 patients with definite NSIP on HRCT had UIP pattern on pathology.

Fibrotic Hypersensitivity Pneumonitis

HRCT findings of fibrotic HP include centrilobular ground-glass nodules; mosaic attenuation and lobular air trapping; and, importantly, mid to upper lobe predominant distribution of fibrosis.[58,69–72] In more advanced cases of fibrotic HP, honeycombing is common, and the HRCT pattern may mimic that of UIP.[58,69,72] Atypical distribution of UIP findings with more than the expected upper lobe involvement may also pose a significant diagnostic challenge (Fig. 7). The associated histopathology may also be difficult and thorough multidisciplinary evaluation may be required to establish the diagnosis.[73,74]

Other Entities Mimicking Idiopathic Pulmonary Fibrosis

UIP pattern on HRCT in patients with CTD is similar to that found in idiopathic UIP and this should be distinguished on a clinical basis. However,

Table 5
Fibrotic lung diseases mimicking IPF on HRCT: clinical and pathologic correlation

Entity	Major Distinctive Features on HRCT	Major Distinctive Features Clinically	Major Distinctive Features on Pathology
NSIP	• More extensive ground-glass opacity • Subpleural sparing • Honeycombing usually absent (seen in advanced cases)	CTD or suggestive symptoms Better prognosis than UIP	Subpleural fibrosis, fibroblast foci, relative absence of any significant inflammatory cell infiltrate
Fibrotic HP	• Centrilobular ground-glass nodules, • Mosaic attenuation • Air trapping • Mid to upper lobe predominant distribution	Exposure to possible antigens Positive sensitivity panel	Centrilobular fibrosis with relative sparing of the septum and pleura, centrilobular interstitial inflammation with extensive peribronchiolar metaplasia, scattered loosely formed granulomas
CTD-related UIP	• May be indistinguishable from IPF • Ancillary findings suggestive of multiorgan involvement (esophagus, pleura, pericardium)	CTD or suggestive symptoms Usually better prognosis than IPF	Marked lymphoid hyperplasia, peribronchiolar metaplasia, follicular bronchiolitis
Asbestosis	Pleural plaques	History of asbestos exposure	Asbestos bodies or fibers
Sarcoidosis	• Perilymphatic nodules • Bulky lymphadenopathy	Other organ involvement	Noncaseating granulomata

Data from Refs.[13,33,35,42,75]

radiologists may suggest the diagnosis from additional findings such as esophageal dilatation, pleural or pericardial effusion or thickening, and findings of pulmonary hypertension. Asbestosis typically has a histologic and HRCT pattern of UIP, and pleural plaque usually aids in diagnosis. Fibrotic sarcoidosis can be distinguished from UIP by the upper lobe and peribronchial predominant distribution and additional HRCT findings, including pulmonary nodules and lymph node enlargement and calcifications (Fig. 8). Familial UIP may have an appearance indistinguishable from IPF, but sometimes lacks basal predominance.[34]

MULTIDISCIPLINARY DIAGNOSIS OF IDIOPATHIC PULMONARY FIBROSIS

If a confident diagnosis of UIP cannot be made on CT, multidisciplinary discussion is often the next

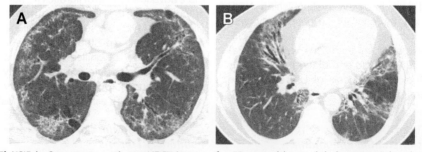

Fig. 6. (*A, B*) NSIP in 2 separate patients. HRCT image of a 53-year-old man (*A*) shows peripheral ground-glass opacity and reticulation with subpleural sparing. Mild traction bronchiectasis is present. HRCT image of a 52-year-old man shows architectural distortion with traction bronchiectasis and ground-glass opacity located predominantly along the bronchovascular bundles.

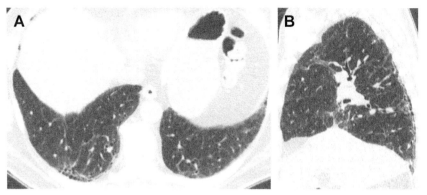

Fig. 7. A 65-year-old man with atypical UIP with relative basal sparing. Axial (*A*) and sagittal reformatted (*B*) HRCT images show subpleural reticulation and honeycombing with relative sparing of the lung bases.

step that may help to establish a diagnosis or establish the need for biopsy.[61,75] Flaherty and colleagues[76] reported that, in a group of 58 patients with diffuse lung disease, after multidisciplinary review of all the available data, radiologists changed their initial diagnosis in 50% of cases, pulmonologists in 30% of cases, and pathologists in 20% of cases. In multiple studies assessing the accuracy of CT for IPF diagnosis, pathology was considered a gold standard. However, it should be kept in mind that there is substantial interobserver variation among pathologists in the assessment of nonneoplastic lung disease.[77] Although multidisciplinary review is considered essential in the diagnosis of interstitial pneumonia, there is no standardized way of arriving at the diagnosis. There are potential setbacks to this approach, one of them being the danger that a dominant personality can strongly influence the diagnosis.

OTHER CONSIDERATIONS
High-Resolution Computed Tomography in Prognosis

Among patients with IIPs, UIP histopathology is associated with the worst prognosis. Patients with IPF who have a definite or possible UIP pattern on HRCT have a shorter survival than those who have indeterminate CT findings.[37,55] However, when HRCT findings are discordant with histopathologic UIP, survival may be slightly better. Patients with NSIP pattern on HRCT and UIP on histopathology (discordant UIP) have survival rates that are modestly better than those of patients with concordant UIP.[55] The extent of honeycombing and pulmonary fibrosis on HRCT has been shown to correlate with prognosis.[78–80] The rate of progression of fibrosis is also an important prognostic factor.[81] DLco, which is an important clinical predictors of mortality, was found to correlate well with baseline HRCT findings.[37]

High-Resolution Computed Tomography in Established Idiopathic Pulmonary Fibrosis

1. Evaluation for acute complications:
   a. Acute exacerbation of fibrosis
   b. Infection
   c. Pneumothorax
   d. Pneumomediastinum
2. Evaluation for chronic complications:
   a. Detection of cancer
   b. Identification of findings suggestive of pulmonary hypertension

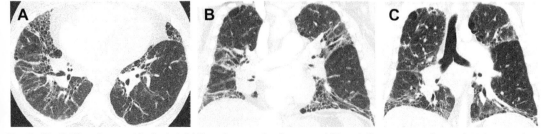

Fig. 8. (*A–C*) Fibrotic sarcoidosis. Axial (*A*) and coronal reformatted (*B* and *C*) contrast-enhanced CT images show extensive peribronchial reticulation, traction bronchiectasis, and honeycombing without a basal or subpleural predominance.

3. Other:
   a. Prognostic value
   b. Assessment of progression
   c. Assessment of response to therapy

Acute exacerbation of idiopathic pulmonary fibrosis

Acute exacerbation (AE) presents as acutely worsened dyspnea (<1-month duration) and hypoxemia with new abnormalities on HRCT. In a series described by Kim and colleagues,[82] the annual incidence of AE was 8.5% and the biannual incidence was 9.6%. In another study by Song and colleagues,[83] 1-year and 3-year incidences were 14.2% and 20.7%, respectively. This complication is estimated to occur in 5% to 10% of patients with IPF every year[84] and carries a very poor prognosis, with an in-hospital mortality of 50%, and 1-year and 5-year survival rates from the initial diagnosis of 56.2% and 18.4%, respectively.[83] The HRCT findings are nonspecific and include new groundglass opacity and consolidation superimposed on underlying pulmonary fibrosis[84–87] (Fig. 9). Infection and pulmonary edema should be excluded. The most common histopathologic pattern of lung injury is DAD followed by organizing pneumonia (OP).[88–90] The distribution of consolidation and ground-glass opacity can be peripheral, patchy, or diffuse. The peripheral and multifocal pattern, which suggests OP as the primary histopathology of acute lung injury, seems to be associated with better prognosis, whereas the diffuse pattern, suggesting DAD, is associated with higher mortality. In patients who survive, some abnormalities resolve; however, fibrosis is likely to progress with increased traction bronchiectasis and reticulation.[90] AE has no definitive precipitating events in most cases, although it has been reported following lung biopsy and bronchiolar lavage. At present, there is no effective treatment of AE, with supportive care being the most important tool. Emerging evidence shows that chronic treatment of IPF may reduce the risk of AE.[82]

Increased risk of pulmonary infection

Patients with IPF have increased risk of pulmonary infection and this should be considered in the differential diagnosis of AE of IPF. Detection of infection may be difficult because of background parenchymal abnormalities. Patients with IPF are prone to aspergillus infection,[91] which most commonly presents as aspergilloma formation in a preexisting cavity. Chronic necrotizing aspergillosis may develop.[92,93] Another common infection is mycobacteria disease. Of note, postprimary pulmonary tuberculosis in the setting of IPF may have atypical imaging findings, including subpleural nodules, masses, and coalescent consolidation.[94]

Spontaneous pneumothorax and pneumomediastinum

Patients with IPF are predisposed to pneumothorax, which occurs in 4% to 6% of patients.[95–97] Pneumothorax likely results from rupture of a subpleural honeycomb cyst into the pleural space. Significant collapse of the lung is unusual given the degree of pleural thickening and stiffness related to fibrosis. However, pneumothorax is usually poorly tolerated because of reduced respiratory reserve. Pneumomediastinum, which is often asymptomatic, most likely results from rapidly increased intrathoracic pressure, such as from cough, leading to alveolar rupture and dissection of gas along the bronchovascular bundles into the mediastinum[91] (Fig. 10).

Increased risk of lung cancer

There is increased incidence of lung cancer in patients with fibrotic lung disease, especially IPF. The reported frequency varies and was calculated at 4.4% in a study by Hubbard and colleagues[98] with an odds ratio of 7.31, and 13.1% in a study by Lee and colleagues.[99] The risk increased with smoking (odds ratio, 2.71), male sex, and age.[100] Synchronous primary lung cancers occur in up to 15% of patients with IPF.[101] In one study,

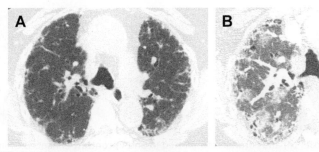

Fig. 9. A 68-year-old woman with AE of IPF. HRCT image at baseline (A) shows subpleural reticulation. HRCT image at the time of acute dyspnea (B) shows patchy ground-glass opacity superimposed on preexisting fibrosis.

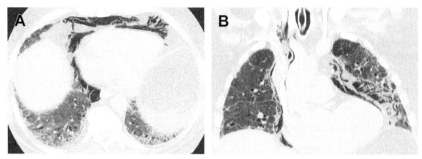

Fig. 10. Pneumomediastinum in a patient with IPF. Axial (*A*) and coronal reformatted (*B*) HRCT images show extensive mediastinal gas tracking cephalad to the neck. Subpleural and basal predominant reticulation is present.

squamous cell carcinoma was the most common histopathologic type,[102] followed by adenocarcinoma. Although lung cancer in the general population has an upper lobe predominance, lung cancer associated with IPF occurs more frequently in the lower lobes[99,103] or with equal distribution between upper and lower lobes.[104,105] With IPF, lung cancers develop most commonly in the peripheral lung and at the junction of fibrotic and normal lung[104–106] (**Fig. 11**). Delay in diagnosis is common. A retrospective study by Yoshida and colleagues[104] showed a 409-day median delay in lung cancer diagnosis in patients with pulmonary fibrosis.

Pulmonary hypertension

The frequency of pulmonary hypertension (PH) in IPF is high and was reported in 32% to 46% of patients referred for lung transplant.[107–111] Although PH in IPF is usually not severe, it is associated with increased mortality, with a 1-year mortality of 28.0% compared with 5.5% for patients without PH. In addition, mean systolic pulmonary artery pressure correlates with decreased survival rate.[112] PH in IPF is thought to be secondary to vasoconstriction from chronic hypoxia and vasculature destruction from fibrosis. However, these factors alone do not fully explain the pathophysiology of PH because there is significant discordance between the degree of fibrosis on HRCT and severity of PH.[107]

High-resolution computed tomography in prognosis and longitudinal monitoring

Quantitative CT scoring of fibrosis can be combined with clinical data and lung function test results to better predict patient-specific mortality. Because of substantial interobserver variation in characterization and visual quantification of fibrosis, several models for quantitative evaluation of the CT data have been developed.[36] Different parameters can be used to quantify the CT fibrosis score, starting from simply mean lung attenuation for assessing lung density (relative amount of soft tissue) to complex texture and fractal analysis. The severity of the CT fibrosis score directly correlates with survival and pulmonary function test results.[37,59,113,114] The semiquantitative CT scoring for the extent of fibrosis in IPF, which includes the gender, age, and physiology (CT-GAP model), was shown to correlate with DLco.[115]

Serial HRCT scanning of patients with IPF is not performed in routine clinical practice and is mostly confined to clinical trials because clinical parameters such as declining pulmonary function testing

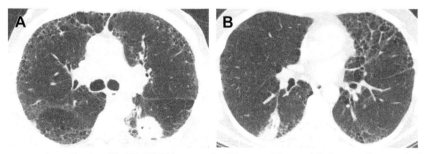

Fig. 11. Lung cancer in patients with IPF. HRCT image of a 57-year old man (*A*) shows a large spiculated mass in the superior segment of the left lower lobe. Subpleural reticulation and honeycombing are present. HRCT image of a 58-year-old man (*B*) shows an elongated mass in the superior right upper lobe, which may be mistaken for focal infection. Subpleural honeycombing is present along with reticulation, with more involvement of the left lung.

and worse performance on the 6-minute walk test indicate disease progression. Additional HRCT scanning of patients with IPF is usually reserved for suspected infection, AE, or other acute complication. Lung cancer screening with CT is not recommended in patients with IPF because of their poor prognosis.

COMBINED PULMONARY FIBROSIS AND EMPHYSEMA

Combined fibrosis and emphysema (CPFE) is a recently recognized entity. Since it was first described as a distinct syndrome by Cottin and colleagues in 2005, it has been increasingly addressed in the literature over the past decade. Radiographically, it consists of upper lobe predominant emphysema and lower lobe predominant fibrosis. Clinically, patients are usually older male current or former smokers and present with severe dyspnea, relatively preserved lung volumes (slightly subnormal spirometry), a profoundly impaired carbon monoxide transfer capacity, and hypoxemia during exercise.[116] In the 2013 revision of the ATS-ERS classification of IIPs, CPFE was described as an example of coexisting patterns of IIP in smokers rather than representing a distinct IIP.[1]

CPFE is a rare entity. In reported studies, CPFE was present in 8% to 51% of patients with IPF,[117] which itself is rare. On a series of 61 patients,[118] the most common CT findings included upper lobe emphysema (centrilobular 97%, paraseptal 93%, and bullae 54%) and lower lobe fibrosis, including honeycombing (95%), reticulations (87%), traction bronchiectasis (69%), ground-glass opacity (66%), and architectural or bronchial distortion (39%) (Fig. 12). A UIP pattern of fibrosis

on HRCT is the most common, but other IIP patterns can also coexist, such as NSIP, DIP, and RB, because of the strong association with smoking.[117-119] Similarly, histopathologic findings in patients with CPFE vary and can include emphysema in addition to UIP, NSIP, RB with fibrosis, and airspace enlargement with fibrosis.[120]

Recognizing CPFE on CT is important because of its different natural history, complications, and high mortality.[120] Survival in patients with CPFE is poor, with reported 5-year survival rates of 35% to 80%,[119] which is better than patients with IPF but worse than patients with emphysema without fibrosis.[121] Major causes of death include cor pulmonale, chronic respiratory failure, AE, and lung cancer.[118]

The poor prognosis these patients have when pulmonary arterial hypertension (PAH) is present is well recognized. Patients with CPFE have a prevalence of PAH ranging between 47% and 90%, which is higher than that of patients with emphysema or IPF alone.[117] Cottin and colleagues[118] described the prevalence at diagnosis in 47% of patients and 55% at follow-up. It is well known that the presence of PH at diagnosis is an independent predictor of survival in these patients. Overall, 5-year survival is 55%, which is slightly better than in patients with IPF, but worse than in patients with emphysema alone. However, when correcting for the presence of PAH, 5-year survival is 75% if no PAH is present, and 25% when PAH is present.[118]

Another well-known complication of patients with CPFE is the strikingly high incidence of lung cancer, reported between 42% and 47%,[121,122] which is higher than in patients with IPF or chronic obstructive pulmonary disease (COPD) alone.[117] In a series of 47 patients with CPFE and lung cancer by Girard and colleagues,[123] 47% of patients had no cancer-related symptoms at the time of diagnosis. The most common histologic type is squamous cell carcinoma, followed by adenocarcinoma. In up to 49% of patients, the cancer abutted pleura, and 43% were located in the lower or middle lobes. The prognosis is poorer than for those with COPD of IPF alone, with overall survival of 10.8 months.[117] Patients with CPFE also have higher risk of developing acute lung injury after treatments such as surgery, radiation, or chemotherapy.[117]

TREATMENT

Treatment of IPF has been challenging and not very effective. Several agents have been used in the past, including corticosteroids, immunosuppressants such as azathioprine,

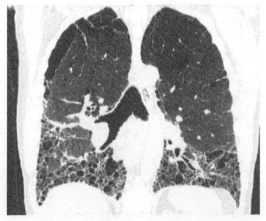

Fig. 12. A 75-year-old man with CPFE. Coronal reformatted HRCT image shows upper lung predominant centrilobular emphysema and basal and subpleural predominant reticulation and honeycombing.

antineoplastics such as cyclophosphamide, and *N*-acetylcysteine.[124] None of them individually or combined have been successful, and in some cases they have even proved harmful.[125] Recent developments in the treatment of IPF include the use of the antifibrotic agents pirfenidone and nintedanib. These agents were earlier approved in Japan and Europe after several international trials. Two phase III trials were then conducted in the US (ASCEND for pirfenidone and INPULSIS for nintedanib). After results showing a slow in the decline of lung function in patients with IPF, these drugs were approved by the US Food and Drug Administration (FDA) for the treatment of IPF in October 2014. A subsequent meta-analysis of 5 randomized controlled trials involving pirfenidone showed a reduction in all-cause and IPF-specific mortality and worsening of IPF. However, no impact on AEs was found.[126]

Pirfenidone is an orally administered pyridine originally studied for its analgesic, antiinflammatory, and antipyretic properties. Subsequently, its antifibrotic properties were discovered.[124] The ASCEND trial showed that, compared with placebo, this drug reduced disease progression, including reduced decline in lung function, exercise tolerance, and progression-free survival in patients with IPF. The most common side effects included gastrointestinal symptoms and photosensitivity rash.[127–129] Nintedanib was originally developed for cancer treatment as an angiostatic factor, but it also shows antifibrotic properties as an intracellular inhibitor of several tyrosine kinases that targets multiple growth factor receptors.[130] The INPULSIS trial compared nintedanib with placebo and met its primary end point of slowing the annual rate of decline in forced vital capacity.[131]

These drugs are currently approved by the FDA without specifying the degree of disease severity. They are also included in the ATS's guidelines for the treatment of IPF.[2] There is hope but also uncertainty regarding the role that these agents will play. For example, the population of patients with IPF enrolled in the phase III trials was small, with only 27% of patients with IPF meeting all the enrollment criteria.[132] Furthermore, the role of these drugs in the treatment of patients who lack a confident IPF diagnosis remains unclear, but it is reasonable to think that slowing disease progression at earlier stages of fibrosis might result in longer survival. Similarly, the role of these drugs in patients with comorbid conditions such as PH and cardiovascular disease has not been well evaluated, because it commonly precludes their enrollment in clinical trials.[130] In addition, both INPULSIS and ASCEND trials lasted 1 year. The long-term effects of pirfenidone and nintedanib in slowing disease progression and the tolerability of their side effects in day-to-day life have yet to be determined. At the same time, there are ongoing studies and trials in different stages evaluating new agents and combinations of agents,[133] so IPF treatment will continue to evolve. In addition, lung transplant is the last option for patients with end-stage fibrosis with the goal being to improve quality of life.

WHAT REFERRING PHYSICIANS NEEDS TO KNOW

- Surgical lung biopsy is not indicated for patients with a definite UIP pattern and a clinical presentation consistent with IPF.
- Although a definite UIP pattern on HRCT usually indicates IPF, multidisciplinary discussion may be required when clinical or pathologic data are discordant.
- Mimics of UIP on HRCT include NSIP, HP, fibrosing sarcoidosis, asbestosis, and drug reaction; UIP pattern can be seen in IPF as well as in CTDs, so thorough clinical evaluation is necessary.
- HRCT findings not only aid in diagnosis but also have prognostic value, with honeycombing being the most specific finding and associated with a worse prognosis.
- Acutely worsened dyspnea and hypoxia in patients with fibrosis may indicate AE of fibrosis, a condition with high mortality; when this is suspected, infection and edema need to be excluded.
- CPFE is a distinct phenotype of IPF in smokers and is associated with extremely poor survival.

SUMMARY

HRCT plays a central role in the multidisciplinary diagnosis of IPF. In patients with a clinical presentation consistent with IPF, HRCT is sufficient to confirm the diagnosis without the need for surgical biopsy. Thus, it is important for radiologists to recognize the characteristic HRCT features of UIP as well as its mimics in order to properly assist in managing patients with fibrotic lung disease. Although HRCT to monitor patients with IPF is not routine in clinical practice, radiologists should be aware of complications that may be encountered at diagnosis or on subsequent imaging studies.

REFERENCES

1. Travis WD, Costabel U, Hansell DM, et al. An official American Thoracic Society/European Respiratory

Society statement: update of the International Multi-disciplinary Classification of the Idiopathic Interstitial Pneumonias. Am J Respir Crit Care Med 2013; 188(6):733–48.

2. Raghu G, Collard HR, Egan JJ, et al. An official ATS/ERS/JRS/ALAT statement: idiopathic pulmonary fibrosis: evidence-based guidelines for diagnosis and management. Am J Respir Crit Care Med 2011;183(6):788–824.

3. Bjoraker JA, Ryu JH, Edwin MK, et al. Prognostic significance of histopathologic subsets in idiopathic pulmonary fibrosis. Am J Respir Crit Care Med 1998;157:199–203.

4. Mapel DW, Hunt WC, Utton R, et al. Idiopathic pulmonary fibrosis: survival in population based and hospital based cohorts. Thorax 1998;53:469–76.

5. Hubbard R, Johnston I, Britton J. Survival in patients with cryptogenic fibrosis alveolitis: a population-based cohort study. Chest 1998;113:396–400.

6. Martinez FJ, Safrin S, Weycker D, et al. The clinical course of patients with idiopathic pulmonary fibrosis. Ann Intern Med 2005;142:963–7.

7. Collard HR, King TE Jr, Bartelson BB, et al. Changes in clinical and physiologic variables predict survival in idiopathic pulmonary fibrosis. Am J Respir Crit Care Med 2003;168:538–42.

8. Ley B, Collard HR, King TE Jr. Clinical course and prediction of survival in idiopathic pulmonary fibrosis. Am J Respir Crit Care Med 2011;183(4): 431–40.

9. Coultas DB, Zumwalt RE, Black WC, et al. The epidemiology of interstitial lung diseases. Am J Respir Crit Care Med 1994;150:967–72.

10. Nalysnyk L, Cid-Ruzafa J, Rotella P, et al. Incidence and prevalence of idiopathic pulmonary fibrosis: review of the literature. Eur Respir Rev 2012;21(126):355–61.

11. Raghu G, Weycker D, Edelsberg J, et al. Incidence and prevalence of idiopathic pulmonary fibrosis. Am J Respir Crit Care Med 2006;174(7): 810–6.

12. Baumgartner KB, Samet JM, Stidley CA, et al. Cigarette smoking: a risk factor for idiopathic pulmonary fibrosis. Am J Respir Crit Care Med 1997; 155:242–8.

13. Antoniou KM, Hansell DM, Rubens MB, et al. Idiopathic pulmonary fibrosis: outcome in relation to smoking status. Am J Respir Crit Care Med 2008; 177:190–4.

14. Kim HC, Ji W, Kim MY, et al. Interstitial pneumonia related to undifferentiated connective tissue disease: pathologic pattern and prognosis. Chest 2015;147(1):165–72.

15. Raghu G, Freudenberger TD, Yang S, et al. High prevalence of abnormal acid gastro-oesophageal reflux in idiopathic pulmonary fibrosis. Eur Respir J 2006;27:136–42.

16. Lee JS, Collard HR, Raghu G, et al. Does chronic microaspiration cause idiopathic pulmonary fibrosis? Am J Med 2010;123(4):304–11.

17. Lee JS. The role of gastroesophageal reflux and microaspiration in idiopathic pulmonary fibrosis. Clin Pulm Med 2014;21(2):81–5.

18. Lee JS, Ryu JH, Elicker BM, et al. Gastroesophageal reflux therapy is associated with longer survival in patients with idiopathic pulmonary fibrosis. Am J Respir Crit Care Med 2011;184(12): 1390–4.

19. Juarez MM, Chan AL, Norris AG, et al. Acute exacerbation of idiopathic pulmonary fibrosis—a review of current and novel pharmacotherapies. J Thorac Dis 2015;7(3):499–519.

20. Mathieson JR, Mayo JR, Staples CA, et al. Chronic diffuse infiltrative lung disease: comparison of diagnostic accuracy of CT and chest radiography. Radiology 1989;171:111–6.

21. Mayo JR. CT evaluation of diffuse infiltrative lung disease: dose considerations and optimal technique. J Thorac Imaging 2009;24(4):252–9.

22. Dodd JD, de Jong PA, Levy RD, et al. Conventional high-resolution CT versus contiguous multidetector CT in the detection of bronchiolitis obliterans syndrome in lung transplant recipients. J Thorac Imaging 2008;23(4):235–43.

23. Kalra MK, Maher MM, Rizzo S, et al. Radiation exposure from chest CT: issues and strategies. J Korean Med Sci 2004;19(2):159–66.

24. Hodnett PA, Naidich DP. Fibrosing interstitial lung disease. A practical high-resolution computed tomography–based approach to diagnosis and management and a review of the literature. Am J Respir Crit Care Med 2013;188(2):141–9.

25. McCollough CH, Chen GH, Kalender W, et al. Achieving routine submillisievert CT scanning: report from the summit on management of radiation dose in CT. Radiology 2012;264(2): 567–80.

26. Vardhanabhuti V, Loader RL, Mitchell GR, et al. Image quality assessment of standard- and low-dose chest CT using filtered back projection, adaptive statistical iterative reconstruction, and novel model-based iterative reconstruction algorithms. Am J Roentgenol 2013;200(3):545–52.

27. Duan X, McCollough C. Risks, benefits, and risk reduction strategies in thoracic CT imaging. Semin Respir Crit Care Med 2014;35(1):83–90.

28. Padole A, Khawaja RDA, Kalra MK, et al. CT radiation dose and iterative reconstruction techniques. Am J Roentgenol 2015;204(4):384–92.

29. Kim Y, Kim YK, Lee BE, et al. Ultra-low-dose CT of the thorax using iterative reconstruction: evaluation of image quality and radiation dose reduction. Am J Roentgenol 2015;204(6):1197–202.

30. Kubo T, Lin P-J P, Stiller W, et al. Radiation dose reduction in chest CT: a review. Am J Roentgenol 2008;190(2):335–43.

31. Christe A, Charimo-Torrente J, Roychoudhury K, et al. Accuracy of low-dose computed tomography (CT) for detecting and characterizing the most common CT-patterns of pulmonary disease. Eur J Radiol 2013;82(3):e142–50.

32. Sverzellati N, Lynch DA, Hansell DM, et al. American Thoracic Society–European Respiratory Society classification of the idiopathic interstitial pneumonias: advances in knowledge since 2002. Radiographics 2015;35(7):1849–71.

33. Sumikawa H, Johkoh T, Ichikado K, et al. Usual interstitial pneumonia and chronic idiopathic interstitial pneumonia: analysis of CT appearance in 92 patients. Radiology 2006;241:258–66.

34. Hunninghake GW, Lynch DA, Galvin JR, et al. Radiologic findings are strongly associated with a pathologic diagnosis of usual interstitial pneumonia. Chest 2003;124:1215–23.

35. Gruden JF. CT in idiopathic pulmonary fibrosis: diagnosis and beyond. Am J Roentgenol 2016; 206(3):495–507.

36. Misumi S, Lynch DA. Idiopathic pulmonary fibrosis/usual interstitial pneumonia. Proc Am Thorac Soc 2006;3(4):307–14.

37. Lynch DA, Godwin JD, Safrin S, et al. High-resolution computed tomography in idiopathic pulmonary fibrosis: diagnosis and prognosis. Am J Respir Crit Care Med 2005;172:488–93.

38. Flaherty KR, Toews GB, Travis WD, et al. Clinical significance of histological classification of idiopathic interstitial pneumonia. Eur Respir J 2002; 19:275–83.

39. Hansell DM, Bankier AA, MacMahon H, et al. Fleischner Society: glossary of terms for thoracic imaging. Radiology 2008;246:697–722.

40. Akira M, Inoue Y, Kitaichi M, et al. Usual interstitial pneumonia and nonspecific interstitial pneumonia with and without concurrent emphysema: thin-section CT findings. Radiology 2009;251(1): 271–9.

41. Watadani T, Sakai F, Johkoh T, et al. Interobserver variability in the CT assessment of honeycombing in the lungs. Radiology 2013;266:936–44.

42. Leung AN, Miller RR, Muller NL. Parenchymal opacification in chronic infiltrative lung diseases: CT-pathologic correlation. Radiology 1993;188: 209–14.

43. Remy-Jardin M, Giraud F, Remy J, et al. Importance of ground-glass attenuation in chronic diffuse infiltrative lung disease: pathologic-CT correlation. Radiology 1993;189:693–8.

44. Nishimura K, Kitaichi M, Izumi T, et al. Usual interstitial pneumonia: histologic correlation with high-resolution CT. Radiology 1992;182:337–42.

45. Jung JI, Kim HH, Jung YJ, et al. Mediastinal lymphadenopathy in pulmonary fibrosis: correlation with disease severity. J Comput Assist Tomogr 2000; 24:706–10.

46. Niimi H, Kang EY, Kwong JS, et al. CT of chronic infiltrative lung disease: prevalence of mediastinal lymphadenopathy. J Comput Assist Tomogr 1996; 20:305–8.

47. Souza CA, Muller NL, Lee KS, et al. Idiopathic interstitial pneumonias: prevalence of mediastinal lymph node enlargement in 206 patients. AJR Am J Roentgenol 2006;186:995–9.

48. Tcherakian C, Cottin V, Brillet PY, et al. Progression of idiopathic pulmonary fibrosis: lessons from asymmetrical disease. Thorax 2011;66(3):226–31.

49. Hunninghake GW, Zimmerman MB, Schwartz DA, et al. Utility of a lung biopsy for the diagnosis of idiopathic pulmonary fibrosis. Am J Respir Crit Care Med 2001;164:193–6.

50. Raghu G, Mageto YN, Lockhart D, et al. The accuracy of the clinical diagnosis of new-onset idiopathic pulmonary fibrosis and other interstitial lung disease: a prospective study. Chest 1999; 116:1168–74.

51. Chung JH, Chawla A, Peljto AL, et al. CT scan findings of probable usual interstitial pneumonitis have a high predictive value for histologic usual interstitial pneumonitis. Chest 2015;147(2):450–9.

52. Kaarteenaho R. The current position of surgical lung biopsy in the diagnosis of idiopathic pulmonary fibrosis. Respir Res 2013;14(1):43.

53. Kaarteenaho R, Kinnula VL. Diffuse alveolar damage: a common phenomenon in progressive interstitial lung disorders. Pulm Med 2011;2011: 531302.

54. Gruden JF, Panse PM, Gotway MB, et al. Diagnosis of usual interstitial pneumonitis in the absence of honeycombing: evaluation of specific CT criteria with clinical follow-up in 38 patients. Am J Roentgenol 2016;206(3):472–80.

55. Flaherty KR, Thwaite EL, Kazerooni EA, et al. Radiological versus histological diagnosis in UIP and NSIP: survival implications. Thorax 2003;58: 143–8.

56. Johkoh T, Muller NL, Cartier Y, et al. Idiopathic interstitial pneumonias: diagnostic accuracy of thin-section CT in 129 patients. Radiology 1999; 211:555–60.

57. Tsubamoto M, Muller NL, Johkoh T, et al. Pathologic subgroups of nonspecific interstitial pneumonia: differential diagnosis from other idiopathic interstitial pneumonias on high-resolution computed tomography. J Comput Assist Tomogr 2005;29:793–800.

58. Silva CI, Müller NL, Lynch DA, et al. Chronic hypersensitivity pneumonitis: differentiation from idiopathic pulmonary fibrosis and nonspecific

interstitial pneumonia by using thin-section CT. Radiology 2008;246:288–97.

59. Sumikawa H, Johkoh T, Colby TV, et al. Computed tomography findings in pathological usual interstitial pneumonia: relationship to survival. Am J Respir Crit Care Med 2008;177(4):433–9.

60. Sverzellati N, Wells AU, Tomassetti S, et al. Biopsy-proved idiopathic pulmonary fibrosis: spectrum of nondiagnostic thin-section CT diagnoses. Radiology 2010;254(3):957–64.

61. Thomeer M, Demedts M, Behr J, et al. Multidisciplinary interobserver agreement in the diagnosis of idiopathic pulmonary fibrosis. Eur Respir J 2008;31(3):585–91.

62. Fell CD, Martinez FJ, Liu LX, et al. Clinical predictors of a diagnosis of idiopathic pulmonary fibrosis. Am J Respir Crit Care Med 2010;181(8):832–7.

63. Kligerman SJ, Groshong S, Brown KK, et al. Nonspecific interstitial pneumonia: radiologic, clinical, and pathologic considerations. Radiographics 2009;29(1):73–87.

64. Silva CI, Müller NL, Hansell DM, et al. Nonspecific interstitial pneumonia and idiopathic pulmonary fibrosis: changes in pattern and distribution of disease over time. Radiology 2008;247(1):251–9.

65. Elliot TL, Lynch DA, Newell JD Jr, et al. High-resolution computed tomography features of nonspecific interstitial pneumonia and usual interstitial pneumonia. J Comput Assist Tomogr 2005;29:339–45.

66. Johkoh T, Muller NL, Colby TV, et al. Nonspecific interstitial pneumonia: correlation between thin-section CT findings and pathologic subgroups in 55 patients. Radiology 2002;225:199–204.

67. Hartman TE, Swensen SJ, Hansell DM, et al. Nonspecific interstitial pneumonia: variable appearance at high-resolution chest CT. Radiology 2000;217:701–5.

68. MacDonald SL, Rubens MB, Hansell DM, et al. Nonspecific interstitial pneumonia and usual interstitial pneumonia: comparative appearances at and diagnostic accuracy of thin-section CT. Radiology 2001;221:600–5.

69. Lynch DA, Newell JD, Logan PM, et al. Can CT distinguish hypersensitivity pneumonitis from idiopathic pulmonary fibrosis? Am J Roentgenol 1995;165:807–11.

70. Hansell DM, Wells AU, Padley SP, et al. Hypersensitivity pneumonitis: correlation of individual CT patterns with functional abnormalities. Radiology 1996;199:123–8.

71. Small JH, Flower CD, Traill ZC, et al. Air-trapping in extrinsic allergic alveolitis on computed tomography. Clin Radiol 1996;51:684–8.

72. Silva CI, Churg A, Mullor NL. Hypersensitivity pneumonitis: spectrum of high-resolution CT and pathologic findings. Am J Roentgenol 2007;188:334–44.

73. Elicker BM, Jones KD, Henry TS, et al. Multidisciplinary approach to hypersensitivity pneumonitis. J Thorac Imaging 2016;31(2):92–103.

74. Smith M, Dalurzo M, Panse P, et al. Usual interstitial pneumonia-pattern fibrosis in surgical lung biopsies: clinical, radiological and histopathological clues to aetiology. J Clin Pathol 2013;66:896–903.

75. Chung JH, Lynch DA. The value of a multidisciplinary approach to the diagnosis of usual interstitial pneumonitis and idiopathic pulmonary fibrosis: radiology, pathology, and clinical correlation. Am J Roentgenol 2016;206(3):463–71.

76. Flaherty KR, King TE Jr, Raghu G, et al. Idiopathic interstitial pneumonia: what is the effect of a multidisciplinary approach to diagnosis? Am J Respir Crit Care Med 2004;170:904–10.

77. Nicholson AG, Addis BJ, Bharucha H, et al. Interobserver variation between pathologists in diffuse parenchymal lung disease. Thorax 2004;59:500–5.

78. Gay SE, Kazerooni EA, Toews GB, et al. Idiopathic pulmonary fibrosis: predicting response to therapy and survival. Am J Respir Crit Care Med 1998;157:1063–72.

79. Nagao T, Nagai S, Hiramoto Y, et al. Serial evaluation of high-resolution computed tomography findings in patients with idiopathic pulmonary fibrosis in usual interstitial pneumonia. Respiration 2002;69:413–9.

80. Shin KM, Lee KS, Chung MP, et al. Prognostic determinants among clinical, thin-section CT, and histopathologic findings for fibrotic idiopathic interstitial pneumonias: tertiary hospital study. Radiology 2008;249:328–37.

81. Hwang JH, Misumi S, Curran-Everett D, et al. Longitudinal follow-up of fibrosing interstitial pneumonia: relationship between physiologic testing, computed tomography changes, and survival rate. J Thorac Imaging 2011;26:209–17.

82. Kim DS. Acute exacerbations in patients with idiopathic pulmonary fibrosis. Respir Res 2013;14:86.

83. Song JW, Hong SB, Lim CM, et al. Acute exacerbation of idiopathic pulmonary fibrosis: incidence, risk factors and outcome. Eur Respir J 2011;37:356–63.

84. Collard HR, Moore BB, Flaherty KR, et al. Acute exacerbations of idiopathic pulmonary fibrosis. Am J Respir Crit Care Med 2007;176(7):636–43.

85. Akira M, Kozuka T, Yamamoto S, et al. Computed tomography findings in acute exacerbation of idiopathic pulmonary fibrosis. Am J Respir Crit Care Med 2008;178(4):372–8.

86. Silva CI, Müller NL, Fujimoto K, et al. Acute exacerbation of chronic interstitial pneumonia: high-resolution computed tomography and pathologic findings. J Thorac Imaging 2007;22:221–0.

87. Bhatti H, Girdhar A, Usman F, et al. Approach to acute exacerbation of idiopathic pulmonary fibrosis. Ann Thorac Med 2013;8(2):71–7.

88. Kim DS, Park JH, Park BK, et al. Acute exacerbation of idiopathic pulmonary fibrosis: frequency and clinical features. Eur Respir J 2006;27(1): 143–50.

89. Parambil JG, Myers JL, Ryu JH. Histopathologic features and outcome of patients with acute exacerbation of idiopathic pulmonary fibrosis undergoing surgical lung biopsy. Chest 2005;128(5): 3310–5.

90. Kligermans SJ, Franks TJ, Galvin JR. From the radiologic pathology archives: organization and fibrosis as a response to lung injury in diffuse alveolar damage, organizing pneumonia, and acute fibrinous and organizing pneumonia. Radiographics 2013;33(7):1951–75.

91. Lloyd CR, Walsh SL, Hansell DM. High-resolution CT of complications of idiopathic fibrotic lung disease. Br J Radiol 2011;84:581–92.

92. Saraceno JL, Phelps DT, Ferro TJ, et al. Chronic necrotizing pulmonary aspergillosis: approach to management. Chest 1997;112:541–8.

93. Roberts CM, Citron KM, Strickland B. Intrathoracic aspergilloma: role of CT in diagnosis and treatment. Radiology 1987;165:123–8.

94. Chung MJ, Goo JM, Im JG. Pulmonary tuberculosis in patients with idiopathic pulmonary fibrosis. Eur J Radiol 2004;52:175–9.

95. Picado C, Gomez de Almeida R, Xaubet A, et al. Spontaneous pneumothorax in cryptogenic fibrosing alveolitis. Respiration 1985;48:77–80.

96. Fujiwara T. Pneumomediastinum in pulmonary fibrosis. Detection by computed tomography. Chest 1993;104:44–6.

97. Franquet T, Gimenez A, Torrubia S, et al. Spontaneous pneumothorax and pneumomediastinum in IPF. Eur Radiol 2000;10:108–13.

98. Hubbard R, Venn A, Lewis S, et al. Lung cancer and cryptogenic fibrosing alveolitis. A population-based cohort study. Am J Respir Crit Care Med 2000;161:5–8.

99. Lee HJ, Im JG, Ahn JM, et al. Lung cancer in patients with idiopathic pulmonary fibrosis: CT findings. J Comput Assist Tomogr 1996;20:979–82.

100. Park J, Kim DS, Shim TS, et al. Lung cancer in patients with idiopathic pulmonary fibrosis. Eur Respir J 2001;17:1216–9.

101. Mizushima Y, Kobayashi M. Clinical characteristics of synchronous multiple lung cancer associated with idiopathic pulmonary fibrosis. A review of Japanese cases. Chest 1995;108:1272–7.

102. Aubry MC, Myers JL, Douglas WW, et al. Primary pulmonary carcinoma in patients with idiopathic pulmonary fibrosis. Mayo Clin Proc 2002;77(8): 763–70.

103. Sakai S, Ono M, Nishio T, et al. Lung cancer associated with diffuse pulmonary fibrosis: CT-pathologic correlation. J Thorac Imaging 2003;18: 67–71.

104. Yoshida R, Arakawa H, Kaji Y. Lung cancer in chronic interstitial pneumonia: early manifestation from serial CT observations. Am J Roentgenol 2012;199:85–90.

105. Matsushita H, Tanaka S, Saiki Y, et al. Lung cancer associated with usual interstitial pneumonia. Pathol Int 1995;45:925–32.

106. Kishi K, Homma S, Kurosaki A, et al. High-resolution computed tomography findings of lung cancer associated with idiopathic pulmonary fibrosis. J Comput Assist Tomogr 2006;30:95–9.

107. Corte TJ, Wort SJ, Wells AU. Pulmonary hypertension in idiopathic pulmonary fibrosis: a review. Sarcoidosis Vasc Diffuse Lung Dis 2009;26:7–19.

108. Hamada K, Nagai S, Tanaka S, et al. Significance of pulmonary arterial pressure and diffusion capacity of the lung as prognosticator in patients with idiopathic pulmonary fibrosis. Chest 2007;131: 650–6.

109. Nadrous HF, Pellikka PA, Krowka MJ, et al. Pulmonary hypertension in patients with idiopathic pulmonary fibrosis. Chest 2005;128:2393–9.

110. Sherner J, Collen J, King CS, et al. Pulmonary hypertension in idiopathic pulmonary fibrosis: epidemiology, diagnosis and therapeutic implications. Curr Respir Care Rep 2012;1(4):233–42.

111. Shorr AF, Wainright JL, Cors CS, et al. Pulmonary hypertension in patients with pulmonary fibrosis awaiting lung transplant. Eur Respir J 2007;30: 715–21.

112. Lettieri CJ, Nathan SD, Barnett SD, et al. Prevalence and outcomes of pulmonary arterial hypertension in advanced idiopathic pulmonary fibrosis. Chest 2006;129:746–52.

113. Best AC, Meng J, Lynch AM, et al. Idiopathic pulmonary fibrosis: physiologic tests, quantitative CT indexes, and CT visual scores as predictors of mortality. Radiology 2008;246(3):935–40.

114. Oda K, Ishimoto H, Yatera K, et al. High-resolution CT scoring system-based grading scale predicts the clinical outcomes in patients with idiopathic pulmonary fibrosis. Respir Res 2014; 15(1):10.

115. Ley B, Elicker BM, Hartman TE, et al. Idiopathic pulmonary fibrosis: CT and risk of death. Radiology 2014;273(2):570–9.

116. Margaritopoulos GA, Harari S, Caminati A, et al. Smoking-related idiopathic interstitial pneumonia: a review. Respirology 2016;21(1):57–64.

117. Lin H, Jiang S. Combined pulmonary fibrosis and emphysema (CPFE): an entity different from emphysema or pulmonary fibrosis alone. J Thorac Dis 2015;7(4):767–79.

118. Cottin V, Nunes H, Brillet PY, et al. Combined pulmonary fibrosis and emphysema: a distinct under-recognised entity. Eur Respir J 2005;26:586–93.

119. Jankowich MD, Rounds SI. Combined pulmonary fibrosis and emphysema syndrome. A review. Chest 2012;141(1):222–31.

120. Madan R, Matalon S, Vivero M. Spectrum of smoking-related lung diseases: imaging review and update. J Thorac Imaging 2016;31(2):78–91.

121. Fujiwara A, Tsushima K, Sugiyama S, et al. Histological types and localizations of lung cancers in patients with combined pulmonary fibrosis and emphysema. Thoracic Cancer 2013;4:354–60.

122. Kitaguchi Y, Fujimoto K, Hanaoka M, et al. Clinical characteristics of combined pulmonary fibrosis and emphysema. Respirology 2010;15:265–71.

123. Girard N, Marchand-Adam S, Naccache JM, et al. Lung cancer in combined pulmonary fibrosis and emphysema: a series of 47 western patients. J Thorac Oncol 2014;9(8):1162–70.

124. Raghu G, Selman M. New antifibrotic treatments indicated for idiopathic pulmonary fibrosis offer hopes and raises questions [Editorial]. Am J Respir Crit Care Med 2015;191(3):252–4.

125. Raghu G, Anstrom KJ, King TE Jr, et al, Idiopathic Pulmonary Fibrosis Clinical Research Network. Prednisone, azathioprine, and N-acetylcysteine for pulmonary fibrosis. N Engl J Med 2012;366:1968–77.

126. Aravena C, Labarca G, Venegas C, et al. Pirfenidone for idiopathic pulmonary fibrosis: a systematic review and meta-analysis. PLoS One 2015;10(8):e0136160.

127. King TE Jr, Bradford WZ, Castro-Bernardini S, et al. A phase 3 trial of pirfenidone in patients with idiopathic pulmonary fibrosis. N Engl J Med 2014;370:2083–92.

128. Taniguchi H, Ebina M, Kondoh Y, et al. Pirfenidone in idiopathic pulmonary fibrosis. Eur Respir J 2010;35:821–9.

129. Noble PW, Albera C, Bradford WZ, et al. Pirfenidone in patients with idiopathic pulmonary fibrosis (CAPACITY): two randomised trials. Lancet 2011;377:1760–9.

130. Spagnolo P, Maher TM, Richeldi L. Idiopathic pulmonary fibrosis: recent advances on pharmacological therapy. Pharmacol Ther 2015;152:18–27.

131. Richeldi L, du Boid RM, Raghu G, et al. Efficacy and safety of nintedanib in idiopathic pulmonary fibrosis. N Engl J Med 2014;370(22):2071–82.

132. King CS, Nathan SD. Practical considerations in the pharmacologic treatment of idiopathic pulmonary fibrosis. Curr Opin Pulm Med 2015;21(5):479–89.

133. Lehtonen ST, Veijola A, Karvonen H, et al. Pirfenidone and nintedanib modulate properties of fibroblasts and myofibroblasts in idiopathic pulmonary fibrosis. Respir Res 2016;17(1):14.

Imaging of Pulmonary Manifestations of Connective Tissue Diseases

 CrossMark

Jitesh Ahuja, MD[a],*, Deepika Arora, MD[b],
Jeffrey P. Kanne, MD[c], Travis S. Henry, MD[d],
J. David Godwin, MD[a]

KEYWORDS

• Connective tissue disease • Interstitial lung disease • Autoimmune lung disease

KEY POINTS

• Connective tissue diseases (CTDs) are a heterogeneous group of systemic inflammatory disorders characterized by the presence of circulating autoantibodies and autoimmune-mediated organ damage.
• The lung is a frequent target and more than one thoracic compartment can be involved, including the airway, lung parenchyma, pulmonary vasculature, pleura, and pericardium.
• Interstitial lung disease (ILD) and pulmonary arterial hypertension are the most common thoracic manifestations, and they increase morbidity and mortality in patients with CTDs.
• The most common histopathologic patterns of ILD are nonspecific interstitial pneumonia, usual interstitial pneumonia, organizing pneumonia, and lymphoid interstitial pneumonia.
• The radiologic and histopathologic features of ILD in patients with CTDs are similar to those with idiopathic ILD. Extrapulmonary manifestations, demographic features, and serology can help distinguish CTD-ILD from idiopathic ILD.

INTRODUCTION

Connective tissue diseases (CTDs), also called collagen vascular diseases, are a heterogeneous group of systemic inflammatory disorders characterized by the presence of circulating autoantibodies (Table 1) and autoimmune-mediated organ damage. The lung is a frequent target, and more than one thoracic compartment can be involved, including the airways, lung parenchyma, pulmonary vasculature, pleura, and pericardium.

The CTDs that often involve the respiratory system are rheumatoid arthritis (RA), scleroderma or system sclerosis (SSc), Sjögren syndrome (SS), polymyositis (PM)/dermatomyositis (DM), systemic lupus erythematosis (SLE), mixed CTD (MCTD), and undifferentiated CTD (UCTD).

Interstitial lung disease (ILD) and pulmonary arterial hypertension are the most common thoracic manifestations, and they increase morbidity and mortality in patients with CTD.[1,2] Thoracic abnormalities usually follow systemic

[a] Department of Radiology, University of Washington, 1959 Northeast Pacific Street, Seattle, WA 98195, USA; [b] Division of Rheumatology, Multicare Health System, Allenmore Medical Center Building A, 1901 South Union Avenue, Suite A221, Tacoma, WA 98405, USA; [c] Department of Radiology, School of Medicine and Public Health, University of Wisconsin, 600 Highland Avenue, Madison, WI 53792, USA; [d] Department of Radiology and Biomedical Imaging, University of California, 505 Parnassus Avenue M391, Box 0628, San Francisco, CA 94143, USA
* Corresponding author. Department of Radiology, University of Washington, 1959 Northeast Pacific Street, Box 357115, Seattle, WA 98195.
E-mail address: ahujaj@uw.edu

Radiol Clin N Am 54 (2016) 1015–1031
http://dx.doi.org/10.1016/j.rcl.2016.05.005
0033-8389/16/$ – see front matter © 2016 Elsevier Inc. All rights reserved.

radiologic.theclinics.com

Table 1
Autoantibodies in CTDs

Autoantibody	CTD
ANA	Various CTDs (SLE, SSc, SS, PM/DM) Nucleolar staining suggests SSc
Anti-dsDNA antibody	SLE
Anti-Ro antibody	SLE, SS
Anti-La antibody	SS, SLE
Anti-topoisomerase I (anti-Scl-70)	SSc
RF	RA, SS
Anti-CCP antibody	RA
Anti-RNP	MCTD
Anti-tRNA synthetases (Jo-1, MDA-5)	PM/DM/ antisynthetase syndrome

Abbreviations: ANA, antinuclear antibody; CCP, cyclic citrullinated peptide; dsDNA, double-stranded DNA; MCTD, mixed connective tissue disease; PM/DM, polymyositis/dermatomyositis; RA, rheumatoid arthritis; RF, rheumatoid factor; RNP, ribonucleoprotein; SLE, systemic lupus erythematosis; SS, Sjögren syndrome; SSc, systemic sclerosis.

manifestations of the CTDs but occasionally precede extrathoracic manifestations by months or even years.[1,3,4]

The pattern and frequency of thoracic diseases vary depending on the underlying CTD (Table 2). The most common histopathologic patterns of ILD are nonspecific interstitial pneumonia (NSIP), usual interstitial pneumonia (UIP), organizing pneumonia (OP), and lymphoid interstitial pneumonia (LIP).

The radiologic and histopathologic features of ILD in patients with CTDs are similar to those with idiopathic interstitial pneumonia.[5,6] However, close evaluation of the chest radiograph and high-resolution computed tomography (HRCT) scans can offer clues to the underlying CTD. For example, arthropathy suggests RA; esophageal dilation and pulmonary artery enlargement out of proportion to lung fibrosis suggest SSc; soft tissue calcification suggests DM or SSc; and pleural or pericardial effusion or thickening suggests SLE.

Extrapulmonary manifestations, demographic features, and serology can help distinguish CTD-ILD from idiopathic interstitial pneumonia.[5,7] Mediastinal lymphadenopathy is frequent in CTD and should not be considered malignant in the absence of known neoplasm. Treatment complications, including drug toxicity and opportunistic infection, can confuse the radiologic appearance and make diagnosis more difficult.

This article focuses on the thoracic manifestations of CTDs and briefly discusses complications caused by treatment.

PATTERNS OF INTERSTITIAL LUNG DISEASE ASSOCIATED WITH CONNECTIVE TISSUE DISEASES
Nonspecific Interstitial Pneumonia

NSIP is the most common pattern of ILD in CTDs,[8,9] and NSIP associated with CTD is far more common than idiopathic NSIP.[10,11] Some patients who are initially thought to have idiopathic NSIP later manifest CTD. Hence, CTDs should be thoroughly investigated in patients who present with an NSIP pattern of ILD without extrathoracic manifestations of CTD.[12,13]

NSIP pattern can occur with any CTD but particularly in SSc, PM/DM, and MCTD.[1,14] Spatial and temporal homogeneity are the pathologic hallmarks of NSIP.[15] Depending on the degree of interstitial inflammation and fibrosis, NSIP is divided into 2 categories, cellular and fibrotic, the latter with a worse prognosis.[15,16] On HRCT, ground-glass opacity (GGO) is the predominant abnormality with mild reticulation and traction bronchiectasis and bronchiolectasis (Table 3). The abnormality is concentrated in lower lobes, often in a peribronchovascular distribution (Fig. 1). Another distinctive feature of NSIP is that fibrosis may to some extent spare the immediately subpleural lung zone; some degree of sparing has been found in 20% to 64% of patients with NSIP.[1,6,12,17–19] Reticulation and traction bronchiectasis and bronchiolectasis increase with more advanced fibrotic NSIP. Honeycombing develops in advanced stages, but is uncommon initially.[6,17]

Usual Interstitial Pneumonia

UIP is the second most common pattern of CTD-ILD and the most common pattern of RA-ILD.[6,17] Pathologically, UIP is characterized by spatial and temporal heterogeneity.[15] Radiologic and pathologic features of UIP in CTDs are similar to those in idiopathic pulmonary fibrosis (IPF), except that fibroblastic foci may be less frequent than in IPF, which may account for the better prognosis of UIP in CTD than in IPF.[20]

HRCT features of UIP include peripheral and lower lobe predominance of reticulation, traction bronchiectasis, and honeycombing (Fig. 2). Coronal reformatting helps to display this distribution. Honeycombing needs to be distinguished from paraseptal emphysema and traction bronchiolectasis. Honeycombing is identified by peripheral

Table 2
Relative prevalence of ILD in connective tissue disease

ILD Pattern	SSc	RA	SLE	PM/DM	MCTD	SS
ILD overall	+++	++	+	+++	++	++
NSIP	+++	++	++	+++	++	+++
UIP	+	+++	+	+	+	+
OP	+	++	+	+++	+	–
LIP	–	+	+	–	–	++
Common ILD Patterns	NSIP >> UIP	UIP > NSIP = OP > LIP	NSIP > UIP = LIP = OP	NSIP = OP > UIP	NSIP > OP = UIP	NSIP > LIP > UIP

Abbreviations: LIP, lymphoid interstitial pneumonia; NSIP, nonspecific interstitial pneumonia; OP, organizing pneumonia; UIP, usual interstitial pneumonia.

Table 3
Typical HRCT findings suggestive of ILD histology

ILD Histology	Typical HRCT Findings
NSIP	Bilateral basal-predominant ground-glass opacities in peribronchovascular distribution with or without subpleural sparing. Reticulation and traction bronchiectasis can be seen with fibrotic NSIP. Honeycombing is rare.
UIP	Peripheral and basal-predominant reticulation with traction bronchiectasis/bronchiolectasis. Architectural distortion, honeycombing, and volume loss in advanced disease.
OP	Areas of GGO or consolidation in basal distribution with peripheral or peribronchovascular predominance. Reverse halo sign (atoll sign) can be seen.
LIP	Ground-glass opacities with scattered thin-walled cysts, primarily in a perivascular distribution. Reticulation and nodules may occur.

clustering of cysts that have well-defined and shared walls. Paraseptal emphysema is more common in upper lungs and emphysematous cystic spaces often retain accompanying blood vessels. The dilated airways of traction bronchiolectasis can be traced proximally to connect to more central airways.[21] GGO may be present but it is not the predominant finding in UIP; it usually indicates early or fine fibrosis rather than interstitial inflammation when it is present in the vicinity of reticulation.[1,17,21]

Organizing Pneumonia

OP can occur in any CTD but is most commonly associated with PM/DM.[1,9,17] On histology, OP is characterized by the presence of granulation tissue in alveoli, alveolar ducts, and small airways.[9,11]

HRCT shows bilateral consolidation with peripheral or peribronchial distribution. Lower lobes are slightly more commonly involved than upper lobes

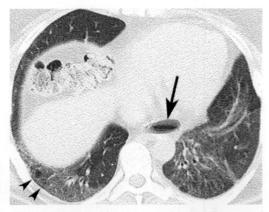

Fig. 1. A 38-year-old woman with scleroderma and NSIP. HRCT shows basal-predominant GGO in a peribronchovascular distribution, with subpleural sparing (*arrowheads*). Esophageal dilation is present (*arrow*).

(Fig. 3). Polygonal or arcadelike opacities indicating a perilobular distribution are also common. Other findings include patchy GGO, large nodular or masslike consolidation, and GGO surrounded by ring-shaped or crescent-shaped consolidation (reverse halo or atoll sign). Bronchial dilation can be seen within the consolidation.[1,17,22,23] OP usually responds to corticosteroid treatment.

Lymphoid Interstitial Pneumonia

LIP is uncommon. It is associated not only with CTD but also with acquired immunodeficiency syndrome and other immunodeficiencies. Among CTDs, LIP is most closely associated with SS but also with SLE and RA.[17,24] On histology, it is characterized by interstitial infiltration and expansion by polyclonal lymphocytes and plasma cells. HRCT shows basal-predominant GGO and thin-walled cysts in peribronchovascular distribution (Fig. 4). Other findings include perilymphatic nodules and interlobular septal thickening. Occasionally, large nodules occur in association with cysts, suggesting lymphoma or amyloidosis, the latter especially if the nodules are calcified or ossified.[1,17,22,25]

SPECIFIC CONNECTIVE TISSUE DISEASES
Rheumatoid Arthritis

RA is the most common CTD, affecting 1% of the population worldwide. RA is more common in women (female/male ratio, 3:1), usually between 25 and 50 years of age.[26] It is characterized by progressive, symmetric, and chronic inflammatory polyarthropathy, especially involving small joints of the hands and feet. Extra-articular manifestations, including thoracic manifestations, are frequent in patients with seropositive and nodular disease. Although articular disease is more common in women, pulmonary manifestations are more common in men.[26] The risk of lung disease is increased

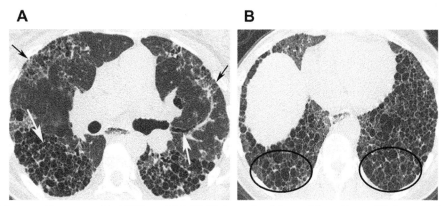

Fig. 2. A 51-year-old woman with MCTD and UIP. HRCT through midlungs (*A*) and bases (*B*) shows peripheral and basal-predominant reticulation (*black arrows*), traction bronchiectasis (*white arrows*), and honeycombing (*circles*).

by cigarette smoking, a high titer of rheumatoid factor (RF), and seropositivity for anticyclic citrullinated peptide.[5]

RA can affect all the components of the respiratory tract. Occasionally it presents with pulmonary disease. Lung involvement, especially RA-ILD, increases morbidity and mortality in patients with RA; mortality is 3 times higher with RA-ILD. Lung disease is second to infection as the most common cause of death in patients with RA.[3,27,28]

Pleural disease including effusion and thickening is the most common thoracic manifestation of RA. Pleural effusion develops in 5% of clinic cases but pleural effusion or thickening is found in 38% to 73% in autopsy series. Pleural effusion is usually small and unilateral; it often resolves spontaneously.[1,6,26,29]

The prevalence of clinically significant ILD in RA is 5%. Unlike other CTDs, in which NSIP is the most common ILD pattern, UIP is the most common ILD pattern in RA, followed by NSIP and OP (**Fig. 5**). Rarely, desquamative interstitial pneumonia and LIP occur with RA.[30–32] The severity of ILD does not always go with the severity of articular disease. In RA, a UIP pattern of ILD carries a worse prognosis than other patterns of ILD. Although CTD-associated ILDs have a better prognosis than idiopathic ILD of the same severity, there is no survival difference between RA-UIP and idiopathic UIP (IPF).[33,34] Histopathologically, CTD-associated ILD has fewer fibroblastic foci, more lymphoid aggregates, and more germinal centers than does idiopathic ILD.[32]

Small airways diseases in RA includes constrictive bronchiolitis (also known as obliterative or fibrotic bronchiolitis) and follicular bronchiolitis. Physiologic evidence of its presence can be seen in 16% to 68% of patients.[35,36] HRCT is more sensitive than pulmonary function testing in revealing small airways diseases in patients with

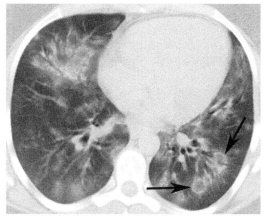

Fig. 3. A 30-year-old woman with polymyositis and OP. Computed tomography (CT) shows bilateral peribronchovascular nodular consolidations, some of which show reverse halo sign or atoll sign (*arrows*).

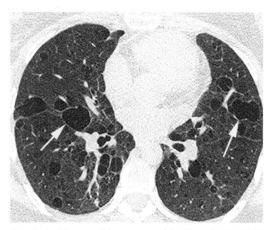

Fig. 4. A 34-year-old woman with SS and LIP. HRCT shows thin-walled cysts (*arrows*) in peribronchovascular distribution in both lungs.

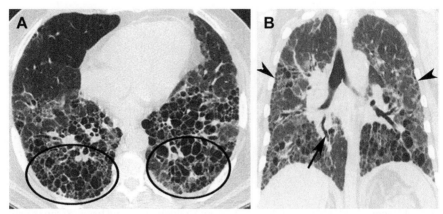

Fig. 5. A 63-year-old man with RA and UIP. Axial (*A*) and coronal reformatted (*B*) HRCT shows peripheral and basal-predominant reticulation (*arrowheads in B*), traction bronchiectasis (*arrow in B*), and honeycombing (*circles in A*).

asymptomatic RA, showing it in up to two-thirds of patients with RA with normal physiologic testing[3,37] (Fig. 6). On histology, constrictive bronchiolitis shows fibrous narrowing and obliteration of small airways. HRCT shows mosaic attenuation on inspiratory images and air trapping on expiratory images. Bronchiectasis and bronchial wall thickening often accompany constrictive bronchiolitis.[37,38]

Follicular bronchiolitis is characterized by lymphoid follicles in a peribronchial and peribronchiolar distribution. HRCT shows small centrilobular nodules and branching shadows of GGO or greater opacity (Fig. 7). Follicular bronchiolitis often responds to corticosteroid therapy, but constrictive bronchiolitis does not respond to therapy and may lead to respiratory failure and death.[36,37]

Cricoarytenoid arthritis is under-recognized, but occurs in up to 75% of patients with RA examined with direct laryngoscopy. Patients present with hoarseness, odynophagia, dysphagia, or globus sensation. It can cause life-threatening airway compromise, especially in the setting of endotracheal intubation.[39,40]

Patients with RA may also have necrobiotic lung nodules, which range from 0.5 to 5 cm in diameter (Fig. 8). They are found on HRCT in up to 20% of patients with RA.[1,41] Rheumatoid nodules are more frequent in men, smokers, and patients with subcutaneous nodules and high RF titer. Lung nodules are usually asymptomatic. Pathologically, they are similar to subcutaneous nodules, with central fibrinoid necrosis and surrounding granulomatous inflammation.[42]

Rheumatoid nodules are usually peripherally located in the mid and upper lung zones. They may cavitate, grow, or resolve spontaneously. Rarely, they rupture into the pleural space and cause pneumothorax, pleural effusion, or empyema. Differential diagnosis includes nodules caused by infection, tumor, and even amyloidosis, and bronchoscopy or biopsy may be required. The association of rheumatoid nodules with pneumoconiosis coal workers' pneumoconiosis is known as Caplan syndrome.[43] However, Caplan syndrome is extremely rare.

The medications used to treat RA can cause pulmonary complications, including ILD, and predispose to opportunistic infection. Penicillamine and

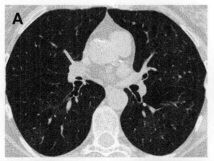
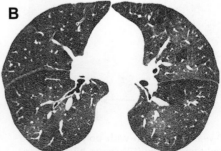

Fig. 6. A 60-year-old woman with RA and constrictive bronchiolitis. Inspiratory (*A*) and expiratory (*B*) HRCT shows mosaic attenuation in both lungs, better seen on expiratory image (*B*), and indicating air trapping.

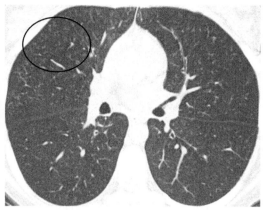

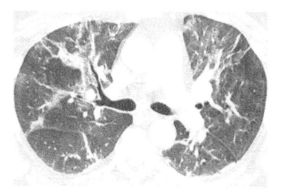

Fig. 9. A 64-year-old man with RA on methotrexate developed OP. HRCT shows peribronchovascular GGO and consolidation in both lungs.

Fig. 7. A 41-year-old woman with RA and follicular bronchiolitis. HRCT shows ill-defined centrilobular nodules in right upper lobe (*circle*).

gold salts can cause constrictive bronchiolitis and diffuse alveolar damage[30,44]; these agents are no longer in common use. Methotrexate can cause OP, hypersensitivity reaction, pulmonary fibrosis, and diffuse alveolar damage (Fig. 9). Patients with preexisting lung disease are more susceptible to methotrexate pulmonary toxicity.[44,45] Pulmonary function tests, chest radiographs, and even HRCT in some cases are sometimes obtained before the patient begins treatment with methotrexate or other immunomodulator drugs and during treatment if new pulmonary symptoms arise. Excluding infection and establishing the temporal relationship between drug treatment and onset of symptoms and radiologic findings help diagnose drug toxicity. Symptoms usually decrease when the offending medication is stopped. Bronchoscopy and biopsy may be required, especially in the acute setting, to make the diagnosis of drug toxicity and exclude other causes of lung disease.

Systemic Sclerosis/Scleroderma

SSc, a multisystem autoimmune disease, is more common in women (male/female ratio of 1:3 to 1:8) and has peak incidence between 45 and 64 years of age.[46] The pathologic triad of inflammation, fibrosis, and vascular damage characterizes this disease.

SSc is categorized as limited or diffuse, based on the degree of cutaneous involvement. The limited form is known as CREST (calcinosis, Raynaud phenomenon, esophageal dysmotility, sclerodactyly, and telangiectasia) syndrome. The two categories have different patterns of organ involvement, clinical manifestations, autoantibody profile, and prognosis. ILD and pulmonary arterial hypertension are the two most common pulmonary manifestations of SSc and are the leading causes of morbidity and mortality. Pulmonary arterial hypertension can result from either pulmonary vasculopathy or pulmonary fibrosis. ILD is more common in patients with diffuse SSc, whereas pulmonary arterial hypertension is more prevalent in the limited form.[1,6,47]

ILD is found on autopsy in up to 75% of patients with SSc, and NSIP is the most common pattern[1,6,48] (Fig. 10); UIP is the second most common pattern, and its prognosis is worse. In the largest study of biopsy-proven SSc-ILD, 77% of the patients had NSIP (mostly fibrotic), and the remainder had UIP.[49,50] On HRCT, cellular NSIP shows GGO in peribronchovascular distribution with lower lobe predominance, often with subpleural sparing. Fibrotic NSIP may have bronchiectasis and bronchiolectasis within GGO. GGO in cellular NSIP corresponds histologically with interstitial

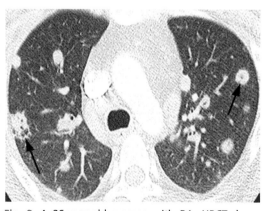

Fig. 8. A 26-year-old woman with RA. HRCT shows well-defined soft tissue nodules in both lungs, some of which have central cavitation (*arrows*).

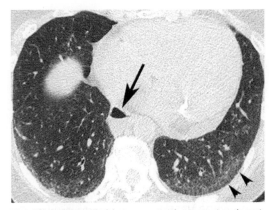

Fig. 10. A 53-year-old woman with systemic sclerosis and NSIP. HRCT shows basal-predominant GGO with subpleural sparing (*arrowheads*). Esophageal dilation is noted (*arrow*).

inflammation and may respond to treatment, whereas GGO in fibrotic NSIP corresponds with fibrosis rather than inflammation and does not respond to treatment[6,17] (**Fig. 11**).

In patients with pulmonary arterial hypertension, radiography or computed tomography (CT) usually shows enlarged central pulmonary arteries, but normal-sized arteries do not exclude the diagnosis (**Fig. 12**). Mosaic attenuation on HRCT reflects the patchy hyperemia and oligemia.[1,51]

Esophageal involvement is an early manifestation of SSc, found in up to 97% of patients.[46] Esophageal dysmotility can lead to aspiration bronchiolitis or pneumonia. HRCT shows centrilobular nodules, consolidation, bronchiectasis, and mucous plugging in the dependent portion of the lungs.

SSc often involves the heart, with myocardial fibrosis, arrhythmia, heart failure, or pericardial disease.[52,53] SSc increases the risk of lung cancer, likely because of pulmonary fibrosis.[54]

Sjögren Syndrome

SS is characterized by T-lymphocyte infiltration of various organs, typically lacrimal and salivary glands and the respiratory tract. Symptoms include xerophthalmia (dry eyes) and xerostomia (dry mouth). Upper airway involvement can manifest as crusting and dryness of the nasal mucosa causing epistaxis or septal perforation; these findings should also promote consideration of granulomatosis with polyangiitis (GPA). SS affects women more often than men (female/male ratio of 9:1), usually in the fourth and fifth decades of life. Most cases of SS are primary, but one-third of cases are secondary; that is, associated with other CTDs such as RA, SLE, or scleroderma.[1,3,55]

ILD is common in SS, most often NSIP, but LIP, UIP, OP, and even amyloidosis also occur[56–58] (**Fig. 13**). When SS impairs the mucous glands of the airways, microbial clearance is impaired, leading to recurrent infection and bronchiectasis. Other airway abnormalities include follicular bronchiolitis and constrictive bronchiolitis. Pleural involvement is uncommon and is almost always associated with secondary SS, particularly in cases with RA or SLE.[1,57]

Patients with SS have a 16-times to 44-times increased risk of lymphoma.[1,59] SS-associated lymphoma usually arises from the salivary glands or mucosa-associated lymphoid tissue of the stomach or lung; it is usually a non-Hodgkin B-cell type and has a good prognosis. Lymphoma should be considered if CT shows large nodules (>1 cm), consolidation, or pleural effusion.[60]

Morbidity in SS is usually caused by impaired function of exocrine glands. Increased mortality is caused by associated disease in patients with secondary SS or by development of lymphoproliferative disorder.[58]

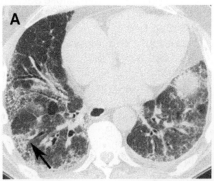
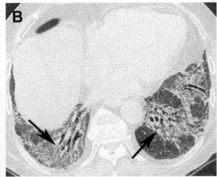

Fig. 11. A 58-year-woman with systemic sclerosis and fibrotic NSIP. HRCT through midlungs (*A*) and bases (*B*) shows basal-predominant GGO in peribronchovascular distribution with traction bronchiectasis (*arrows*).

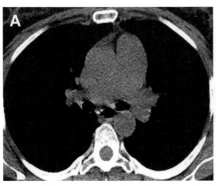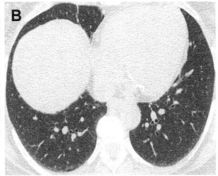

Fig. 12. A 53-year-old woman with scleroderma and pulmonary hypertension. CT with soft tissue (*A*) and lung (*B*) windows shows dilated main pulmonary artery (*A*) in the absence of pulmonary fibrosis (*B*).

Systemic Lupus Erythematosis

SLE has a wide range of immunologic and clinical manifestations. It affects mostly women (female/male ratio of 6–9:1) of reproductive age, with a predilection for the African American population in the United States.[61]

Pleural disease is the most common thoracic manifestation. Pleuritic chest pain, fever, cough, and dyspnea are typical. Pleural effusion, unilateral or bilateral, and usually small, occurs in 30% to 50% of patients with SLE (Fig. 14). The diagnosis of lupus pleuritis is established by pleural fluid serology, with high antinuclear antibody (ANA) titer and higher ANA titers in the pleural fluid than in the blood serum.[62] Pericardial effusion and cardiomegaly occur in 35% of patients with SLE[53,63] (see Fig. 14).

Infection causes a lot of morbidity and mortality in patients with SLE, one of the most common being community-acquired pneumonia (Fig. 15). However, several atypical infections are important, including those caused by *Pneumocystis jiroveci*, *Cytomegalovirus*, *Aspergillus*, *Nocardia*, and mycobacteria in patients on high-dose corticosteroids or other immunosuppressive drugs.[64,65]

Acute lupus pneumonitis occurs in 14% of patients with SLE and is the presenting manifestation of SLE in about half of them.[66] Clinically and radiologically, acute lupus pneumonitis resembles infectious pneumonia. HRCT shows patchy consolidation or GGO, with or without pleural effusion (Fig. 16). Infection must be excluded before corticosteroids or immunosuppressive drugs are given. Mortality in acute lupus pneumonitis is as high as 50%, and half of the surviving patients develop chronic lung abnormalities.[66,67]

Diffuse alveolar hemorrhage (DAH) is another severe but rare complication of SLE; it can mimic acute lupus pneumonitis or infection. Its prevalence is 2% to 5.4% of patients with SLE.[68] HRCT shows bilateral consolidation, GGO, and interlobular septal thickening, predominantly in central mid and lower lung zones, with relative sparing of the periphery[1,6,17] (Fig. 17). DAH should be suspected in patient with SLE presenting with sudden onset of dyspnea, new diffuse opacities on radiographs or CT, and decreased hematocrit, with or without hemoptysis. Bronchoalveolar lavage is required to exclude infection and confirm DAH. Mortality in DAH is about 50%.[68]

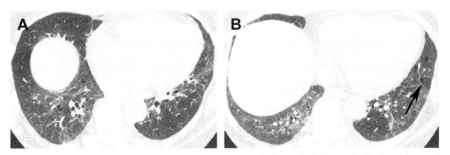

Fig. 13. A 63-year-old woman with SS and LIP. HRCT at two levels (*A* and *B*) through the lung bases shows basal-predominant GGO bilaterally and a few cysts in the left lower lobe (*arrow in B*).

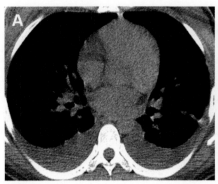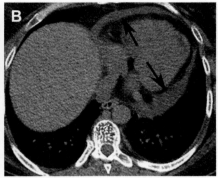

Fig. 14. Two different patients with SLE. CT of a 31-year-old woman (*A*) shows bilateral pleural effusions, and CT of a 49-year-old woman (*B*) shows pericardial effusion (*arrows*).

In contrast with other CTDs, ILD is uncommon in SLE, affecting only about 3% of cases. NSIP is the most common histologic pattern.[69] Airway disease is also infrequent.

Shrinking lung syndrome (SLS) is a rare, but probably underdiagnosed, cause of respiratory disease in patients with SLE.[70,71] SLS is characterized by progressive loss of lung volume without underlying lung fibrosis or pleural disease.[71] Weakness of the respiratory muscles (including the diaphragm) is a hallmark of SLS, but the exact cause is unclear.[72] Possible mechanisms include a primary myopathy of the respiratory muscles, phrenic nerve palsy, or diffuse diaphragm fibrosis.[73]

Patients with SLS present with progressive dyspnea over weeks to months, with or without pleuritic chest pain. Physical examination is often notable for rapid, shallow breathing, use of accessory ventilator muscles, and paradoxic abdominal wall movement.[74] PFTs show low lung volume and restriction. Imaging findings include low lung volume with elevation of the hemidiaphragms and basal atelectasis, in the absence of significant ILD or pleural disease.[72–76] Comparison with earlier chest radiographs shows the decrease in lung volume (**Fig. 18**), and fluoroscopy of the diaphragm (sniff test) may show decreased diaphragmatic excursion.[77] In one case of confirmed SLS at our institution, CT showed thinning of the diaphragmatic crura (see **Fig. 18**). Although the finding of crus thinning provides objective evidence of diaphragm wasting, it does not reveal whether the cause is neurologic or myopathic. Thus, by observing low lung volume and possibly diaphragm muscle thinning, radiologists may be able to suggest the diagnosis of SLS. Prompt recognition is important because high-dose corticosteroid treatment can reduce morbidity.[73,74]

Some patients with SLE have recurrent venous or arterial thrombosis caused by antiphospholipid antibodies, with risk of pulmonary embolism, stroke, and pregnancy-related mortality such as

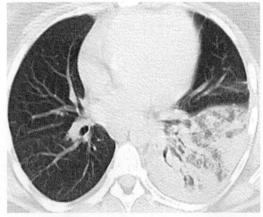

Fig. 15. A 33-year-old woman with SLE and community-acquired pneumonia. HRCT shows consolidation in the left lower lobe.

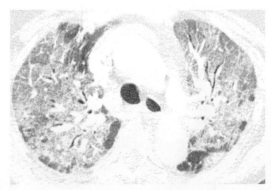

Fig. 16. A 71-year-old woman with SLE and acute lupus pneumonitis. HRCT shows diffuse GGO in both lungs.

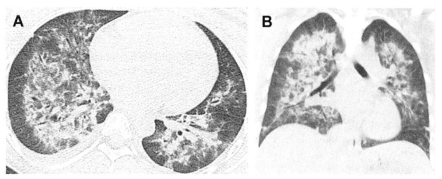

Fig. 17. A 20-year-old woman with SLE and DAH. Axial (*A*) and coronal reformatted (*B*) HRCT shows consolidation predominantly in a central distribution, with peripheral sparing.

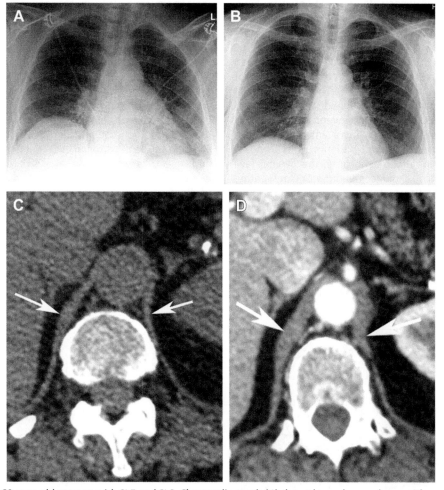

Fig. 18. A 60-year-old woman with SLE and SLS. Chest radiograph (*A*) shows lower lung volume with new vascular crowding and basal atelectasis compared with baseline radiograph 3 years before (*B*). Axial CT image (*C*) shows thinning of the diaphragmatic crura (*arrows*), a new finding from prior CT (*D*). No fibrosis was visible on lung windows (not shown) of the CT scan.

preeclampsia, HELLP (hemolysis, elevated liver enzyme levels, low platelet counts) syndrome, and miscarriage (Fig. 19). Rarely, chronic pulmonary thromboembolic disease and pulmonary hypertension develop.[78]

Polymyositis and Dermatomyositis

PM and DM are idiopathic myopathies characterized by inflammation in proximal skeletal muscles. PM/DM manifests as proximal muscles weakness that evolves over several weeks or months. DM is distinguished from PM by cutaneous manifestations, including heliotrope rash on the eyelids, Gottron papules over the knuckles, mechanic's hands, V sign, and shawl sign. PM/DM is more common in women than in men (female/male ratio, 2:1) and has a bimodal age incidence, with the first peak during childhood (10–15 years) and the second peak during adulthood (35–65 years).[79] Underlying malignancy (carcinoma of the lung, breast, colon, or cervix) should be suspected with late-onset disease (>50 years of age), more frequently with DM than PM.[80]

Thoracic manifestations occur in more than 50% of cases and are a common cause of morbidity and mortality.[79,81] They include ILD, aspiration syndromes caused by pharyngeal muscle weakness, and hypoventilation or respiratory failure caused by involvement of respiratory muscles.[81] Some patients with PM/DM have antisynthetase syndrome, the clinical features of which include inflammatory myopathy, ILD, fever, inflammatory arthritis, Raynaud phenomenon, mechanic's hands, esophageal dysmotility, and antisynthetase antibodies on serology.[82] Anti–Jo-1 is the most common antisynthetase antibody, and its presence is strongly associated with ILD. About 50% to 70% of patients who are anti–Jo-1 positive develop ILD, but only 10% of patients who are negative

develop ILD.[82,83] The recently identified anti-MDA5 (melanoma differentiation-associated gene 5) antibodies are associated with clinically amyopathic PM/DM, rapidly progressive ILD, severe skin manifestations, and poor prognosis.[84]

NSIP and OP are the most common patterns of ILD in patients with PM/DM (Fig. 20) and they frequently coexist. UIP is less common, and, rarely, acute interstitial pneumonia occurs with histologic pattern of diffuse alveolar damage.[1,17,85] As with other collagen vascular diseases, ILD may precede clinical myositis and skin lesions. Airway and pleural involvement and pulmonary arterial hypertension are rare in PM/DM.

Mixed Connective Tissue Disease

MCTD is a distinct clinical entity with features of SLE, SSc, RA, or PM/DM with high-titer anti-ribonucleoprotein antibodies. It affects women (female/male ratio, 9:1) in the second and third decades. Common clinical features include Raynaud phenomenon, inflammatory arthritis, serositis (pleuritis and pericarditis), myositis, and esophageal dysfunction.[86,87]

Thoracic manifestations occur in 20% to 80% of patients,[8,87] the most common of which are ILD and pulmonary arterial hypertension. ILD occurs in 20% to 60% of patients, and NSIP is the most common histopathologic pattern (Fig. 21), with UIP and LIP less common.[1,6,87] Esophageal dysmotility and gastroesophageal reflux are common, and they promote aspiration syndromes. Some investigators have suggested that chronic gastroesophageal reflux is a factor in the pathogenesis of ILD.[88]

Pulmonary arterial hypertension occurs in 10% to 45% of patients,[47] and it indicates a bad prognosis.[89] As with SSc, pulmonary arterial hypertension usually indicates vasculopathy (World Health Organization [WHO] class I) rather than underlying

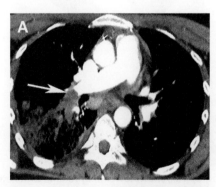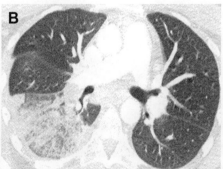

Fig. 19. A 33-year-old woman with SLE. CT with soft tissue (A) and lung (B) window settings shows occlusive thromboembolism in the interlobar right pulmonary artery (arrow in A). The large GGO in the right lower lobe (B) likely represents pulmonary hemorrhage from the acute pulmonary embolism.

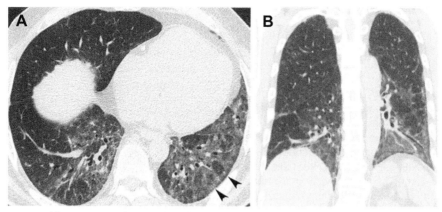

Fig. 20. A 55-year-old man with polymyositis and NSIP. Axial (*A*) and coronal reformatted (*B*) HRCT shows basal-predominant GGO with subpleural sparing (*arrowheads*).

ILD (WHO class III). Pleural thickening or effusion occurs in less than 10% of patients, usually in association with predominant clinical features of SLE. Less common thoracic manifestations are alveolar hemorrhage, thromboembolism, and respiratory muscle dysfunction.[6,47]

Undifferentiated Connective Tissue Disease

UCTD is defined as an autoimmune disease that is manifested by positive ANA and signs and symptoms of CTD that persist for at least 3 years, but that does not meet criteria that would allow it to be classified as a defined CTD. Some cases evolve into a defined CTD, usually within 5 years (early or evolving UCTD). Cases that do not develop a defined CTD (stable UCTD) are usually mild, with no major organ involvement. Another set of patients may have single-organ involvement (eg, lung, nervous system, or liver), with positive ANA and nonspecific clinical manifestations. About a third of patients affected by idiopathic NSIP have clinical manifestations suggesting UCTD; some

investigators have suggested the term lung-dominant-CTD to describe these cases, characterized by lung involvement, mild extrapulmonary symptoms, and positive ANA.[90,91]

NEWER BIOLOGIC AGENTS

In the last decade, many new biologic agents have proved effective in treating autoimmune diseases, particularly RA. These agents include the tumor necrosis factor inhibitors infliximab, etanercept, adalimumab, certolizumab, and golimumab; an interleukin (IL)-6 receptor inhibitor, tocilizumab; an IL-1 antagonist, anakinra; a T-cell blocker, abatacept; a B cell–depleting antibody, rituximab; and a Janus kinase inhibitor, tofacitinib.

These biologic agents can cause infectious and noninfectious pulmonary complications, such as reactivation of latent pulmonary tuberculosis, sarcoidlike reactions, and (rarely) ILD or exacerbation of preexisting ILD. Usually the benefits exceed the risks in treating patients with preexisting ILD.[92,93]

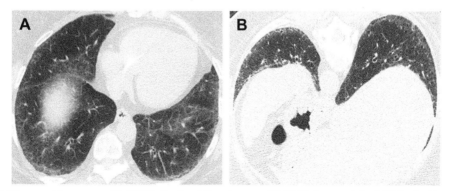

Fig. 21. A 68-year-old woman with MCTD. Supine (*A*) and prone (*B*) HRCT shows subtle GGO in the lung bases on supine image, which persists on prone image, indicating early ILD.

SUMMARY

CTDs are a heterogeneous group of systemic auto-immune disorders with a wide spectrum of pulmonary manifestations, including ILD, pleural disease, airway disease, and pulmonary hypertension. Lung manifestations may precede the systemic manifestations by months or years. Clinical and radiologic features of CTD-ILD are similar to those of idiopathic interstitial pneumonias. Radiologic clues on imaging, extrapulmonary manifestations, and serology help distinguish CTD-ILD from idiopathic interstitial pneumonia. Infections and treatment complications can add to the radiographic findings. Bronchoscopy and biopsy may be required to evaluate infection or drug toxicity. A multidisciplinary approach, with participation by pulmonologists, rheumatologists, radiologists, and pathologists, is often needed for effective evaluation and management of patients with CTDs.

REFERENCES

1. Capobianco J, Grimberg A, Thompson BM, et al. Thoracic manifestations of collagen vascular diseases. Radiographics 2012;32(1):33–50.
2. Woodhead F, Wells AU, Desai SR. Pulmonary complications of connective tissue diseases. Clin Chest Med 2008;29(1):149–64.
3. Olson AL, Brown KK, Fischer A. Connective tissue disease-associated lung disease. Immunol Allergy Clin N Am 2012;32(4):513–36.
4. Vij R, Strek ME. Diagnosis and treatment of connective tissue disease-associated interstitial lung disease. Chest 2013;143(3):814–24.
5. Bryson T, Sundaram B, Khanna D, et al. Connective tissue disease-associated interstitial pneumonia and idiopathic interstitial pneumonia: similarity and difference. Semin Ultrasound CT MR 2014;35(1):29–38.
6. Franquet T. High-resolution CT of lung disease related to collagen vascular disease. Radiol Clin North Am 2001;39(6):1171–87.
7. Mittoo S, Gelber AC, Christopher-Stine L, et al. Ascertainment of collagen vascular disease in patients presenting with interstitial lung disease. Respir Med 2009;103(8):1152–8.
8. Kim EA, Lee KS, Johkoh T, et al. Interstitial lung diseases associated with collagen vascular diseases: radiologic and histopathologic findings. Radiographics 2002;22:S151–65.
9. Tansey D, Wells AU, Colby TV, et al. Variations in histological patterns of interstitial pneumonia between connective tissue disorders and their relationship to prognosis. Histopathology 2004;44(6):585–96.
10. Cottin V. Significance of connective tissue diseases features in pulmonary fibrosis. Eur Respir Rev 2013;22(129):273–80.
11. Silva CI, Muller NL. Interstitial lung disease in the setting of collagen vascular disease. Semin Roentgenol 2010;45(1):22–8.
12. Travis WD, Hunninghake G, King TE Jr, et al. Idiopathic nonspecific interstitial pneumonia: report of an American Thoracic Society project. Am J Respir Crit Care Med 2008;177(12):1338–47.
13. Park IN, Jegal Y, Kim DS, et al. Clinical course and lung function change of idiopathic nonspecific interstitial pneumonia. Eur Respir J 2009;33(1):68–76.
14. Kligerman SJ, Groshong S, Brown KK, et al. Nonspecific interstitial pneumonia: radiologic, clinical, and pathologic considerations. Radiographics 2009;29(1):73–87.
15. American Thoracic Society, European Respiratory Society. American Thoracic Society/European Respiratory Society international multidisciplinary consensus classification of the idiopathic interstitial pneumonias. This joint statement of the American Thoracic Society (ATS), and the European Respiratory Society (ERS) was adopted by the ATS Board of Directors, June 2001 and by the ERS Executive Committee, June 2001. Am J Respir Crit Care Med 2002;165(2):277–304.
16. Travis WD, Matsui K, Moss J, et al. Idiopathic nonspecific interstitial pneumonia: prognostic significance of cellular and fibrosing patterns: survival comparison with usual interstitial pneumonia and desquamative interstitial pneumonia. Am J Surg Pathol 2000;24(1):19–33.
17. Lynch DA. Lung disease related to collagen vascular disease. J Thorac Imaging 2009;24(4):299–309.
18. Silva CI, Muller NL, Lynch DA, et al. Chronic hypersensitivity pneumonitis: differentiation from idiopathic pulmonary fibrosis and nonspecific interstitial pneumonia by using thin-section CT. Radiology 2008;246(1):288–97.
19. Silva CI, Muller NL, Hansell DM, et al. Nonspecific interstitial pneumonia and idiopathic pulmonary fibrosis: changes in pattern and distribution of disease over time. Radiology 2008;247(1):251–9.
20. Song JW, Do KH, Kim MY, et al. Pathologic and radiologic differences between idiopathic and collagen vascular disease-related usual interstitial pneumonia. Chest 2009;136(1):23–30.
21. Lynch DA, Huckleberry JM. Usual interstitial pneumonia: typical and atypical high-resolution computed tomography features. Semin Ultrasound CT MR 2014;35(1):12–23.
22. Mueller-Mang C, Grosse C, Schmid K, et al. What every radiologist should know about idiopathic interstitial pneumonias. Radiographics 2007;27(3):595–615.
23. Lynch DA, Travis WD, Muller NL, et al. Idiopathic interstitial pneumonias: CT features. Radiology 2005;236(1):10–21.

24. Swigris JJ, Berry GJ, Raffin TA, et al. Lymphoid interstitial pneumonia: a narrative review. Chest 2002; 122(6):2150–64.

25. Carrillo J, Restrepo CS, Rosado de Christenson M, et al. Lymphoproliferative lung disorders: a radiologic-pathologic overview. Part I: reactive disorders. Semin Ultrasound CT MR 2013;34(6):525–34.

26. Massey H, Darby M, Edey A. Thoracic complications of rheumatoid disease. Clin Radiol 2013; 68(3):293–301.

27. Olson AL, Swigris JJ, Sprunger DB, et al. Rheumatoid arthritis-interstitial lung disease-associated mortality. Am J Respir Crit Care Med 2011;183(3): 372–8.

28. Sihvonen S, Korpela M, Laippala P, et al. Death rates and causes of death in patients with rheumatoid arthritis: a population-based study. Scand J Rheumatol 2004;33(4):221–7.

29. Bouros D, Pneumatikos I, Tzouvelekis A. Pleural involvement in systemic autoimmune disorders. Respiration 2008;75(4):361–71.

30. Kim DS. Interstitial lung disease in rheumatoid arthritis: recent advances. Curr Opin Pulm Med 2006;12(5):346–53.

31. Kim EJ, Elicker BM, Maldonado F, et al. Usual interstitial pneumonia in rheumatoid arthritis-associated interstitial lung disease. Eur Respir J 2010;35(6): 1322–8.

32. Lee HK, Kim DS, Yoo B, et al. Histopathologic pattern and clinical features of rheumatoid arthritis-associated interstitial lung disease. Chest 2005; 127(6):2019–27.

33. Park JH, Kim DS, Park IN, et al. Prognosis of fibrotic interstitial pneumonia: idiopathic versus collagen vascular disease-related subtypes. Am J Respir Crit Care Med 2007;175(7):705–11.

34. Kim EJ, Collard HR, King TE Jr. Rheumatoid arthritis-associated interstitial lung disease: the relevance of histopathologic and radiographic pattern. Chest 2009;136(5):1397–405.

35. White ES, Tazelaar HD, Lynch JP 3rd. Bronchiolar complications of connective tissue diseases. Semin Respir Crit Care Med 2003;24(5):543–66.

36. Hayakawa H, Sato A, Imokawa S, et al. Bronchiolar disease in rheumatoid arthritis. Am J Respir Crit Care Med 1996;154(5):1531–6.

37. Perez T, Remy-Jardin M, Cortet B. Airways involvement in rheumatoid arthritis: clinical, functional, and HRCT findings. Am J Respir Crit Care Med 1998;157(5 Pt 1):1658–65.

38. Aquino SL, Webb WR, Golden J. Bronchiolitis obliterans associated with rheumatoid arthritis: findings on HRCT and dynamic expiratory CT. J Comput Assist Tomogr 1994;18(4):555–8.

39. Brazeau-Lamontagne L, Charlin B, Levesque RY, et al. Cricoarytenoiditis: CT assessment in rheumatoid arthritis. Radiology 1986;158(2):463–6.

40. Lawry GV, Finerman ML, Hanafee WN, et al. Laryngeal involvement in rheumatoid arthritis. A clinical, laryngoscopic, and computerized tomographic study. Arthritis Rheum 1984;27(8):873–82.

41. Cortet B, Flipo RM, Remy-Jardin M, et al. Use of high resolution computed tomography of the lungs in patients with rheumatoid arthritis. Ann Rheum Dis 1995;54(10):815–9.

42. Hakala M, Paakko P, Huhti E, et al. Open lung biopsy of patients with rheumatoid arthritis. Clin Rheumatol 1990;9(4):452–60.

43. Caplan A. Certain unusual radiological appearances in the chest of coal-miners suffering from rheumatoid arthritis. Thorax 1953;8(1):29–37.

44. Silva CI, Muller NL. Drug-induced lung diseases: most common reaction patterns and corresponding high-resolution CT manifestations. Semin Ultrasound CT MR 2006;27(2):111–6.

45. Imokawa S, Colby TV, Leslie KO, et al. Methotrexate pneumonitis: review of the literature and histopathological findings in nine patients. Eur Respir J 2000; 15(2):373–81.

46. Coral-Alvarado P, Pardo AL, Castano-Rodriguez N, et al. Systemic sclerosis: a world wide global analysis. Clin Rheumatol 2009;28(7):757–65.

47. Crestani B. The respiratory system in connective tissue disorders. Allergy 2005;60(6):715–34.

48. Fujita J, Yoshinouchi T, Ohtsuki Y, et al. Non-specific interstitial pneumonia as pulmonary involvement of systemic sclerosis. Ann Rheum Dis 2001;60(3): 281–3.

49. Bouros D, Wells AU, Nicholson AG, et al. Histopathologic subsets of fibrosing alveolitis in patients with systemic sclerosis and their relationship to outcome. Am J Respir Crit Care Med 2002; 165(12):1581–6.

50. Solomon JJ, Fischer A. Connective tissue disease-associated interstitial lung disease: a focused review. J Intensive Care Med 2015;30(7):392–400.

51. Grosse C, Grosse A. CT findings in diseases associated with pulmonary hypertension: a current review. Radiographics 2010;30(7):1753–77.

52. Strollo D, Goldin J. Imaging lung disease in systemic sclerosis. Curr Rheumatol Rep 2010;12(2): 156–61.

53. Ruano CA, Lucas RN, Leal CI, et al. Thoracic manifestations of connective tissue diseases. Curr Probl Diagn Radiol 2015;44(1):47–59.

54. Marasini B, Conciato L, Belloli L, et al. Systemic sclerosis and cancer. Int J Immunopathol Pharmacol 2009;22(3):573–8.

55. Mayberry JP, Primack SL, Muller NL. Thoracic manifestations of systemic autoimmune diseases: radiographic and high-resolution CT findings. Radiographics 2000;20(6):1623–35.

56. Ito I, Nagai S, Kitaichi M, et al. Pulmonary manifestations of primary Sjogren's syndrome: a clinical,

radiologic, and pathologic study. Am J Respir Crit Care Med 2005;171(6):632–8.

57. Matsuyama N, Ashizawa K, Okimoto T, et al. Pulmonary lesions associated with Sjogren's syndrome: radiographic and CT findings. Br J Radiol 2003; 76(912):880–4.

58. Parambil JG, Myers JL, Lindell RM, et al. Interstitial lung disease in primary Sjogren syndrome. Chest 2006;130(5):1489–95.

59. Kassan SS, Thomas TL, Moutsopoulos HM, et al. Increased risk of lymphoma in sicca syndrome. Ann Intern Med 1978;89(6):888–92.

60. Honda O, Johkoh T, Ichikado K, et al. Differential diagnosis of lymphocytic interstitial pneumonia and malignant lymphoma on high-resolution CT. AJR Am J Roentgenol 1999;173(1):71–4.

61. Pons-Estel GJ, Alarcon GS, Scofield L, et al. Understanding the epidemiology and progression of systemic lupus erythematosus. Semin Arthritis Rheum 2010;39(4):257–68.

62. Good JT Jr, King TE, Antony VB, et al. Lupus pleuritis. Clinical features and pleural fluid characteristics with special reference to pleural fluid antinuclear antibodies. Chest 1983;84(6):714–8.

63. Fenlon HM, Doran M, Sant SM, et al. High-resolution chest CT in systemic lupus erythematosus. AJR Am J Roentgenol 1996;166(2):301–7.

64. Kinder BW, Freemer MM, King TE Jr, et al. Clinical and genetic risk factors for pneumonia in systemic lupus erythematosus. Arthritis Rheum 2007;56(8): 2679–86.

65. Pego-Reigosa JM, Medeiros DA, Isenberg DA. Respiratory manifestations of systemic lupus erythematosus: old and new concepts. Best Pract Res Clin Rheumatol 2009;23(4):469–80.

66. Cheema GS, Quismorio FP Jr. Interstitial lung disease in systemic lupus erythematosus. Curr Opin Pulm Med 2000;6(5):424–9.

67. Matthay RA, Schwarz MI, Petty TL, et al. Pulmonary manifestations of systemic lupus erythematosus: review of twelve cases of acute lupus pneumonitis. Medicine (Baltimore) 1975;54(5):397–409.

68. Zamora MR, Warner ML, Tuder R, et al. Diffuse alveolar hemorrhage and systemic lupus erythematosus. Clinical presentation, histology, survival, and outcome. Medicine (Baltimore) 1997;76(3):192–202.

69. Weinrib L, Sharma OP, Quismorio FP Jr. A long-term study of interstitial lung disease in systemic lupus erythematosus. Semin Arthritis Rheum 1990;20(1):48–56.

70. Gheita TA, Azkalany GS, El-Fishawy HS, et al. Shrinking lung syndrome in systemic lupus erythematosus patients; clinical characteristics, disease activity and damage. Int J Rheum Dis 2011;14(4): 361–8.

71. Hoffbrand BI, Beck ER. "Unexplained" dyspnoea and shrinking lungs in systemic lupus erythematosus. Br Med J 1965;1(5445):1273–7.

72. Burns NS, Stevens AM, Iyer RS. Shrinking lung syndrome complicating pediatric systemic lupus erythematosus. Pediatr Radiol 2014;44(10): 1318–22.

73. Gheita TA, El-Mofty S, Fawzy SM, et al. Shrinking lung syndrome in systemic lupus erythematosus patients with dyspnea. Egypt Rheumatologist 2012; 34(4):179–83.

74. Warrington KJ, Moder KG, Brutinel WM. The shrinking lungs syndrome in systemic lupus erythematosus. Mayo Clin Proc 2000;75(5):467–72.

75. Singh R, Huang WQ, Menon Y, et al. Shrinking lung syndrome in systemic lupus erythematosus and Sjogren's syndrome. J Clin Rheumatol 2002;8(6): 340–5.

76. Pillai S, Mehta J, Levin T, et al. Shrinking lung syndrome presenting as an initial pulmonary manifestation of SLE. Lupus 2014;23(11):1201–3.

77. Allen D, Stoller JK, Minai OA. A 45-year-old woman with systemic lupus erythematosus and progressive dyspnea. Chest 2007;131(4):1252–5.

78. Love PE, Santoro SA. Antiphospholipid antibodies: anticardiolipin and the lupus anticoagulant in systemic lupus erythematosus (SLE) and in non-SLE disorders. Prevalence and clinical significance. Ann Intern Med 1990;112(9):682–98.

79. Dalakas MC, Hohlfeld R. Polymyositis and dermatomyositis. Lancet 2003;362(9388):971–82.

80. Hill CL, Zhang Y, Sigurgeirsson B, et al. Frequency of specific cancer types in dermatomyositis and polymyositis: a population-based study. Lancet 2001;357(9250):96–100.

81. Schwarz MI. The lung in polymyositis. Clin Chest Med 1998;19(4):701–12, viii.

82. Solomon J, Swigris JJ, Brown KK. Myositis-related interstitial lung disease and antisynthetase syndrome. J Bras Pneumol 2011;37(1):100–9.

83. Friedman AW, Targoff IN, Arnett FC. Interstitial lung disease with autoantibodies against aminoacyl-tRNA synthetases in the absence of clinically apparent myositis. Semin Arthritis Rheum 1996; 26(1):459–67.

84. Ceribelli A, Fredi M, Taraborelli M, et al. Prevalence and clinical significance of anti-MDA5 antibodies in European patients with polymyositis/dermatomyositis. Clin Exp Rheumatol 2014;32(6):891–7.

85. Douglas WW, Tazelaar HD, Hartman TE, et al. Polymyositis-dermatomyositis-associated interstitial lung disease. Am J Respir Crit Care Med 2001; 164(7):1182–5.

86. Sharp GC, Irvin WS, Tan EM, et al. Mixed connective tissue disease–an apparently distinct rheumatic disease syndrome associated with a specific antibody to an extractable nuclear antigen (ENA). Am J Med 1972;52(2):148–59.

87. Bodolay E, Szekanecz Z, Devenyi K, et al. Evaluation of interstitial lung disease in mixed connective

tissue disease (MCTD). Rheumatology (Oxford) 2005;44(5):656–61.

88. Fagundes MN, Caleiro MT, Navarro-Rodriguez T, et al. Esophageal involvement and interstitial lung disease in mixed connective tissue disease. Respir Med 2009;103(6):854–60.

89. Burdt MA, Hoffman RW, Deutscher SL, et al. Long-term outcome in mixed connective tissue disease: longitudinal clinical and serologic findings. Arthritis Rheum 1999;42(5):899–909.

90. Mosca M, Tani C, Carli L, et al. Undifferentiated CTD: a wide spectrum of autoimmune diseases. Best Pract Res Clin Rheumatol 2012;26(1):73–7.

91. Mosca M, Tani C, Vagnani S, et al. The diagnosis and classification of undifferentiated connective tissue diseases. J Autoimmun 2014;48–49:50–2.

92. Hadjinicolaou AV, Nisar MK, Bhagat S, et al. Non-infectious pulmonary complications of newer biological agents for rheumatic diseases–a systematic literature review. Rheumatology (Oxford) 2011; 50(12):2297–305.

93. Roubille C, Haraoui B. Interstitial lung diseases induced or exacerbated by DMARDS and biologic agents in rheumatoid arthritis: a systematic literature review. Semin Arthritis Rheum 2014;43(5): 613–26.

Imaging of Hypersensitivity Pneumonitis

Andrea L. Magee, MD[a],*, Steven M. Montner, MD[a],
Aliya Husain, MD[b], Ayodeji Adegunsoye, MD[b],
Rekha Vij, MD[c], Jonathan H. Chung, MD[a]

KEYWORDS

- Hypersensitivity pneumonitis • Interstitial lung disease • Parenchymal lung disease
- High-resolution computed tomography

KEY POINTS

- Hypersensitivity pneumonitis (HP) is a complex syndrome of diffuse parenchymal lung disease caused by inhalation of and sensitization to an ever-expanding list of aerosolized antigens. Notably, environmental exposures, including metal dusts, wood dust, avian antigens, and vegetable and animal dusts are also associated with an increased risk of developing idiopathic pulmonary fibrosis.
- Lower rates of HP occur in smokers as compared with matched nonsmokers.
- Histopathologically, HP features a triad of predominantly lymphocytic interstitial infiltrate, cellular bronchiolitis, and poorly formed non-necrotizing granulomas.
- There is a lack of consensus regarding diagnostic criteria for HP, and diagnosis requires a multidisciplinary approach involving clinicians, radiologists, and pathologists.
- The classic high-resolution computed tomography appearance of HP features upper-lung–predominant pulmonary changes including ground-glass opacities, poorly defined centrilobular nodules, and lobular areas of decreased attenuation representing air-trapping. The characteristic constellation of findings is termed the headcheese sign.

INTRODUCTION

Hypersensitivity pneumonitis (HP) is a diffuse parenchymal lung disease caused by inhalation of and sensitization to an ever-expanding list of aerosolized antigens.[1] HP develops in a minority of antigenic exposure cases, and although the factors responsible for such highly variable susceptibility remain elusive, genetic predisposition and misdirected immune modulatory processes have been long suspected in the pathophysiology of HP. Animal studies using in vivo and in vitro techniques have provided clues to some of the alterations in the function of alveolar macrophages, respiratory epithelial cells, and lymphocytes, which contribute to the pathogenesis of HP.[2–5]

Robust epidemiologic information is severely lacking in HP, in part due to nonconsensus regarding diagnostic criteria as well as the complex nature of collecting data on a disease that varies with the changing seasons, and that is heavily influenced by local customs, including

The authors have nothing to disclose.

[a] Department of Radiology, The University of Chicago, 5841 South Maryland Avenue, MC2026, Chicago, IL 60637, USA; [b] Department of Pathology, The University of Chicago, 5841 South Maryland Avenue, #6101, Chicago, IL 60637, USA; [c] Department of Pulmonology & Critical Care, The University of Chicago, 5841 South Maryland Avenue, MC6076, Chicago, IL 60637, USA
* Corresponding author.
E-mail address: Andrea.Magee@uchospitals.edu

radiologic.theclinics.com

smoking and occupational practices.[6] In 1994, Coultas and colleagues[7] estimated that the annual incidence of interstitial lung diseases (ILDs) in the Bernalillo County, New Mexico, population to be approximately 30 per 100,000 per year, with HP accounting for fewer than 2% of these cases. In 2001, these data were compared with those collected by ILD registries in Belgium, Germany, and Italy, with this aggregate analysis suggesting that HP may represent anywhere between 1.5% and 13.0% of all ILD cases.[8]

Epidemiologic data suggest that HP shows a slight female preponderance and occurs more frequently in nonsmokers, with one study demonstrating a smoking rate of only 2% in the HP population.[9,10] A large cohort study found that patients with HP are less likely to be current smokers but are equally likely to be former smokers when compared with the general population.[11] This is in opposition to idiopathic pulmonary fibrosis, which is more common in men and in smokers.

Antigens reported to cause HP are categorized by antigen subtype in **Table 1**.[6,12–18] Most of the inciting antigens in HP are smaller than 5 μm in size, a diameter that permits inhalation into the tracheobronchial tree and deposition at the alveolar level.[14] Inhaled particles larger than 10 μm are retained by the oropharyngeal and nasopharyngeal mucous membranes, and conversely, particles smaller than 0.1 μm are small enough to be inhaled and subsequently exhaled without being deposited.[19]

NORMAL ANATOMY AND IMAGING

High-resolution computed tomography (HRCT) is the imaging modality of choice for examination of patients with ILD. Thin-section CT images (0.625-mm to 1.5-mm slice thickness) are

Table 1
Antigens reported to cause HP

Antigen Subtype	Examples	Exposure Sources	Resultant Disease
Bacteria	*Saccharopolyspora rectivirgula* *Thermoactinomyces vulgaris, Absidia corymbifera*	Moldy hay, grain, silage	Farmer's lung
Fungi, yeast	*Aspergillus* sp	Moldy hay, grain	Farmer's lung
		Moldy compost and mushrooms	Mushrooms worker's lung
	Trichosporon cutaneum	Contaminated homes	Summer-type HP
	Penicillium sp	Moldy cork	Suberosis
		Moldy cheese or cheese casings	Cheese washer's lung
		Dry sausage dust in salami factories	Chacinero lung
	Alternaria sp	Contaminated oak, cedar, and mahogany dust; pine and spruce pulp	Woodworker's lung
Mycobacteria	*Mycobacterium avium* complex	Mold on ceiling or walls, tub water	Hot tub lung
		Mist from pool water, sprays and fountains	Swimming pool lung
Animal proteins	Proteins in avian droppings and serum and on feathers	Parakeets, pigeons, parrots, cockatiels, ducks, chickens, turkeys	Pigeon breeder's lung Bird fancier's lung
	Animal fur dust	Animal pelts	Furrier's lung
	Rats, gerbils	Urine, serum, pelt proteins	Laboratory worker's lung
	Avian proteins	Feather beds, pillows, duvets	Feather duvet lung
	Silkworm proteins	Dust from silkworm larvae and cocoons	Silk production HP
Chemicals	Diisocyanates, toluene, trimellitic anhydride	Polyurethane foams, spray paints, dyes, glues, varnishes, lacquer	Chemical worker's lung
	Pyrethrum	Insecticide	Pyrethrum pneumonitis

Abbreviation: HP, hypersensitivity pneumonitis.

collected with a high spatial frequency reconstruction algorithm, using multidetector volumetric acquisition with additional volumetric contiguous axial images for expiration and prone series. This has replaced the earlier method, which involved acquisition of HRCT images at 10-mm to 20-mm intervals through the thorax, which limits evaluation of focal abnormalities.[20] The evaluation of multiple reconstructions permits thorough characterization of patchy or multifocal disease, better evaluation of the extent of disease, and improved identification of ancillary findings, such as pulmonary nodules or bronchiolitis.[21] Most ILD HRCT protocols included low-dose prone and expiratory phase imaging to evaluate dependent pulmonary opacities and to assess for air-trapping, respectively.[22]

PATHOLOGY AND IMAGING FINDINGS

HP is often categorized into acute, subacute, and chronic stages; however, there is considerable overlap in the presentation of patients in each stage. To meet the challenge of classifying patients with HP, 1 study performed cluster analysis and showed that a 2-cluster solution best fit the data from a set of 199 patients with HP, with 1 cluster of patients displaying more recurrent systemic systems and lesser abnormalities on chest radiograph when compared with the second cluster of patients who displayed more clubbing, hypoxemia, restrictive pulmonary function test (PFT) patterns, and fibrosis seen on CT.[23] For the time being, however, the 3-stage scheme persists among clinicians and within the literature.

Acute HP results from intermittent high-intensity antigenic exposure, with symptoms occurring 2 to 9 hours after antigen exposure and with resolution within 1 to 12 days of antigen withdrawal.[14,24,25] Symptoms range from myalgia, cough, and dyspnea to florid pulmonary edema requiring respiratory support.[25,26] Physical examination in acute HP reveals tachypnea, diffuse fine rales, and a characteristic high-pitched end-inspiratory wheeze known as a "squawk," which is thought to be the manifestation of rapid oscillation during opening of small airways in deflated areas of the lung.[27–29]

Subacute HP results from continuous low-intensity antigen exposure, repeated acute attacks, or in some cases may be the manifestation of long-standing undiagnosed acute HP.[13,30] Symptoms in subacute HP tend to be milder and more insidious when compared with acute HP, although associated cyanosis, fatigue, anorexia, and weight loss may require hospitalization.[24,26] Physical examination in subacute HP often reveals bibasilar inspiratory crackles and tachypnea. Wheezing is less common in subacute HP than in acute HP.

Chronic HP may occur as a progression from acute or subacute HP, or may represent a distinct etiology resulting from ongoing low-level exposure without any acute episodes. Symptoms often reported by patients with chronic HP include progressive dyspnea on exertion, fatigue and malaise, cough, and weight loss. Chronic HP may evolve to pulmonary fibrosis or even emphysema in some cases, but the factors producing these 2 such disparate outcomes are not yet understood.[14]

Pathology

Lung biopsy is not required for diagnosis of HP, but has utility in ambiguous cases.[31] In acute HP, histopathology shows nonspecific findings of acute lung injury, which include peribronchovascular fibrin deposition and interstitial accumulation of neutrophils, lymphocytes, plasma cells, and macrophages.[32,33] Alveolar spaces may contain proteinaceous exudates, edema, or hemorrhage.

The histologic changes of subacute HP occur at the level of the terminal bronchioles and alveoli and consist of a classic histologic triad of a predominantly lymphocytic interstitial infiltrate (**Fig. 1**), cellular bronchiolitis, and poorly formed non-necrotizing granulomas (see **Fig. 1**; **Fig. 2**).[12,34–36] The characteristic lymphocytic infiltrate likely develops through the interplay of heightened recruitment through upregulation of alveolar macrophage costimulatory molecules, oligoclonal expansion of lymphocyte gene segments producing local proliferation, and increased longevity of these cells through alterations in numerous apoptotic pathways.[37–40] Rarely, well-

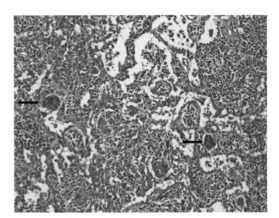

Fig. 1. Lung biopsy from a patient with acute exacerbation of HP shows a chronic inflammatory infiltrate composed mainly of lymphocytes in both the interstitium and the alveoli. Several multinucleated giant cells (*arrows*) are also present.

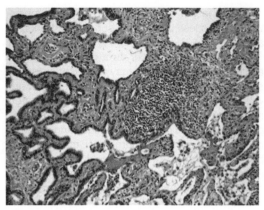

Fig. 2. Medium-power photomicrograph shows an area of bronchiolar metaplasia (*left*) and a lymphoid aggregate (*center*) in the same patient.

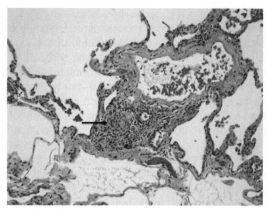

Fig. 4. Medium-power micrograph shows poorly formed granuloma in a perivascular location (*arrow*).

formed granulomas may be seen, but if these are numerous then alternate diagnoses should be considered.[36]

Histopathology in chronic HP consistently shows chronic bronchiolitis, with varying degrees of patchy fibrosis, fibroblastic foci (Fig. 3), and occasional poorly formed granulomas (Fig. 4).[31] The classic poorly formed granulomas are not ubiquitously present, with 1 study showing them in only 58% of cases and others reporting them in as few as 50% of cases.[31,41] When present, they are most commonly seen in the peribronchiolar tissue (see Fig. 3; Fig. 5). Giant cells are usually present in conjunction with granulomas, and often contain cholesterol clefts within their cytoplasm (Fig. 6).[41]

Imaging

The chest radiograph is of limited utility in confirming a diagnosis of HP, and is felt to have greater

clinical significance in ruling out other diagnoses in question.[26] Up to 20% of patients with HP will have no abnormalities on chest radiograph.[42] When abnormalities are noted, the most common pattern of findings is nodular or reticulonodular ground-glass nodules with sparing of the lung bases.[43] Chronic HP often manifests as nonspecific upper-lung zone predominant fibrotic changes such as honeycombing and reticular opacities.

HRCT is preferred in the radiologic evaluation of HP. In acute HP, HRCT may be normal or may show diffuse ground-glass or centrilobular ground-glass nodules.[44] Subacute HP often features ground-glass opacity (Fig. 7), poorly defined

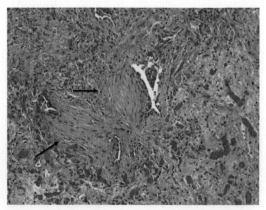

Fig. 3. Medium-power photomicrograph shows a large area of fibrosis within which there are 2 fibroblastic foci (*arrows*) containing bluish myxoid stroma.

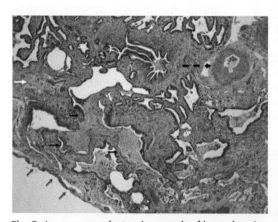

Fig. 5. Low-power photomicrograph of lung showing extensive interstitial fibrosis (*solid white arrow*) and honeycomb change (*short black arrows*) in a patient with chronic HP. Complete destruction of alveoli is seen, with only mucus-filled, dilated airspaces lined by bronchial epithelial cells. There is also secondary pulmonary hypertension, as demonstrated by the presence of a thick walled pulmonary arterial branch (*dashed black arrow*). Pleural surface is indicated by red arrows.

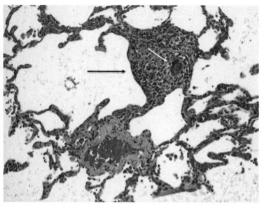

Fig. 6. Medium-power photomicrograph of lung biopsy in a patient with subacute HP showing non-necrotizing granuloma (*black arrow*) with multinucleated giant cells (*white arrow*).

centrilobular nodules, and areas of air-trapping at the level of the secondary pulmonary lobule with mid-lung and upper-lung zone predominance (Fig. 8), although a diffuse pattern is also not uncommon.[45] Expiratory phase imaging in subacute HP often features lobular areas of decreased attenuation representing air-trapping (Fig. 9). Air-trapping may be seen in up to 75% of patients with HP, and has been shown to correlate with obstructive pattern findings on PFTs, including reduced forced expiratory volume in 1 second (FEV1)/forced vital capacity (FVC) ratio and reduced FEV25 to 75.[46] One study found that in up to 13% of subacute HP cases, thin-walled cysts with diameter smaller than 15 mm are present (Fig. 10).[47]

Given the importance of air-trapping in the diagnosis of HP, identifying probable air-trapping on nonexpiratory CT scans is a useful skill. Obviously, the most accurate way to assess air-trapping is to include expiratory CT to the protocol such that it can be compared with inspiratory CT scans. Focal

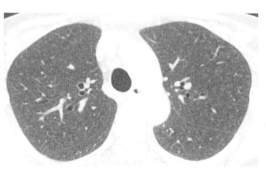

Fig. 7. Axial CT in a patient with bird fancier's disease shows diffuse centrilobular ground-glass opacities within the lungs with centrilobular predominance.

areas of lung that do not increase in attenuation with expiration are representative of air-trapping; however, many chest CT scans are not performed with expiratory phase CT and, therefore, possible or probable air-trapping must be inferred based on inspiratory images. On inspiratory imaging, significant air-trapping usually manifests as mosaic attenuation (well-demarcated areas of variable lung attenuation) (Fig. 11A). Mosaic attenuation may be due to air-trapping in the setting of small airways diseases, vascular diseases such pulmonary hypertension, and especially pulmonary arterial hypertension, and parenchymal infiltration including pulmonary edema, infection, hemorrhage, and pulmonary fibrosis. CT findings suggestive of air-trapping as a cause of mosaic attenuation include bronchial wall thickening, bronchiectasis, mucus plugging that suggests large airway disease, and in contrast includes direct signs of small airways diseases, including tree-in-bud and centrilobular nodules (Fig. 11B).

Mosaic attenuation is not exclusive to HP, and must be considered carefully when present on HRCT in a patient with suspected HP. This pattern of attenuation can be seen in patients with small airways diseases, such as bronchiolitis, in large airway disease, such as bronchiectasis or asthma, and in vascular pathologies, including chronic thromboembolic pulmonary hypertension.[48]

In chronic HP, fibrotic changes, such as septal thickening, traction bronchiectasis, and honeycombing, are seen, classically, in a peribronchovascular distribution with a mid-lung and upper-lung zone predominance, although lower and peripheral lung distribution also may be seen.[14,49] The presence and the extent of fibrotic changes are of strong clinical interest, as the extent of pulmonary fibrosis has been shown to positively correlate with increased mortality in patients with HP.[50] Several studies have shown that honeycombing and traction bronchiectasis associated with fibrotic changes are better able to predict mortality than PFTs.[51–53] Lung consolidation may be seen in chronic HP, but is felt to represent superimposed infection, and is not intrinsically related to HP pathophysiology.

The headcheese sign is relatively specific for HP, and consists of a constellation of ground-glass opacities, air-trapping, and normal intervening lung with geographic (abrupt) margination (Fig. 12). The headcheese sign reflects both the infiltrative (ground-glass opacity) and obstructive (air-trapping) elements of HP. The abrupt changes in lung parenchymal density are caused by the margins of secondary pulmonary lobules. The headcheese pattern can on occasion be seen in sarcoidosis, respiratory bronchiolitis, mycoplasma

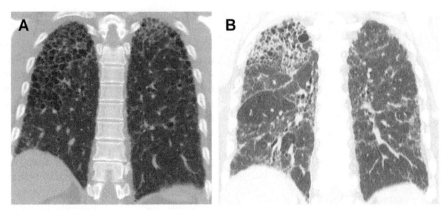

Fig. 8. Coronal CT reformats (*A*, *B*) in 2 separate patients with HP show upper-lung zone predominant reticular fibrosis, subpleural honeycombing, and traction bronchiectasis. The second image (*B*) shows mosaic attenuation with concomitant air-trapping.

pneumonia, and desquamative interstitial pneumonitis.[54]

The prognostic utility of radiologic findings in HP, particularly those indicating parenchymal fibrosis, is often critical in assessment of patients who cannot tolerate a lung biopsy.[44,50] In histologic evaluation, the fibroblastic focus is thought to represent active lung injury in the setting of fibrotic lung disease, and profusion of fibroblastic foci is felt to be a valid marker of continued antigenic exposure and physiologic decline.[55,56] The extent of traction bronchiectasis in patients with chronic HP has been recently shown by multivariate regression analysis to be a significant independent predictor of increased fibroblastic foci, providing a valuable imaging correlate for this histopathologic marker of active lung injury.[57]

DIAGNOSTIC CRITERIA

The diagnostic criteria for HP are not widely agreed on. In 1989, Richerson and colleagues[16] proposed that the constellation of PFT findings, a

known exposure with the presence of a corresponding antibody, and chest radiographic abnormalities have diagnostic utility in identifying cases of HP. In 1997, Schuyler and Cormier[58] proposed a set of major and minor criteria, stating that a patient who fulfills 4 major criteria and 2 minor criteria may have HP, assuming similar diseases have been excluded. Major criteria consist of appropriate symptoms, evidence of exposure, compatible radiologic findings, lymphocytosis on bronchoalveolar lavage (BAL), compatible histologic findings, and reproduction of symptoms following exposure. Minor criteria consisted of bibasilar rales, decreased diffusing capacity, and hypoxemia, either at rest or on exertion.[58]

In 2003, the HP study, a prospective multicenter cohort study, developed a clinical prediction rule for HP through evaluation of 661 patients. Six statistically significant predictors of active HP (exposure to a known offending antigen, symptoms 4–8 hours after exposure, positive precipitating antibodies, inspiratory crackles, recurrent symptoms, and weight loss, listed in order of

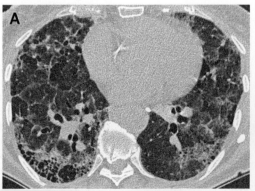
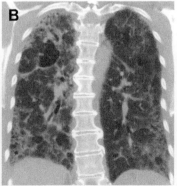

Fig. 9. Axial (*A*) and coronal (*B*) expiratory phase CT showing fibrotic changes of HP with superimposed finding of air-trapping in this patient with known HP.

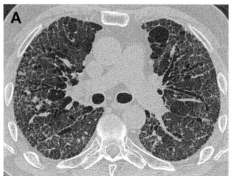
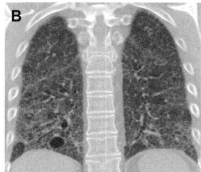

Fig. 10. Axial (A) and coronal (B) CT show predominantly subpleural fibrotic changes, including honeycombing and traction bronchiectasis typical of fibrotic HP with superimposed focal cystic regions.

descending positive predictive value) were identified through regression analyses. This clinical model concluded that the presence of all 6 predictors confers a 98% probability of HP.[15]

In the absence of firm diagnostic criteria, the diagnosis of HP is reached through the collection of supporting data. A multidisciplinary approach, involving clinical, radiographic, and pathologic perspectives, is essential in navigating the often broad differential considerations that must be considered in a patient with suspected HP.[59] Testing for serum precipitins to common antigens, specific inhalation challenge, PFTs, BAL, and lung biopsy can be used in diagnostic evaluation of a patient with suspected HP.

There is debate regarding the clinical utility of testing for specific antibodies in the workup on HP. The HP study showed that the presence of serum precipitins has utility as a predictor of HP, with an odds ratio of 5.3, but numerous studies have demonstrated positive precipitins in asymptomatic patients who have had incidental or ongoing exposure to common HP-inciting antigens. For instance, 54% of asymptomatic dairy farmers assessed in 1 study tested positive for precipitins to *Micropolyspora faeni*

antigens.[15,31,60–62] Testing for precipitins is widely regarded as only a confirmatory test.

Specific inhalation challenge (SIC) is controlled exposure of a patient to a nebulized antigenic inhalation under medical supervision. A positive result requires a 15% decrease in FVC, a 20% decrease in diffusion capacity for carbon monoxide (DLCO), or a 10% to 15% decrease in FVC accompanied by a 0.5°C increase in core body temperature within 24 hours of antigenic inhalation. One study found that with these criteria, SIC had a sensitivity of 73% and a specificity of 84% in diagnosing HP, but notes frequent false negatives and advises that it be used as only a confirmatory test.[63,64]

PFT in HP often shows resting hypoxemia and restrictive-pattern findings with reduced DLCO.[12,35] Findings are useful in guiding treatment, particularly in indicating whether or not a patient may benefit from corticosteroid therapy, but have limited utility in distinguishing HP from other pulmonary diseases.[26] PFT is useful in monitoring changes in the pulmonary functioning of patients with HP over time, with significant decreases in total lung capacity and DLCO seen in acute exacerbations.[65] Not surprisingly, PFT findings have

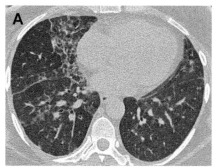
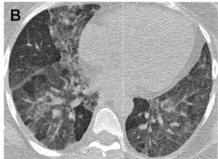

Fig. 11. Inspiratory phase imaging (A) in this patient with HP demonstrates mosaic attenuation and patchy pulmonary fibrosis. Expiratory phase imaging (B) demonstrates superimposed air-trapping.

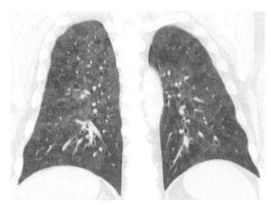

Fig. 12. Coronal CT reformatted image shows the headcheese sign, featuring sharp geographic margination along the edges of the secondary pulmonary lobules, which feature 3 distinct levels of attenuation representing normal, ground-glass opacity, and hyperinflated regions of lung. This sign in the subacute or chronic setting is highly suggestive of HP.

been shown to correlate with changes in the appearance of patients' chest CT examination. The presence of ground-glass opacities has been shown to correlate positively with FEV1/FVC ratio. The presence of a pulmonary reticular pattern correlates negatively with residual volume, and correlates positively with FEV1/FVC ratio. And decreased attenuation on CT shows strong positive correlation to residual volume (RV) and the RV/total lung capacity (TLC) ratio, consistent with an explanation of air-trapping for both findings.[66]

The American Thoracic Society guidelines define lymphocytosis in BAL fluid as exceeding 15% lymphocytes.[67] BAL in patients with HP shows an increase in overall cellularity as well as a characteristic lymphocytosis.[56,68] However, during an acute HP exacerbation, BAL fluid may show a greater proportion of neutrophils relative to lymphocytes.[65]

DIFFERENTIAL DIAGNOSIS
Subacute Hypersensitivity Pneumonitis

The differential diagnosis for subacute HP includes respiratory bronchiolitis, atypical (viral) infection, pulmonary hemorrhage, aspiration, and, rarely, metastatic calcification. Of these, the most common alternative consideration is respiratory bronchiolitis, given the often indolent presentation of both conditions. The imaging appearance of HP and respiratory bronchiolitis are nearly identical, especially when presenting with centrilobular ground-glass nodularity. Presence of associated air-trapping is more suggestive of HP than respiratory bronchiolitis; however, smoking also may lead

to small airways diseases, which would manifest as air-trapping on chest CT. That being said, a large degree of air-trapping with concomitant centrilobular ground-glass nodularity is highly suggestive of HP. One of the most helpful differentiators is the clinical history of smoking. As aforementioned, smoking is relatively protective in the setting of HP while being the causative agent in almost all patients with a respiratory bronchiolitis.

Respiratory bronchiolitis is extremely common in smokers, and by definition, is asymptomatic. Patients who have clinical and/or physiologic abnormalities with respiratory bronchiolitis are considered to have respiratory bronchiolitis ILD. Most patients who smoke do not develop respiratory bronchiolitis ILD, suggesting that other factors play a role in the development of this more severe condition. Patients with respiratory bronchiolitis ILD usually present in middle age with indolent symptoms of mild cough and/or dyspnea. PFTs usually demonstrate a mixed obstructive restrictive pattern (although often with more restriction) with a reduction in diffusion capacity.

Chronic Hypersensitivity Pneumonitis

The differential diagnosis for fibrotic HP includes idiopathic pulmonary fibrosis (IPF), nonspecific interstitial pneumonia (NSIP), and systemic etiologies such as sarcoidosis.

IPF is a chronic fibrosing idiopathic ILD that occurs more commonly in the sixth and seventh decades of life, is common among smokers, and shows male predominance.[69] Notably, environmental exposures, including metal dusts, wood dust, avian antigens, and vegetable and animal dusts are associated with an increased risk of developing IPF.[70] IPF is characterized by radiologic and pathologic features known as the usual interstitial pneumonitis (UIP) pattern. IPF is indistinguishable from HP in terms of nonspecific clinical presentation and pulmonary function testing, which shows restrictive pattern and decreased DLCO.[35] The UIP pattern on HRCT is characterized by a basilar or peripheral distribution of reticular opacities, with subpleural fibrosis, traction bronchiectasis, and honeycombing (Fig. 13). Up to 70% of patients with IPF will have mediastinal lymphadenopathy.[71] Both UIP and HP may feature honeycombing, traction bronchiectasis, and irregular reticulations on CT. The presence of micronodules, a peribronchovascular distribution of findings, multilobar decreased attenuation, and sparing of the lung bases favor HP over UIP.[41,59,70]

NSIP is a chronic inflammatory infiltrative process, which most commonly presents with cough

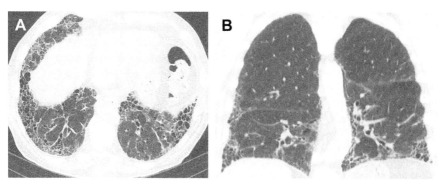

Fig. 13. Axial (A) CT in a case of UIP shows peripheral reticular abnormality, traction bronchiectasis, and honeycombing. Coronal (B) CT reformat shows honeycombing and reticular opacities in a subpleural and basilar distribution.

and progressive dyspnea, and occurs most commonly in nonsmokers. NSIP shows a female predominance. PFTs in NSIP show a restrictive pattern. Like HP, NSIP may show HRCT findings of patchy ground-glass opacities with reticular opacities and honeycombing present to a highly variable extent (**Fig. 14**).[72] Unlike HP, however, there is a lower lung zone predominance in NSIP of up to 94% (**Fig. 15**).[21,49]

HP may mimic UIP and NSIP on imaging. Upper-lung zone predominance is more common in chronic HP than in UIP or NSIP. Lower lung zone predominance was found in 1 study in 83% of patients with UIP/IPF and 94% of patients with NSIP, and was seen in 31% of chronic patients with HP, demonstrating that although often upper-lung predominant, HP is not uncommonly basilar predominant.[49] This study also demonstrated that peripheral predominance of abnormalities was less common in HP than in UIP/IPF and NSIP. HP, IPF, and NSIP are characterized by a peribronchovascular distribution of abnormalities on HRCT.[49] The features that best differentiate

chronic HP from IPF and NSIP are the presence of lobular areas of decreased attenuation, centrilobular and peribronchovascular distribution of nodules, and mid-lung and upper-lung zone predominance.[49]

Sarcoidosis is a multisystem granulomatous disease, which features a nonspecific clinical presentation and a female predominance. PFTs can show obstruction, restriction, or both. HRCT features common to both HP and sarcoidosis include ground-glass opacities, mosaic perfusion, and upper-lobe–predominant fibrosis (**Fig. 16**). Architectural distortion with traction bronchiectasis and honeycombing are commonly observed with fibrotic progression of the disease.[73] Bilateral hilar lymphadenopathy with a symmetric perilymphatic micronodular pattern is highly specific for sarcoidosis.[59,74] The presence of well-formed nonnecrotic granulomas on pathology strongly favors sarcoidosis over HP.

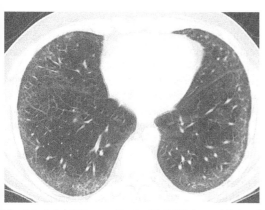

Fig. 14. Axial CT in a patient with NSIP shows bilateral lower-lung–predominant fine reticular abnormality and ground-glass opacity with subpleural sparing.

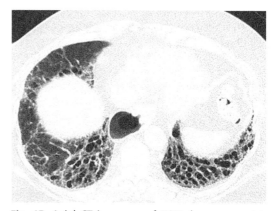

Fig. 15. Axial CT in a case of NSIP shows symmetric lower-lung–predominant reticular abnormality, exuberant traction bronchiectasis, and ground-glass opacity, as well as a dilated esophagus in this patient with underlying collagen vascular disease.

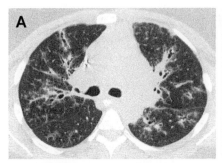 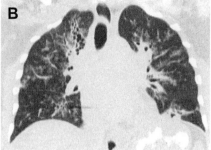

Fig. 16. Axial (*A*) and coronal (*B*) CTs in a patient with sarcoidosis show bilateral upper-lung and middle-lung zone reticulonodular opacities and changes of pulmonary fibrosis.

PEARLS AND PITFALLS

- HP is a complex syndrome of diffuse parenchymal lung disease caused by inhalation of and sensitization to an ever-expanding list of aerosolized antigens.[1] Notably, environmental exposures, including metal dusts, wood dust, avian antigens, and vegetable and animal dusts are also associated with an increased risk of developing IPF.
- Lower rates of HP occur in smokers as compared with matched nonsmokers.
- Histopathologically, HP features a triad of predominantly lymphocytic interstitial infiltrate, cellular bronchiolitis, and poorly formed non-necrotizing granulomas.
- There is a lack of consensus regarding diagnostic criteria for HP, and diagnosis requires a multidisciplinary approach involving clinicians, radiologists, and pathologists.
- The classic HRCT appearance of HP features upper-lung–predominant pulmonary changes, including ground-glass opacities, poorly defined centrilobular nodules, and lobular areas of decreased attenuation representing air-trapping. The characteristic constellation of findings is termed the headcheese sign.

WHAT THE REFERRING PHYSICIAN NEEDS TO KNOW

Because of the nonspecific clinical presentation, laboratory findings, and radiologic findings in HP, a high degree of clinical suspicion is essential in avoiding delays in diagnosis. Early diagnosis of HP and prompt intervention can slow the progression of irreversible parenchymal damage, and can preserve patients' quality of life. A study using a regression model to compare health-related quality of life between patients with HP and IPF found that patients with HP experienced poorer quality of life in 8 of 8 evaluated domains, including physical functioning, emotional functioning, mental health, and vitality.[69]

Mortality data are thought to grossly underreport the reality of HP, as these data are largely collected from death certificates, which frequently code cause of death as acute causes, some of which may be related to ILD, such as respiratory failure. A study evaluating all-cause mortality in patients with HP found 5-year survival for patients with HP was 82%, as compared with 93% in the demographically matched control group. The hazard ratio of 2.17 increased to 2.98 when adjustments were made for age, sex, and smoking.[11] Another study revealed through univariate analysis that older age, male gender, presence of crackles on auscultation, higher FEV1/FEV ratio, desaturation during exercise, and presence of fibrosis on HRCT were statistically significant predictors of mortality in HP. Multivariate analysis revealed that age, oxygen saturation during exercise, and radiologic fibrosis remained significant.[75]

Although HP occurs less frequently in smokers, it can take a more severe clinical course in this subset of patients. Cigarette smoke exposes the lung parenchyma to high concentrations of reactive oxygen species, and rodent studies have demonstrated that the oxidative stress induced on alveolar macrophages induces macrophage death in a dose-dependent and time-dependent manner.[76] A study evaluating BAL fluid results in patients with HP has shown a near-complete lack of macrophage costimulatory molecule expression in smokers, and a decreased percentage of lymphocytes constituting BAL fluid cellularity in smokers when compared with nonsmokers, suggesting active inhibition of alveolar macrophage activity in smokers.[37]

Primary prevention of HP has practical limitations, as educating healthy individuals in high-risk groups, such as farmers, to the hazards of antigenic exposures and recommended avoidance techniques is inherently difficult.

Secondary prevention, consisting of elimination and avoidance of the offending antigen, is more practically implemented. Avoidance of antigenic triggers can halt progression of the disease process, as demonstrated by a 2-week in-hospital avoidance trial, which showed statistically significant improvements in vital capacity and leukocytosis after short-duration antigen avoidance.[77] Antigen determination requires thoughtful history-taking with consideration of the patient's environmental and occupational experiences. Although the temporal relationship between exposure and development of symptoms is highly variable, which complicates the physician's task of correlating the two, the endeavor is worthwhile, as the ability to identify an inciting antigen has been shown to be independently associated with improved survival in HP.[78] Use of corticosteroids is appropriate for acute symptomatic relief or in patients who are noncandidates for life-saving transplantation, but it should be noted that long-term outcome in patients with chronic HP does not seem to be impacted by corticosteroid use. Lung or heart/lung transplantation is the only life-saving measure in HP, with 1 retrospective cohort study reporting 5-year postoperative survival rates of 89%. Unfortunately, recurrence of HP occurs in up to 6% of patients posttransplant.[79] The pathophysiology of this recurrence is not yet understood, but components of environmental exposure and continued antigenic stimulation are felt to be critical.

SUMMARY

The management of HP depends on early identification of the disease process, which is complicated by its nonspecific clinical presentation in addition to variable and diverse laboratory and radiologic findings. HP is the result of exposure and sensitization to myriad aerosolized antigens. HP develops in the minority of antigenic exposures, and conversely has been documented in patients with no identifiable exposure, complicating the diagnostic algorithm significantly. Physicians must have a high degree of clinical suspicion; alas, many cases of HP go misdiagnosed or undiagnosed. Key imaging findings, including a constellation of changes seen on HRCT known as the headcheese sign, can contribute greatly to the diagnostic challenge, but a multidisciplinary approach is essential in this endeavor. Prompt diagnosis and early intervention are critical in slowing the progression of irreversible parenchymal damage, and additionally in preserving the quality of life of affected patients.

REFERENCES

1. Demedts M, Wells AU, Antó JM, et al. Interstitial lung diseases: an epidemiological overview. Eur Respir J Suppl 2001;32:2S–16S.
2. Keskinen P, Ronni T, Matikainen S, et al. Regulation of HLA class I and II expression by interferons and influenza A virus in human peripheral blood mononuclear cells. Immunology 1997;91(3):421–9.
3. Dakhama A, Hegele RG, Laflamme G, et al. Common respiratory viruses in lower airways of patients with acute hypersensitivity pneumonitis. Am J Respir Crit Care Med 1999;159(4 Pt 1):1316–22.
4. Wang SZ, Hallsworth PG, Dowling KD, et al. Adhesion molecule expression on epithelial cells infected with respiratory syncytial virus. Eur Respir J 2000; 15(2):358–66.
5. Cormier Y, Israel-Assayag E. The role of viruses in the pathogenesis of hypersensitivity pneumonitis. Curr Opin Pulm Med 2000;6(5):420–3.
6. Bourke SJ, Dalphin JC, Boyd G, et al. Hypersensitivity pneumonitis: current concepts. Eur Respir J Suppl 2001;32:81S–92S.
7. Coultas DB, Zumwalt RE, Black WC, et al. The epidemiology of interstitial lung diseases. Am J Respir Crit Care Med 1994;150(4):967–72.
8. Thomeer MJ, Costabe U, Rizzato G, et al. Comparison of registries of interstitial lung diseases in three European countries. Eur Respir J Suppl 2001;32: 114S–8S.
9. Hanak V, Golbin JM, Ryu JH. Causes and presenting features in 85 consecutive patients with hypersensitivity pneumonitis. Mayo Clin Proc 2007; 82(7):812–6.
10. Mooney JJ, Elicker BM, Urbania TH, et al. Radiographic fibrosis score predicts survival in hypersensitivity pneumonitis. Chest 2013;144(2):586–92.
11. Solaymani-Dodaran M, West J, Smith C, et al. Extrinsic allergic alveolitis: incidence and mortality in the general population. QJM 2007;100(4):233–7.
12. Spagnolo P, Rossi G, Cavazza A, et al. Hypersensitivity pneumonitis: a comprehensive review. J Investig Allergol Clin Immunol 2015;25(4):237–50 [quiz follow 250].
13. Selman M, Buendia-Roldan I. Immunopathology, diagnosis, and management of hypersensitivity pneumonitis. Semin Respir Crit Care Med 2012; 33(5):543–54.
14. Selman M. Hypersensitivity pneumonitis: a multifaceted deceiving disorder. Clin Chest Med 2004;25(3): 531–47, vi.
15. Lacasse Y, Selman M, Costabel U, et al. Clinical diagnosis of hypersensitivity pneumonitis. Am J Respir Crit Care Med 2003;168(8):952–8.
16. Richerson HB, Bernstein IL, Fink JN, et al. Guidelines for the clinical evaluation of hypersensitivity pneumonitis. Report of the Subcommittee on

Hypersensitivity Pneumonitis. J Allergy Clin Immunol 1989;84(5 Pt 2):839–44.

17. Morell F, Cruz MJ, Gómez FP, et al. Chacinero's lung—hypersensitivity pneumonitis due to dry sausage dust. Scand J Work Environ Health 2011; 37(4):349–56.

18. Guillot M, Bertoletti L, Deygas N, et al. Dry sausage mould hypersensitivity pneumonitis: three cases. Rev Mal Respir 2008;25(5):596–600 [in French].

19. Akira M, Suganuma N. Acute and subacute chemical-induced lung injuries: HRCT findings. Eur J Radiol 2014;83(8):1461–9.

20. Remy-Jardin M, Campistron P, Amara A, et al. Usefulness of coronal reformations in the diagnostic evaluation of infiltrative lung disease. J Comput Assist Tomogr 2003;27(2):266–73.

21. Sverzellati N, Lynch DA, Hansell DM, et al. American Thoracic Society-European Respiratory Society Classification of the idiopathic interstitial pneumonias: advances in knowledge since 2002. Radiographics 2015;35(7):1849–71.

22. Small JH, Flower CD, Traill ZC, et al. Air-trapping in extrinsic allergic alveolitis on computed tomography. Clin Radiol 1996;51(10):684–8.

23. Lacasse Y, Selman M, Costabel U, et al. Classification of hypersensitivity pneumonitis: a hypothesis. Int Arch Allergy Immunol 2009;149(2):161–6.

24. Girard M, Lacasse Y, Cormier Y. Hypersensitivity pneumonitis. Allergy 2009;64(3):322–34.

25. Agostini C, Trentin L, Facco M, et al. New aspects of hypersensitivity pneumonitis. Curr Opin Pulm Med 2004;10(5):378–82.

26. Lacasse Y, Cormier Y. Hypersensitivity pneumonitis. Orphanet J Rare Dis 2006;1:25.

27. Earis JE, Marsh K, Pearson MG, et al. The inspiratory "squawk" in extrinsic allergic alveolitis and other pulmonary fibroses. Thorax 1982;37(12):923–6.

28. Forgacs P. The functional basis of pulmonary sounds. Chest 1978;73(3):399–405.

29. Forgacs P. Crackles and wheezes. Lancet 1967; 2(7508):203–5.

30. Selman M, Pardo A, King TE Jr. Hypersensitivity pneumonitis: insights in diagnosis and pathobiology. Am J Respir Crit Care Med 2012;186(4): 314–24.

31. Trahan S, Hanak V, Ryu JH, et al. Role of surgical lung biopsy in separating chronic hypersensitivity pneumonia from usual interstitial pneumonia/idiopathic pulmonary fibrosis: analysis of 31 biopsies from 15 patients. Chest 2008;134(1):126–32.

32. Cordier JF. Challenges in pulmonary fibrosis. 2: Bronchiolocentric fibrosis. Thorax 2007;62(7): 638–49.

33. Hariri LP, Mino-Kenudson M, Shea B, et al. Distinct histopathology of acute onset or abrupt exacerbation of hypersensitivity pneumonitis. Hum Pathol 2012;43(5):660–8.

34. Costabel U, Bonella F, Guzman J. Chronic hypersensitivity pneumonitis. Clin Chest Med 2012;33(1): 151–63.

35. Jeong YJ, Lee KS, Chung MP, et al. Chronic hypersensitivity pneumonia and pulmonary sarcoidosis: differentiation from usual interstitial pneumonia using high-resolution computed tomography. Semin Ultrasound CT MR 2014;35(1):47–58.

36. Castonguay MC, Ryu JH, Yi ES, et al. Granulomas and giant cells in hypersensitivity pneumonitis. Hum Pathol 2015;46(4):607–13.

37. Israel-Assayag E, Dakhama A, Lavigne S, et al. Expression of costimulatory molecules on alveolar macrophages in hypersensitivity pneumonitis. Am J Respir Crit Care Med 1999; 159(6):1830–4.

38. Facco M, Trentin L, Nicolardi L, et al. T cells in the lung of patients with hypersensitivity pneumonitis accumulate in a clonal manner. J Leukoc Biol 2004;75(5):798–804.

39. Laflamme C, Israel-Assayag E, Cormier Y. Apoptosis of bronchoalveolar lavage lymphocytes in hypersensitivity pneumonitis. Eur Respir J 2003;21(2):225–31.

40. Semenzato G, Agostini C, Zambello R, et al. Lung T cells in hypersensitivity pneumonitis: phenotypic and functional analyses. J Immunol 1986;137(4): 1164–72.

41. Takemura T, Akashi T, Kamiya H, et al. Pathological differentiation of chronic hypersensitivity pneumonitis from idiopathic pulmonary fibrosis/usual interstitial pneumonia. Histopathology 2012;61(6): 1026–35.

42. Hodgson MJ, Parkinson DK, Karpf M. Chest X-rays in hypersensitivity pneumonitis: a metaanalysis of secular trend. Am J Ind Med 1989;16(1):45–53.

43. Monkare S, Ikonen M, Haahtela T. Radiologic findings in farmer's lung. Prognosis and correlation to lung function. Chest 1985;87(4):460–6.

44. Tateishi T, Ohtani Y, Takemura T, et al. Serial high-resolution computed tomography findings of acute and chronic hypersensitivity pneumonitis induced by avian antigen. J Comput Assist Tomogr 2011; 35(2):272–9.

45. Remy-Jardin M, Remy J, Wallaert B, et al. Subacute and chronic bird breeder hypersensitivity pneumonitis: sequential evaluation with CT and correlation with lung function tests and bronchoalveolar lavage. Radiology 1993;189(1): 111–8.

46. Chung MH, Edinburgh KJ, Webb EM, et al. Mixed infiltrative and obstructive disease on high-resolution CT: differential diagnosis and functional correlates in a consecutive series. J Thorac Imaging 2001;16(2):69–75.

47. Franquet T, Hansell DM, Senbanjo T, et al. Lung cysts in subacute hypersensitivity pneumonitis. J Comput Assist Tomogr 2003;27(4):475–8.

48. Kligerman SJ, Henry T, Lin CT, et al. Mosaic attenuation: etiology, methods of differentiation, and pitfalls. Radiographics 2015;35(5): 1360–80.

49. Silva CI, Müller NL, Lynch DA, et al. Chronic hypersensitivity pneumonitis: differentiation from idiopathic pulmonary fibrosis and nonspecific interstitial pneumonia by using thin-section CT. Radiology 2008;246(1):288–97.

50. Hanak V, Golbin JM, Hartman TE, et al. High-resolution CT findings of parenchymal fibrosis correlate with prognosis in hypersensitivity pneumonitis. Chest 2008;134(1):133–8.

51. Walsh SL, Sverzellati N, Devaraj A, et al. Connective tissue disease related fibrotic lung disease: high resolution computed tomographic and pulmonary function indices as prognostic determinants. Thorax 2014;69(3):216–22.

52. Walsh SL, Sverzellati N, Devaraj A, et al. Chronic hypersensitivity pneumonitis: high resolution computed tomography patterns and pulmonary function indices as prognostic determinants. Eur Radiol 2012;22(8):1672–9.

53. Siemienowicz ML, Kruger SJ, Goh NS, et al. Agreement and mortality prediction in high-resolution CT of diffuse fibrotic lung disease. J Med Imaging Radiat Oncol 2015;59(5):555–63.

54. Chong BJ, Kanne JP, Chung JH. Headcheese sign. J Thorac Imaging 2014;29(1):W13.

55. Churg A, Sin DD, Everett D, et al. Pathologic patterns and survival in chronic hypersensitivity pneumonitis. Am J Surg Pathol 2009;33(12): 1765–70.

56. Takemura T, Akashi T, Ohtani Y, et al. Pathology of hypersensitivity pneumonitis. Curr Opin Pulm Med 2008;14(5):440–54.

57. Walsh SL, Wells AU, Sverzellati N, et al. Relationship between fibroblastic foci profusion and high resolution CT morphology in fibrotic lung disease. BMC Med 2015;13:241.

58. Schuyler M, Cormier Y. The diagnosis of hypersensitivity pneumonitis. Chest 1997;111(3): 534–6.

59. Elicker BM, Jones KD, Henry TS, et al. Multidisciplinary approach to hypersensitivity pneumonitis. J Thorac Imaging 2015;31(2):92–103.

60. Costabel U, Bross KJ, Marxen J, et al. T-lymphocytosis in bronchoalveolar lavage fluid of hypersensitivity pneumonitis. Changes in profile of T-cell subsets during the course of disease. Chest 1984; 85(4):514–22.

61. Cormier Y, Bélanger J, Beaudoin J, et al. Abnormal bronchoalveolar lavage in asymptomatic dairy farmers. Study of lymphocytes. Am Rev Respir Dis 1984;130(6):1046–9.

62. Fenoglio CM, Reboux G, Sudre B, et al. Diagnostic value of serum precipitins to mould antigens in active hypersensitivity pneumonitis. Eur Respir J 2007;29(4):706–12.

63. Munoz X, Morell F, Cruz MJ. The use of specific inhalation challenge in hypersensitivity pneumonitis. Curr Opin Allergy Clin Immunol 2013;13(2):151–8.

64. Munoz X, Sánchez-Ortiz M, Torres F, et al. Diagnostic yield of specific inhalation challenge in hypersensitivity pneumonitis. Eur Respir J 2014;44(6): 1658–65.

65. Miyazaki Y, Tateishi T, Akashi T, et al. Clinical predictors and histologic appearance of acute exacerbations in chronic hypersensitivity pneumonitis. Chest 2008;134(6):1265–70.

66. Hansell DM, Wells AU, Padley SP, et al. Hypersensitivity pneumonitis: correlation of individual CT patterns with functional abnormalities. Radiology 1996;199(1):123–8.

67. Meyer KC, Raghu G, Baughman RP, et al. An official American Thoracic Society clinical practice guideline: the clinical utility of bronchoalveolar lavage cellular analysis in interstitial lung disease. Am J Respir Crit Care Med 2012; 185(9):1004–14.

68. D'Ippolito R, Chetta A, Foresi A, et al. Induced sputum and bronchoalveolar lavage from patients with hypersensitivity pneumonitis. Respir Med 2004;98(10):977–83.

69. Lubin M, Chen H, Elicker B, et al. A comparison of health-related quality of life in idiopathic pulmonary fibrosis and chronic hypersensitivity pneumonitis. Chest 2014;145(6):1333–8.

70. Raghu G. Idiopathic pulmonary fibrosis: guidelines for diagnosis and clinical management have advanced from consensus-based in 2000 to evidence-based in 2011. Eur Respir J 2011;37(4): 743–6.

71. Souza CA, Müller NL, Lee KS, et al. Idiopathic interstitial pneumonias: prevalence of mediastinal lymph node enlargement in 206 patients. AJR Am J Roentgenol 2006;186(4): 995–9.

72. Kligerman SJ, Groshong S, Brown KK, et al. Nonspecific interstitial pneumonia: radiologic, clinical, and pathologic considerations. Radiographics 2009;29(1):73–87.

73. Patterson KC, Strek ME. Pulmonary fibrosis in sarcoidosis. Clinical features and outcomes. Ann Am Thorac Soc 2013;10(4):362–70.

74. Nunes H, Uzunhan Y, Gille T, et al. Imaging of sarcoidosis of the airways and lung parenchyma and correlation with lung function. Eur Respir J 2012;40(3):750–65.

75. Lima MS, Coletta EN, Ferreira RG, et al. Subacute and chronic hypersensitivity pneumonitis: histopathological patterns and survival. Respir Med 2009; 103(4):508–15.

76. Aoshiba K, Tamaoki J, Nagai A. Acute cigarette smoke exposure induces apoptosis of alveolar macrophages. Am J Physiol Lung Cell Mol Physiol 2001; 281(6):L1392–401.

77. Tsutsui T, Miyazaki Y, Okamoto T, et al. Antigen avoidance tests for diagnosis of chronic hypersensitivity pneumonitis. Respir Investig 2015;53(5): 217–24.

78. Fernandez Perez ER, Swigris JJ, Forssén AV, et al. Identifying an inciting antigen is associated with improved survival in patients with chronic hypersensitivity pneumonitis. Chest 2013;144(5): 1644–51.

79. Kern RM, Singer JP, Koth L, et al. Lung transplantation for hypersensitivity pneumonitis. Chest 2015; 147(6):1558–65.

Clinical-Radiologic-Pathologic Correlation of Smoking-Related Diffuse Parenchymal Lung Disease

Seth Kligerman, MD[a],*, Teri J. Franks, MD[b],
Jeffrey R. Galvin, MD[a],[c]

KEYWORDS

- Smoking • Fibrosis • Emphysema • Langerhans cell • Respiratory bronchiolitis
- Desquamative interstitial pneumonia

KEY POINTS

- Cigarette smoking is considered the paradigm for chronic obstructive pulmonary disease because it causes injury, both permanent and reversible, to the large airways, small airways, and alveoli.
- Acute lung injury in the form of acute eosinophilic pneumonia can be seen in new-onset smokers, smokers who quit and restart smoking, and also the smokers who increase their daily use of cigarettes.
- The imaging and pathologic findings in pulmonary Langerhans cell histiocytosis evolve over time because the disease exists on a spectrum ranging from cellular to later fibrotic disease.
- Respiratory bronchiolitis and desquamative interstitial pneumonia represent a pathologic continuum, although the imaging findings can appear quite different.
- Fibrosis is a common finding in smoking-related lung disease and can range from mild alveolar wall fibrosis to diffuse nonspecific interstitial pneumonia and, in some cases, usual interstitial pneumonia.

INTRODUCTION

The smoke emerging from the mouthpiece of a cigarette is an aerosol containing about 10^{10} particles per milliliter.[1] This smoke is composed of more than 5000 types of chemicals, gases, and particulate matter that is both toxic and carcinogenic.[2] The direct toxicity of cigarette smoke and the body's subsequent response to this lung injury leads to a wide array of pathologic manifestations and disease states that lead to both reversible and irreversible injury to the large airways, small airways, alveolar walls, and alveolar spaces. This articles discusses these various forms of injury and how the pathologic manifestations lead to specific findings on computerized tomography (CT).

CHRONIC OBSTRUCTIVE PULMONARY DISEASE

Chronic obstructive pulmonary disease (COPD) represents a spectrum of disorders that lead to

The authors have nothing to disclose.
The views expressed in this article are those of the author and do not necessarily reflect the official policy or position of the Department of Defense, nor the US Government (T.J. Franks).
[a] Department of Diagnostic Radiology and Nuclear Medicine, University of Maryland School of Medicine, 22 South Greene Street, Baltimore, MD 21231, USA; [b] Department of Defense, Defense Health Agency, Joint Pathology Center, 606 Stephen Sitter Avenue, Silver Spring, MD 20910-1290, USA; [c] Department of Thoracic Radiology, American Institute for Radiologic Pathology, 1010 Wayne Avenue, Suite 320, Silver Spring, MD 20910, USA
* Corresponding author.
E-mail address: skligerman@umm.edu

Radiol Clin N Am 54 (2016) 1047–1063
http://dx.doi.org/10.1016/j.rcl.2016.05.010
0033-8389/16/$ – see front matter © 2016 Elsevier Inc. All rights reserved.

radiologic.theclinics.com

physiologic airflow limitation that is not entirely reversible.[3] Although there are various entities that can lead to COPD, cigarette smoking is considered the paradigm for this physiologic process because it causes injury, both permanent and reversible, to the large airways, small airways, and alveoli.[4] Because COPD is a physiologic abnormality, it should not be diagnosed on anatomic imaging. However, the underlying processes that lead to COPD in smokers, including large airways disease, small airways diseases, and emphysema can be qualitatively and quantitatively assessed on imaging, most notably on CT.[5]

Inflammation of the large airways, or bronchitis, is a common clinical manifestation seen in patients who are smokers and is secondary to an innate immune response to the inhaled toxic particles and gases.[6] This immune response is mediated by various populations of T-cells, macrophages, and neutrophils that lead to the overproduction and hypersecretion of mucus from goblet cells in both the large and small airways.[7,8] In addition to the luminal narrowing from the mucus, the toxins also cause thickening, inflammation, and fibrosis of the bronchial and bronchiolar walls.[9] This leads to a further reduction in luminal diameter as well as a predisposition toward expiratory collapse of both the large and small airways.[8,10] All of these findings lead to dynamic airflow obstruction. On imaging, the walls of the large airways will be thickened and endobronchial mucus plugging may be visualized (**Figs. 1–3**).[11] Although there are numerous software programs that allow for the quantitative measurement of airway wall thickness using variable techniques, in most institutions this is a qualitative assessment and thus can be subjective.[12–15]

However, the injury to the airways goes beyond luminal narrowing. A study using pathologic findings and micro-CT correlation has shown a dramatic reduction in the number of small airways or obliteration or fibrosis of the lumen of small airways between 2 mm and 2.5 mm in diameter in smokers with even mild COPD compared with nonsmoking subjects.[10] In the lungs of subjects with centrilobular emphysema (CLE), there was, on average, a 99.7% reduction in the terminal bronchiolar cross-sectional area and an 89% reduction in the total number of terminal bronchioles per lung compared with nonsmoking control subjects. This injury leads to dilation and destruction of the centrilobular space, which surrounds the proximal respiratory bronchioles just downstream from the terminal bronchioles. It is this injury to the small airways, and not the emphysema itself, that is most responsible for the progression COPD.[16] Similar to bronchial wall thickening, the degree of small airways injury can be indirectly quantified through expiratory imaging, although this is beyond the scope of this article.[15,17]

Emphysema is the most common radiologic finding associated with cigarette smoking and is defined as the permanent enlargement of the airspaces distal to the terminal bronchioles. Various subtypes of emphysema exist but CLE is the most common subtype and has a well-proven association with cigarette smoking.[18,19] In CLE, more central alveoli adjacent to the small airways are dilated but the more peripheral alveoli adjacent to the septum that mark the boundary of the secondary pulmonary lobule are conspicuously spared (see **Fig. 2**). However, in severe disease, this classic pattern of CLE often becomes distorted because either the entire lobule appears to

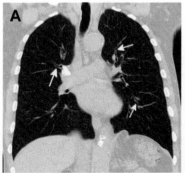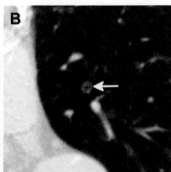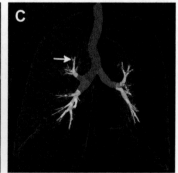

Fig. 1. Bronchial wall thickening due to cigarette smoking in an 80-year-old man. (*A*) Coronal image from a chest CT shows diffuse thickening of the bronchial walls (*arrows*). In most instances this is subjectively graded. (*B*) Coronal oblique image though a subsegmental bronchus in the anterior segment of the left upper lobe (*arrow*) demonstrates the ability of specialized computer software to analyze the bronchial lumen and wall thickness. (*C*) With these data, the software can generate a color-coded VRI map depicting various measurements including wall thickness. The airways coded yellow, orange, and red are more severely thickened (*arrow*).

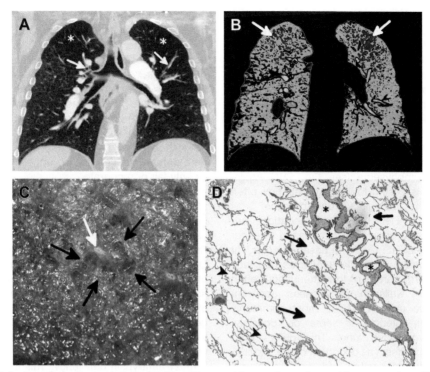

Fig. 2. Radiologic-pathologic correlation of CLE in a 61-year-old man who underwent lung transplant. (*A*) Coronal CT image shows moderate upper lobe predominant CLE (*asterisks*). The large airways are thickened (*arrows*) due to coexistent bronchial inflammation. (*B*) CT density map highlights the areas with a CT attenuation of -950 HU (Hounsfield units) or less as shades of blue (*arrows*) signifying areas of emphysema that composed 32% of the lung volume. (*C*) Gross image from the right upper lobe shows extensive CLE (*black arrows*), which can be seen surrounding the pulmonary artery (*white arrow*). The respiratory bronchiole is too small to be visualized. (*D*) Low-power hematoxylin-eosin stain (H&E) stain shows the emphysematous spaces (*arrows*) most pronounced surrounding the terminal bronchioles (*asterisks*). Alveoli closer to the periphery of the secondary lobule (*arrowheads*) are more normal in size.

be involved or adjacent foci of CLE coalesce to form larger hyperlucent lesions.[20]

Based on these variations in severity, the Fleischner Society recently published a guideline for the scoring of CLE as trace; mild; moderate; confluent; or, in the worst cases, as advanced destructive emphysema (ADE).[20] Trace, mild, and moderate CLE are defined as centrilobular

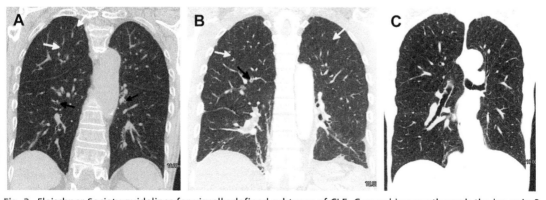

Fig. 3. Fleischner Society guidelines for visually defined subtypes of CLE. Coronal images through the lungs in 3 smokers show (*A*) minimal centrilobular lucencies occupying less than 0.5% of a lung zone (*white arrows*) defined as trace CLE. Bronchial wall thickening signifying associated bronchial disease (*black arrows*) (*B*) Scattered centrilobular lucencies (*white arrows*) involving 0.5% to 5% of a lung zone separated by large regions of normal lung and defined as mild CLE. Associated bronchial disease (*black arrow*). (*C*) More numerous centrilobular lucencies occupying more than 5% of any lung zone defined as moderate CLE.

lucencies involving less than 0.5%, between 0.5% and 5%, and more than 5% of a lung zone, respectively (see **Fig. 3**). Because these percentages are often based on visual approximation, it is to be expected that inter-reader variability will exist. Quantitative measures of emphysema can be assessed through numerous software programs that evaluate the CT attenuation of the lungs. Although various algorithms exist, the most widely accepted is the direct measurement of voxel attenuation with an attenuation of −950 HU or less, signifying an area of emphysema (see **Fig. 2**).[12] Again, although this is a useful tool, it is unclear how often this is used by radiologists in daily practice.

Based on the Fleischer recommendations, severe emphysema should be categorized as either confluent or ADE (**Fig. 4**).[20] In cases of confluent CLE, centrilobular or lobular lucencies coalesce to become larger areas of low attenuation, often without visible walls. In some cases, apparent walls may be present. These most commonly represent the interlobular septa or, possibly, adjacent compressed lung. This differs from ADE, which manifests as distortion of the underlying pulmonary architecture and vasculature with expansion of the entire secondary lobule. This extensive destruction, and apparent distortion and expansion of the entire secondary lobule, is identical to the imaging findings seen with panlobular emphysema (PLE). Many papers have used this term to describe the most severe form of upper lobe predominant emphysema, although it is

unclear if they represent a separate pathologic processes or the end stage of CLE.[5,21,22] However, this pattern of destruction may or may not actually represent pathologic PLE and, therefore, ADE is the preferred term recommended by Fleischner Society.[20] Although this classification system can help define the extent and severity of disease, patterns may overlap and previous studies using less well-defined classifications have shown the inter-observer agreement in regard to the presence and severity of emphysema as only fair or moderate.[5,23,24]

Pathologically, PLE is the result of destruction of alveolar walls of the entire secondary pulmonary lobule (**Fig. 5**). This type of emphysema is classically most severe in the lower lung zones.[21,25,26] Similar to ADE, the underlying architecture of the lung is distorted and the peripheral vasculature is often small.[20] However, in severe cases of PLE, normal interspersed lung is often absent. In cases of milder PLE, the disease may be difficult to detect both pathologically and radiologically.

There are various causes of PLE, such as intravenous Ritalin abuse, but it is typically associated with α1-antitrypsin deficiency. This is a common but under-recognized autosomal dominant genetic condition with more than 120 alleles identified predominantly involving white men.[27–29] The development of PLE in this population is highly associated with smoking and the development of PLE in nonsmokers is relatively uncommon. Therefore, many nonsmoking patients may go

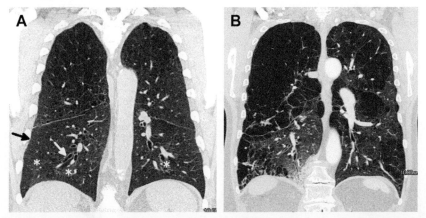

Fig. 4. Fleischner Society guidelines for visually defined subtypes of severe CLE. (A) Coronal image in a 55-year-old male smoker shows confluent CLE with coalescent centrilobular lucencies without extensive hyperexpansion of the secondary pulmonary lobule or distortion of the pulmonary architecture. In addition, there is lower lobe predominant ground glass opacity (*asterisks*) with reticulation (*black arrow*) and bronchiectasis (*white arrow*) due to coexistent desquamative interstitial pneumonia and an nonspecific interstitial pneumonia (NSIP) pattern of fibrosis as seen on explant. (B) Coronal image in a 68-year-old male smoker with ADE shows panlobular lucencies with distortion of the underlying pulmonary architecture and hyperexpansion of the secondary pulmonary lobules.

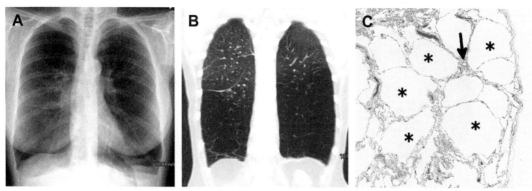

Fig. 5. PLE in a 43-year-old woman with α-1 antitrypsin deficiency. (A) Posterior anterior (PA) radiograph shows marked hyperinflation with lower lung predominant lucencies. (B) Coronal CT image shows lower lobe predominant emphysema, which involves entire secondary pulmonary lobules. No normal lung architecture is seen in the lower lobes. (C) Low-power photomicrograph though a section of the left lower lobe shows emphysematous destruction (asterisks) of the entire secondary pulmonary lobule. The respiratory bronchiole is seen in the center of the lobule (arrow).

undiagnosed unless other manifestations of this genetic condition, such as liver disease, occur.[30,31] Emphysema in patients with α1-antitrypsin deficiency has several pathogenic mechanisms. The α1-antitrypsin protein has both antiproteolytic and anti-inflammatory properties that protect the lungs against neutrophilic proteases and inflammatory mediators, such as IL-8, that are overexpressed in various causes of lung inflammation, most notably smoking.[27] Due to the genetic abnormality, patients with emphysema secondary to α1-antitrypsin deficiency often present at a younger age. Typically, patients will have lower-lung predominant PLE; however, up to one-third of patients have upper lobe predominant findings (see Fig. 4).[28]

Paraseptal or perilobular emphysema is secondary to enlargement of the alveolar ducts and sacs at the periphery of the secondary lobule (Fig. 6).[32–34] Although this type of emphysema can on occasion be seen in nonsmokers, most patients with this finding are smokers and it often coexists with other forms of emphysema.[35] On imaging, the disease is most striking along the subpleural portion of the lung with foci of low attenuation separated by thickened interlobular septa and associated fibrosis.[20] These thickened septa often give this subtype of emphysema well-defined walls. In addition, although they can occur in all forms of emphysema, the development of bulla, defined as a focal lucency measuring greater than 1 cm in diameter with a sharply demarcated thin wall less than or equal to 1 mm in diameter, is common in paraseptal emphysema and can lead to spontaneous pneumothorax.[34,36] In addition, they can become quite large, leading to severe compression of the remaining lung, further hampering pulmonary function (Fig. 7).

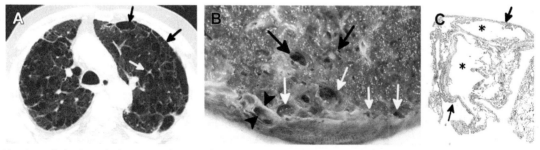

Fig. 6. Radiologic-pathologic correlation of paraseptal emphysema in a 69-year-old man who underwent lung transplant. (A) Axial image through the upper lobe shows extensive CLE (white arrow) as well as peripheral paraseptal emphysema (black arrows). (B) Gross specimen from the right upper lobe shows subpleural foci of paraseptal emphysema (white arrows) in addition to multiple areas of CLE (black arrows). An air collection in the pleural space, known as a bleb, is also present (black arrowheads). (C) Low-power photomicrograph shows subpleural airspace enlargement (asterisks) underlying the pleura and interlobular septa (arrows) consistent with paraseptal emphysema.

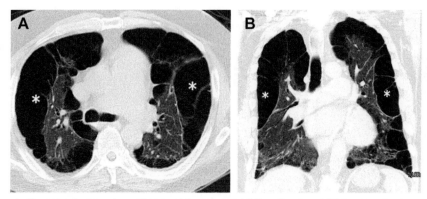

Fig. 7. Severe bullous emphysema in a 46-year-old man. Axial (*A*) and coronal (*B*) images show upper lobe predominant bullae (*asterisks*) along the subpleural surface of the lung. The size and number of the bullae lead to compression of the underlying less involved lung.

ACUTE EOSINOPHILIC PNEUMONIA

Most of the histologic findings seen in the lungs associated with smoking are related to the chronic inhalation of toxins. However, in rare instances, an acute lung injury can be seen in cigarette smokers in the form of acute eosinophilic pneumonia (AEP). Eosinophils are bone marrow–derived cells that are an important constituent of the immune system. They are most prevalent in tissues exposed to the outside environment, namely the gastrointestinal tract, genitourinary tract, and lung.[37] Through the action of intracytoplasmic granules, which are composed of cationic proteins (major basic protein, eosinophilic cationic protein, eosinophil-derived neurotoxin, eosinophil peroxidase), cytokines (numerous interleukins and tumor necrosis factor), and lipid mediators (leukotrienes), these cells serve as a potent defense against parasites, fungi, and other organisms.[38] In addition to the direct ability to damage tissue, the components of these eosinophilic granules can also lead to upregulation of mast cell function, T-cell proliferation, increased vascular permeability, and smooth muscle contraction.[39,40] Therefore, it is not surprising that, although they serve as a potent defense, abnormally increased proliferation and activation of eosinophils can lead to extensive tissue damage, as in the case AEP.

There are many causes of AEP, including infection, drug reaction, and immunologic diseases.[41] One important and increasingly recognized cause is cigarette smoking. The exact cause is not understood but the link is well established. Numerous studies have shown that 3 subpopulations of smokers are most at risk of developing AEP: new-onset smokers, smokers who quit and restart smoking, and also the smokers who increase their daily use of cigarettes.[40,42,43] In some studies, nearly all subjects who developed AEP were current smokers who followed 1 of these trends. In addition, withdrawal of cigarettes and treatment with steroids led to rapid clearing and subsequent smoking provocation tests performed in a controlled environment over 4 hours led to the redevelopment of AEP.[43]

The damage caused by the eosinophils at the level of the basement membranes of the capillary endothelium and alveolar epithelium leads to a leakage of fluid, blood, and proteinaceous material into the air spaces. Histologically, this process leads to diffuse alveolar damage with prominent interstitial and alveolar eosinophils (**Fig. 8**).[44] Therefore, the imaging findings on both radiograph and CT are often nonspecific and include lower lung predominant or diffuse consolidation, ground glass opacity, scattered nodules, and septal thickening along with pleural effusions.[45,46] The axial distribution tends to be more peripheral or random with a central predominance being uncommon. The differential diagnosis includes many more common entities, including fluid overload, acute respiratory distress syndrome, pneumonia, or pulmonary hemorrhage. Clinically, patients are acutely febrile, hypoxemic, and often require intubation due to the severity of the disease.[47] The diagnosis is rarely made by imaging but rather by the presence of an increased number of eosinophils on bronchoalveolar lavage or diffuse alveolar damage with eosinophils on lung biopsy. Once the diagnosis is made, steroids lead to the rapid resolution of this immunologic process and relapse after steroid cessation is rare.[46,48]

PULMONARY LANGERHANS CELL HISTIOCYTOSIS

Langerhans cells are a normal subpopulation of bone marrow–derived antigen-presenting cells, a subset of dendritic cells that are located in

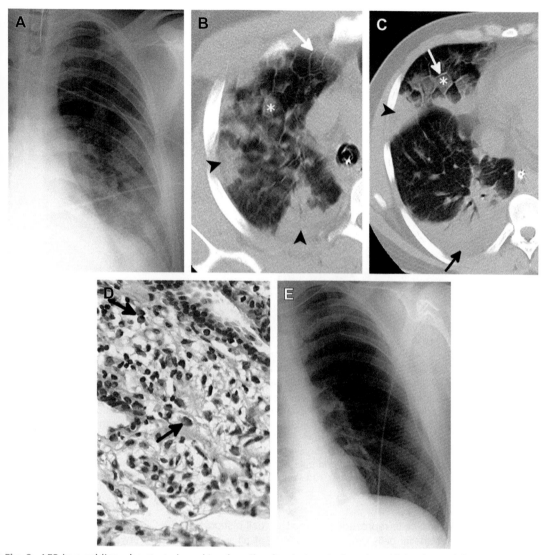

Fig. 8. AEP in a soldier who started smoking heavily after being deployed to Afghanistan. (*A*) Portable radiograph through the left hemithorax shows mid and lower lung, peripheral predominant consolidation, and ground glass opacity. A layering effusion is present. The patient is intubated and a chest tube is present. Axial images through the right lung at the level of the distal trachea (*B*) and lung bases (*C*) show peripheral predominant consolidation (*arrowheads*), ground glass opacity (*asterisks*), septal thickening (*white arrows*), and a pleural effusion (*black arrow*). (*D*) After a lack of improvement on antibiotics, the patient underwent a bronchoscopic biopsy, which showed findings of diffuse alveolar damage and numerous eosinophils (*arrows*). After the diagnosis of AEP was made, the patient was started on corticosteroids. (*E*) Within 36 hours of starting the corticosteroids, the chest radiograph returned to normal.

only a few places in the body, including the skin, tracheobronchial mucosa, lymph nodes, and thymus.[49] In the respiratory system, they serve as a primary line of defense against inhaled antigens to which the airways are constantly exposed. These cells have a characteristic appearance. They are large cells with reniform clefted nuclei and pale eosinophilic cytoplasm with indistinct cell borders (**Fig. 9**).[50] On electron

microscopy, the characteristic finding in Langerhans cells is the presence of pentalaminar rod-shaped cytoplasmic inclusions called Birbeck granules or X-bodies.[51] Langerhans cells have a strong presence of CD1a antigen, which allows for accurate identification on immunohistochemistry. Although positive staining for the intracellular S100 glycoprotein can also be seen in Langerhans cells, it is not specific to this cell type.

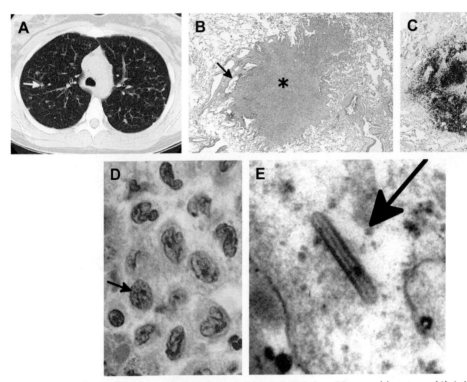

Fig. 9. Nodular form of pulmonary Langerhans cell histiocytosis in a 38-year-old woman. (*A*) Axial image from a CT scan shows numerous bizarre shaped, stellate nodules throughout the upper lobes (*arrow*). The lower lobes were normal. (*B*) Low-power H&E stain from an open lung biopsy shows a conglomeration of Langerhans cells, eosinophils, plasma cells, pigmented cells, and lymphocytes forming discrete bronchiolocentric stellate nodule (*asterisk*) around a respiratory bronchiole (*arrow*). (*C*) CD1a antigen stain turns the Langerhans cells with the nodule brown, confirming the diagnosis. (*D*) High-power H&E stain shows the Langerhans cells (*arrow*), which are large cells with reniform clefted nuclei and pale eosinophilic cytoplasm with indistinct cell borders. (*E*) Electron microscopy image shows a pentalaminar, rod-shaped intracytoplasmic inclusion body (*arrow*) in the Langerhans cell called Birbeck granule or X-body.

Although Langerhans cells represent a normal constituent of the epithelial cells of the tracheobronchial tree, the number of Langerhans cells in the lung is increased in smokers.[52] The exact cause of this is not well understood but it is thought to be secondary to direct and indirect activation and migration of Langerhans cells caused by the antigenic stimulation and subsequent inflammation induced by cigarette smoking. When exposed to these antigens, a variety of cells, including epithelial cells and macrophages, produce numerous cytokines and chemokines, such as tumor necrosis factor-alpha (TNF-α), granulocyte–macrophage colony stimulating factor (GM-CSF), chemokine ligand 20 (CCL20), transforming growth factor-β (TGF-β), and osteopontin, which are crucial for the differentiation, migration, and activation of Langerhans cells.[53,54]

Although the number of Langerhans cells is increased in smokers, only a small percentage of smokers actually develop the clinical, pathologic, and radiologic findings of pulmonary Langerhans cell histiocytosis (PLCH). In a large study looking at all subjects who underwent open lung biopsy for chronic lung disease, PLCH was only diagnosed in 3.4% of subjects.[55] Therefore, some genetic component is also likely necessary for development of PLCH and mutations in v-Raf murine sarcoma viral oncogene homolog B (BRAF), v-Raf murine sarcoma 3611 viral oncogene homolog (ARAF), and mitogen-activated protein kinase 1(MAP2K1) have been seen in both PLCH and systemic forms of Langerhans cell histiocytosis.[54] There is debate about whether PLCH represents a polyclonal reactive process due to inflammation or a clonal proliferation similar to a malignancy. Although a monoclonal neoplastic-like proliferation is characteristic of patients with systemic disease,[56,57] most studies evaluating PLCH in smokers suggest that it represents a polyclonal inflammatory reaction.[50,58]

Although only a small percentage of cigarette smokers will develop PLCH, essentially all patients with PLCH are cigarette smokers or have been exposed to second-hand cigarette smoke.[52,59] Like most inhalational injuries, PLCH is upper lobe predominant. A wide age range is described but most patients who develop PLCH are often 20 to 40 years of age and gender distribution is relatively equal, although the disease is more commonly described in white patients.[60] About 75% of patients are symptomatic at presentation but the symptoms are usually nonspecific and include dyspnea and cough.[59] Constitutional symptoms, such as fever, night-sweats, and weight loss, can be seen in up to one-third of patients. Pneumothorax, which occurs in approximately 15% of patients, may be the presenting finding.[53]

The pathologic and imaging findings in PLCH evolve over time because the disease exists on a spectrum ranging from cellular to fibrotic disease. As the Langerhans cells are activated, they coalesce around the terminal and respiratory bronchioles. Over time, a conglomeration of Langerhans cells, eosinophils, plasma cells, lymphocytes, polymorphonuclear neutrophils, and pigmented cells form discrete bronchiolocentric nodules around the small airways (see **Fig. 9**).[61] On CT these appear as stellate nodules, usually measuring less than 1 cm in diameter.[53,60,61] Over time, these bronchiolocentric nodules begin to cavitate with the areas of cavitation reflecting dilatation of bronchioles.[61] On CT, these appear as cavitary nodules, usually measuring less than 1 cm in diameter, with relatively irregular and thickened walls (**Fig. 10**).[53] Over time, these cystic areas can coalesce and form cysts that may be many centimeters in diameter. As fibrous tissue

continuous to surround the cavity, the cavity is nearly completely replaced with confluent fibrous tissue that is devoid of Langerhans cells.[62] This scarring leads to prominent paracicatricial air space enlargement. On CT, the combination of cystic change and paracicatricial airspace enlargement can mimic severe emphysema, although pathologically the entities look quite distinct (**Fig. 11**).[60] However, because this is a smoking-related injury, coexistent CLE is invariably present. An interesting concept with PLCH is that various stages of this pathologic process can occur along a single bronchiole as the lesions propagate along the bronchiolar axis in both proximal-to-distal and distal-to-proximal directions.[61] Therefore, contiguous cysts and nodules seen on imaging may represent the involvement of a single small airway and not separate lesions. Given its characteristic CT findings, open lung biopsy is often not necessary for the diagnosis.

The primary treatment of PLCH is smoking cessation. Interestingly, most patients will demonstrate either stabilization or regression of their parenchymal findings with or without smoking cessation.[60] Up to 25% of patients will progress to diffuse cystic lung disease requiring transplantation for survival and the diagnosis of PLCH may not be made until lung transplantation.

RESPIRATORY BRONCHIOLITIS AND DESQUAMATIVE INTERSTITIAL PNEUMONIA

Inhalation of toxic particles associated with cigarette smoking leads to various immune responses. Depending on the type immune response and the

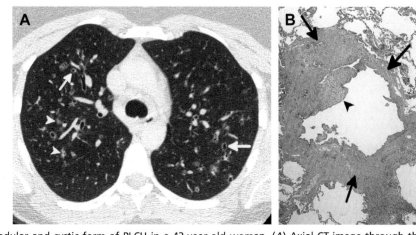

Fig. 10. Nodular and cystic form of PLCH in a 43-year-old woman. (*A*) Axial CT image through the upper lobe shows many bizarrely shaped airway centered nodules (*arrowheads*). Some of these nodules demonstrate foci of cavitation (*arrows*). (*B*) Medium-power photomicrograph shows that the Langerhans nodule has undergone cavitation (*arrows*) and surrounds the respiratory bronchiole, which can be identified by respiratory epithelium (*arrowhead*). This cavitation explains the findings on CT.

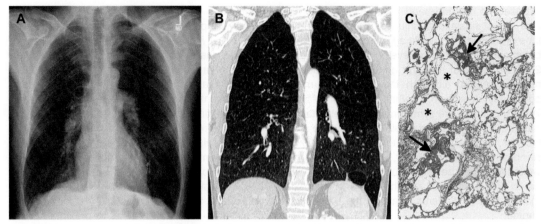

Fig. 11. End-stage PLCH. (*A*) PA radiograph demonstrates marked hyperinflation and lucency. (*B*) Coronal CT in a 48-year-old man shows diffuse upper lobe predominant lucencies with some relative basilar sparing. The imaging manifestations were thought to represent severe confluent emphysema. (*C*) Low-power photomicrograph shows paucicellular stellate scars (*arrows*) with surrounding paracicatricial emphysema (*asterisks*), a finding pathognomonic for PLCH.

cell populations involved, different forms of lung injury can be seen. One of the ubiquitous responses seen in cigarette smoking is respiratory bronchiolitis (RB). RB occurs due to the increased production of macrophages that are created in an attempt to remove many of the inhaled particles and volatiles that make it past the more proximal defenses.[63,64] Macrophages in the distal bronchioles and alveoli around the respiratory bronchioles phagocytize these particles giving them a finely granular, yellow-brown cytoplasmic pigment, referred to as smokers' macrophages. The presence of these smokers' macrophages in the respiratory bronchioles and adjacent alveoli

is termed RB by pathologists. It is seen in nearly all smokers who undergo lung biopsy and may persist even after decades of cessation of smoking (Fig. 12).[65,66] However, only a small percentage of smokers who undergo a CT scan will have the classic imaging findings associated with this pervasive histologic finding.[67]

Given that macrophages are centered on the respiratory bronchiole and adjacent alveoli, it is no surprise that, if present, the CT findings most associated with RB are centrilobular nodules (see Fig. 12).[68] Interestingly, similar to many other inhalational lung diseases, although most of the toxic particles are inhaled into the lower lobes, the

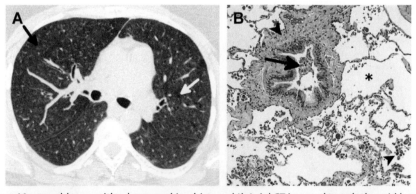

Fig. 12. RB in a 44-year-old man with a long smoking history. (*A*) Axial CT image through the mid lung zone demonstrates diffuse, ill-defined centrilobular nodules (*black arrow*). A few foci of emphysema are present (*white arrow*). Given the smoking history and findings of emphysema, a prospective diagnosis of RB was made. Due to worsening symptoms and restrictive physiology, the patient underwent an open lung biopsy. (*B*) Medium-power photomicrograph shows focal submucosal fibrosis of the respiratory bronchiole (*upper arrowhead*), which is filled with smokers' macrophages (*black arrow*). CLE is seen surrounding the respiratory bronchiole (*asterisk*). In addition, some smokers' macrophages are present in the surrounding airspaces (*lower arrowhead*). Given the clinical, imaging, and histologic findings, a consensus diagnosis of RB-ILD was made.

better-developed lymphatic system in the lower lobes allows for improved clearance of both the particles and the macrophages, leading to an upper lobe predominant pattern.[69] The centrilobular nodules in RB are often ill-defined or hazy, with an imaging appearance similar to the inflammatory subacute phase of hypersensitivity pneumonitis (HP), which makes sense because both represent inhalational injuries with a prominent immune response. The 2 entities, however, are histologically distinct.[68] Because smoking is considered somewhat protective against HP, a history of smoking or the presence of emphysema on CT is an important clue to differentiate between the causes.[70]

RB-interstitial lung disease (RB-ILD) represents a clinical-radiologic-pathologic (CRP) consensus diagnosis in those with the histologic and imaging findings of RB in conjunction with clinical findings of cough and shortness of breath, and pulmonary function abnormalities that can manifest as restrictive, obstructive, or mixed patterns.[71] Importantly, despite some early studies that tried to separate RB and RB-ILD into different histologic and radiologic types, these are the same histologic and radiologic entity and are only separated from each other based on clinical findings.[65,72]

When smokers' macrophages diffusely fill the alveoli, the histologic term desquamative interstitial pneumonia (DIP) is often used.[73] However, the histologic, imaging, and clinical separation between RB and DIP is not black and white.[74] It should be no surprise that many patients with RB will have areas of DIP and nearly all patients with DIP will have coexistent RB. The question then arises in regard to the attempted histologic

separation between these 2 processes that in essence represent a continuum of the same process, namely the overproduction and migration of macrophages in the distal bronchioles and alveoli due to smoking. There have been attempts to separate these entities and some histologic criteria have been established, although they are not well-defined. In one paper, compared with DIP, subjects with the RB histologically had primarily bronchiolocentric findings with less interstitial fibrosis.[75] Nonetheless, alveolar wall and peribronchiolar fibrosis can occur in RB.[65] In another paper, DIP was defined by the presence of pigmented macrophages diffusely involving alveolar spaces in at least 1 low-magnification field without a bronchiolocentric distribution and accompanied by diffuse alveolar septal thickening due to alveolar septal inflammation with or without fibrosis.[76] However, this can be subjective and can vary depending on the site of biopsy.

Despite histologic overlap between RB and DIP, the imaging manifestations in those with the CRP consensus diagnosis of RB-ILD and DIP are often different. Nonetheless, the imaging findings can overlap and, in general, a prospective diagnosis can be difficult.[77] Unlike almost all other inhalation lung injuries, DIP tends to be a lower-lobe predominant process, although the reason for this is unclear. In general, patients with DIP often show extensive but lower lobe predominant ground glass opacity interspersed with more normal areas of lung, often creating a mosaic attenuation (**Fig. 13**).[68,78,79] Emphysema usually presents and imaging findings of RB can be seen. In addition, small cystic structures occur in many cases and may represent foci of emphysema or true

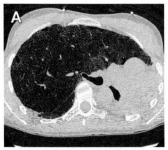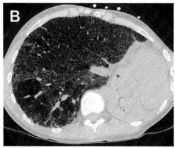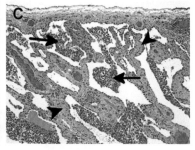

Fig. 13. DIP and fibrosis in a 45-year-old woman with a history of left pneumonectomy for lung cancer. Axial images through the mid (A) and lower (B) lung zones show lower lobe predominant ground glass opacity with cystic changes. There are well-defined areas of sparing, creating a mosaic attenuation. Well-defined areas of centrilobular and paraseptal emphysema are best seen in (A). Areas of reticulation and bronchiectasis are also present but mild. (C) Low-power photomicrograph from the right lower lobe after right lung transplant shows pigmented smokers' macrophages filling the alveolar spaces (*arrows*) and a nonspecific interstitial pneumonia pattern of fibrosis (*arrowheads*). Additionally, areas of emphysema, respiratory bronchiolitis, and air space enlargement with fibrosis are also present but more pronounced in the upper lobes. All of these histologic findings can be seen with severe smoking-related diffuse parenchymal lung disease.

cysts. Findings of fibrosis (see later discussion) are often present.[80]

The outcomes of cases with the CRP consensus diagnosis of RB-ILD and DIP can vary. Physiologic impairments in people with RB-ILD can stabilize or improve but physiologic impairment may progress even with smoking cessation and possible introduction of steroids. Even in the instance of progression, mortality secondary to RB-ILD is rare.[71] In DIP, coexistent areas of pulmonary fibrosis may be seen because smoking is a common cause of fibrosis (see later discussion). Therefore, although most people with DIP can improve with smoking cessation and steroids, those with fibrosis may progress despite therapy and may progress to fulminant respiratory failure requiring a lung transplant for survival (**Fig. 14**). Nonetheless, the true outcomes of these processes are not entirely clear. First, there is a relative lack of large studies describing the imaging findings in patients with pathologically proven DIP, despite that fact that imaging findings suggestive of the diagnosis are not that uncommon (see **Fig. 4**A). This is likely related to the relatively low percentage of patients with nonmalignancy-related, smoking-related lung diseases who undergo open lung biopsy. In most cases only those who are very symptomatic or have extensive parenchymal disease undergo open lung biopsy. This is the subset of patients who are more likely to have worse outcomes. On the other hand, many with more mild to moderate clinical and radiologic manifestations suggestive of DIP never undergo an invasive procedure and thus the true incidence is likely higher and the outcomes better than reported in the literature.

SMOKING-RELATED INTERSTITIAL FIBROSIS

In 1963, Auerbach and colleagues[81] described in great detail the prevalence of alveolar wall fibrosis in smokers. Despite this article being published more than 60 years ago, there has been renewed interest in this common histologic finding and many papers have been published over the last decade describing that smoking can lead to various degrees of pulmonary fibrosis ranging from patchy alveolar wall fibrosis to diffuse alveolar wall fibrosis in a nonspecific interstitial pneumonia (NSIP) pattern, and even to a usual interstitial pneumonia pattern of fibrosis.[75,81–83] Unfortunately, this single histologic finding has been given various names including RB-ILD with fibrosis, airspace enlargement with fibrosis, and smoking-related interstitial fibrosis.[72,84,85] Patients with both emphysema, airway injury, and fibrosis may be quite dyspneic although spirometry findings may be normal due to the combined restrictive physiology seen with fibrosis and obstructive physiology seen with small airways diseases.[82] The key to diagnosis is both the physiologic reduction in diffusing capacity and findings on CT. Although imaging findings can significantly vary depending on the severity of injury, findings of fibrosis are invariably present. In more mild cases, hazy areas of ground glass opacity and reticulation are interspersed with other findings of smoking-related injury, which can include emphysema, RB, and DIP. Foci of CLE may be more well-defined due to the alveolar wall fibrosis (**Fig. 15**). As the degree of fibrosis progresses, there is increased lower-lobe predominant ground glass opacity, reticulation, and traction bronchiectasis,

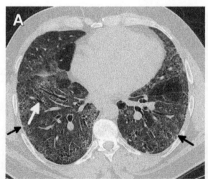
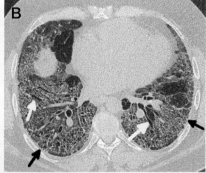

Fig. 14. Progression of DIP and pulmonary fibrosis in a 55-year-old male smoker. (*A*) Axial CT image through the lower lobes from 2012 shows lower lobe predominant ground glass opacity with scattered cystic changes. In addition, there is mild reticulation (*black arrows*) and bronchiectasis (*white arrows*), signifying underlying fibrosis. Open lung biopsy showed DIP and a NSIP of fibrosis. (*B*) Axial CT image from 2015 at the same level as the scan obtained in 2013 shows progressive fibrosis with worsening reticulation (*black arrows*) and bronchiectasis (*white arrows*). Explant showed DIP combined with severely fibrotic NSIP.

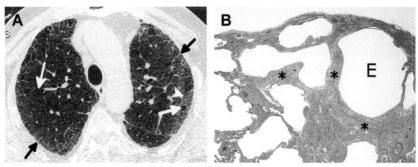

Fig. 15. Airway wall fibrosis associated with smoking in a 67-year-old male smoker. (A) Axial CT image through the upper lobes shows CLE (*white arrows*) and reticulation (*black arrows*). Patchy ground glass opacity is present (*arrowhead*). The areas of CLE with the areas of ground glass opacity appear to have more well-defined walls. (B) Low-power photomicrograph from the left upper lobe shows diffuse alveolar wall fibrosis (*asterisks*) with associated areas of emphysema (E). The fibrotic alveolar walls lead to both the ground glass opacity as well as to the better defined walls of the emphysematous spaces on CT. This common finding has been given many terms and is currently referred to as airspace enlargement with fibrosis. However, this is not a distinct disease but 1 of the many histologic findings in the spectrum of smoking-relate diffuse parenchymal lung.

which usually represent NSIP histologically (see **Fig. 14**). In general, some degree of fibrosis is a common finding in people but the severity and histology varies. The development of numerous terms is confusing because it suggests that these are separate diseases, even though they represent a continuum of a single pathologic process, namely alveolar wall fibrosis, in patients who smoke.

In addition to alveolar wall fibrosis, smoking is a well-defined risk factor for idiopathic pulmonary fibrosis (IPF). The term combined pulmonary fibrosis and emphysema syndrome has been used to describe people with both lower lobe fibrosis and emphysema on imaging and histology (**Fig. 16**).[86,87] Because most people who develop IPF are smokers, the 2 coexistent diseases are not unexpected and it is unclear why a separate term is necessary describe this population. In addition, this term is used interchangeably in

patients with IPF and emphysema, and in those with severe alveolar wall fibrosis causing NSIP and emphysema.

SUMMARY

Smoking involves the inhalation of toxic particles that lead to various histologic findings. These include emphysema, direct and indirect injury to the large and small airways, PLCH, RB, DIP, and alveolar wall fibrosis. Depending on both the patient and the extent and severity of the injury, some or all of these histologic findings can be seen on imaging (**Fig. 17**). However, there is a tendency to divide them into separate disease entities even though they represent various manifestations of a single process. Therefore, it is best to think of them as different manifestations of smoking-

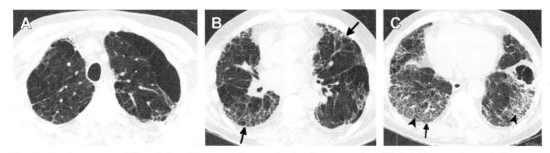

Fig. 16. Emphysema and fibrosis in a 67-year-old man who is a heavy smoker. (A) Axial image through the upper lobes show extensive centrilobular, paraseptal, and bullous emphysema. (B) Axial image through the mid lung zone again shows extensive emphysema with areas of peripheral reticulation (*arrows*). (C) Axial image though the lower lobes shows peripheral predominant pulmonary fibrosis with reticulation (*arrow*) and traction bronchiectasis (*arrowheads*). Transplant showed a combination of severe emphysema in the upper lobes and a usual interstitial pneumonia pattern of fibrosis in the lower lobes. This has been termed combined emphysema with fibrosis.

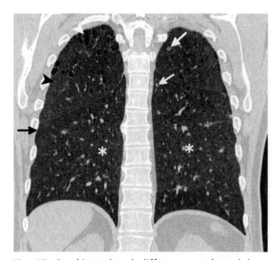

Fig. 17. Smoking-related diffuse parenchymal lung disease. Coronal image in a 52-year-old man who smokes 2 packs per day shows upper lobe predominant CLE (*white arrowhead*), a few scattered centrilobular nodules (*black arrowhead*) due to RB, ill-defined mid and upper lung predominant bronchocentric nodules (*white arrows*) due to PLCH, lower lobe predominant ground glass opacity with cystic changes (*asterisks*) and reticulation (*black arrow*) due to a combination of DIP and alveolar wall fibrosis. All of these findings were confirmed on open lung biopsy, and the constellation of findings on CT and histology are that of smoking-related diffuse parenchymal lung disease.

related diffuse parenchymal lung disease rather than separate disease processes.

REFERENCES

1. Hecht SS. Tobacco smoke carcinogens and lung cancer. J Natl Cancer Inst 1999;91(14): 1194–210.
2. Talhout R, Schulz T, Florek E, et al. Hazardous compounds in tobacco smoke. Int J Environ Res Public Health 2011;8(2):613–28.
3. Viegi G, Pistelli F, Sherrill DL, et al. Definition, epidemiology and natural history of COPD. Eur Respir J 2007;30(5):993–1013.
4. Yoshida T, Tuder RM. Pathobiology of cigarette smoke-induced chronic obstructive pulmonary disease. Physiol Rev 2007;87(3):1047–82.
5. Sverzellati N, Lynch DA, Pistolesi M, et al. Physiologic and quantitative computed tomography differences between centrilobular and panlobular emphysema in copd. Chronic Obstr Pulm Dis (Miami) 2014;1(1):125–32.
6. MacNee W, Tuder RM. New paradigms in the pathogenesis of chronic obstructive pulmonary disease I. Proc Am Thorac Soc 2009;6(6):527–31.
7. Macnee W. Pathogenesis of chronic obstructive pulmonary disease. Clin Chest Med 2007;28(3): 479–513, v.
8. Kim V, Criner GJ. Chronic bronchitis and chronic obstructive pulmonary disease. Am J Respir Crit Care Med 2013;187(3):228–37.
9. Adesina AM, Vallyathan V, Mcquillen EN, et al. Bronchiolar Inflammation and fibrosis associated with smoking - a morphological cross-sectional population analysis. Am Rev Respir Dis 1991;143(1):144–9.
10. McDonough JE, Yuan R, Suzuki M, et al. Small-airway obstruction and emphysema in chronic obstructive pulmonary disease. N Engl J Med 2011;365(17):1567–75.
11. Grenier PA, Beigelman-Aubry C, Fetita C, et al. New frontiers in CT imaging of airway disease. Eur Radiol 2002;12(5):1022–44.
12. Matsuoka S, Yamashiro T, Washko GR, et al. Quantitative CT assessment of chronic obstructive pulmonary disease. Radiographics 2010;30(1):55–66.
13. Coxson HO. Quantitative computed tomography assessment of airway wall dimensions: current status and potential applications for phenotyping chronic obstructive pulmonary disease. Proc Am Thorac Soc 2008;5(9):940–5.
14. Okazawa M, Muller N, McNamara AE, et al. Human airway narrowing measured using high resolution computed tomography. Am J Respir Crit Care Med 1996;154(5):1557–62.
15. Litmanovich DE, Hartwick K, Silva M, et al. Multidetector computed tomographic imaging in chronic obstructive pulmonary disease: emphysema and airways assessment. Radiol Clin North Am 2014; 52(1):137–54.
16. Hogg JC, Chu F, Utokaparch S, et al. The nature of small-airway obstruction in chronic obstructive pulmonary disease. N Engl J Med 2004;350(26): 2645–53.
17. Schroeder JD, McKenzie AS, Zach JA, et al. Relationships between airflow obstruction and quantitative CT measurements of emphysema, air trapping, and airways in subjects with and without chronic obstructive pulmonary disease. AJR Am J Roentgenol 2013;201(3):W460–70.
18. Satoh K, Kobayashi T, Misao T, et al. CT assessment of subtypes of pulmonary emphysema in smokers. Chest 2001;120(3):725–9.
19. Foster WL Jr, Pratt PC, Roggli VL, et al. Centrilobular emphysema: CT-pathologic correlation. Radiology 1986;159(1):27–32.
20. Lynch DA, Austin JH, Hogg JC, et al. CT-Definable subtypes of chronic obstructive pulmonary disease: a statement of the fleischner society. Radiology 2015;277(1):192–205.
21. Anderson AE Jr, Foraker AG. Centrilobular emphysema and panlobular emphysema: two different diseases. Thorax 1973;28(5):547–50.

22. Mitchell RS, Silvers GW, Goodman N, et al. Are centrilobular emphysema and panlobular emphysema two different diseases? Hum Pathol 1970; 1(3):433–41.

23. Barr RG, Berkowitz EA, Bigazzi F, et al. A combined pulmonary-radiology workshop for visual evaluation of COPD: study design, chest CT findings and concordance with quantitative evaluation. Copd 2012;9(2):151–9.

24. Bankier AA, De Maertelaer V, Keyzer C, et al. Pulmonary emphysema: subjective visual grading versus objective quantification with macroscopic morphometry and thin-section CT densitometry. Radiology 1999;211(3):851–8.

25. Shaker SB, Stavngaard T, Stolk J, et al. Alpha1-antitrypsin deficiency. 7: computed tomographic imaging in alpha1-antitrypsin deficiency. Thorax 2004; 59(11):986–91.

26. Hogg JC, Senior RM. Chronic obstructive pulmonary disease - part 2: pathology and biochemistry of emphysema. Thorax 2002;57(9):830–4.

27. Stoller JK, Aboussouan LS. A review of alpha1-antitrypsin deficiency. Am J Respir Crit Care Med 2012;185(3):246–59.

28. Parr DG, Stoel BC, Stolk J, et al. Pattern of emphysema distribution in alpha1-antitrypsin deficiency influences lung function impairment. Am J Respir Crit Care Med 2004;170(11):1172–8.

29. Stern EJ, Frank MS, Schmutz JF, et al. Panlobular pulmonary emphysema caused by i.v. injection of methylphenidate (Ritalin): findings on chest radiographs and CT scans. AJR Am J Roentgenol 1994; 162(3):555–60.

30. Seersholm N, Kok-Jensen A. Clinical features and prognosis of life time non-smokers with severe alpha 1-antitrypsin deficiency. Thorax 1998;53(4): 265–8.

31. Fairbanks KD, Tavill AS. Liver disease in alpha 1-antitrypsin deficiency: a review. Am J Gastroenterol 2008;103(8):2136–41 [quiz: 2142].

32. Takahashi M, Fukuoka J, Nitta N, et al. Imaging of pulmonary emphysema: a pictorial review. Int J Chron Obstruct Pulmon Dis 2008;3(2):193–204.

33. Thurlbeck WM. The pathobiology and epidemiology of human emphysema. J Toxicol Environ Health 1984;13(2–3):323–43.

34. The definition of emphysema. Report of a National Heart, Lung, and Blood Institute, Division of Lung Diseases workshop. Am Rev Respir Dis 1985; 132(1):182–5.

35. Mets OM, van Hulst RA, Jacobs C, et al. Normal range of emphysema and air trapping on CT in young men. AJR Am J Roentgenol 2012;199(2): 336–40.

36. Jordan KG, Kwong JS, Flint J, et al. Surgically treated pneumothorax. Radiologic and pathologic findings. Chest 1997;111(2):280–5.

37. Kato M, Kephart GM, Talley NJ, et al. Eosinophil infiltration and degranulation in normal human tissue. Anatomical Rec 1998;252(3):418–25.

38. Tefferi A, Patnaik MM, Pardanani A. Eosinophilia: secondary, clonal and idiopathic. Br J Haematol 2006;133(5):468–92.

39. Rothenberg ME, Hogan SP. The eosinophil. Annu Rev Immunol 2006;24:147–74.

40. Cottin V, Cordier JF. Eosinophilic lung diseases. Immunol Allergy Clin N Am 2012;32(4):557–86.

41. Obadina ET, Torrealba JM, Kanne JP. Acute pulmonary injury: high-resolution CT and histopathological spectrum. Br J Radiol 2013;86(1027):20120614.

42. Shorr AF, Scoville SL, Cersovsky SB, et al. Acute eosinophilic pneumonia among US Military personnel deployed in or near Iraq. JAMA 2004; 292(24):2997–3005.

43. Uchiyama H, Suda T, Nakamura Y, et al. Alterations in smoking habits are associated with acute eosinophilic pneumonia. Chest 2008;133(5):1174–80.

44. Tazelaar HD, Linz LJ, Colby TV, et al. Acute eosinophilic pneumonia: histopathologic findings in nine patients. Am J Respir Crit Care Med 1997;155(1):296–302.

45. Daimon T, Johkoh T, Sumikawa H, et al. Acute eosinophilic pneumonia: Thin-section CT findings in 29 patients. Eur J Radiol 2008;65(3):462–7.

46. Hayakawa H, Sato A, Toyoshima M, et al. A clinical study of idiopathic eosinophilic pneumonia. Chest 1994;105(5):1462–6.

47. Philit F, Etienne-Mastroianni B, Parrot A, et al. Idiopathic acute eosinophilic pneumonia: a study of 22 patients. Am J Respir Crit Care Med 2002;166(9): 1235–9.

48. Jhun BW, Kim SJ, Kim K, et al. Outcomes of rapid corticosteroid tapering in acute eosinophilic pneumonia patients with initial eosinophilia. Respirology 2015;20(8):1241–7.

49. Chu T, Jaffe R. The normal Langerhans cell and the LCH cell. Br J Cancer Suppl 1994;23:S4–10.

50. Yousem SA, Colby TV, Chen YY, et al. Pulmonary Langerhans' cell histiocytosis: molecular analysis of clonality. Am J Surg Pathol 2001;25(5):630–6.

51. Vassallo R, Ryu JH, Colby TV, et al. Pulmonary Langerhans'-cell histiocytosis. N Engl J Med 2000; 342(26):1969–78.

52. Tazi A. Adult pulmonary Langerhans' cell histiocytosis. Eur Respir J 2006;27(6):1272–85.

53. Suri HS, Yi ES, Nowakowski GS, et al. Pulmonary langerhans cell histiocytosis. Orphanet J Rare Dis 2012;7:16.

54. Gupta N, Vassallo R, Wikenheiser-Brokamp KA, et al. Diffuse cystic lung disease. Part I. Am J Respir Crit Care Med 2015;191(12):1354–66.

55. Gaensler EA, Carrington CB. Open biopsy for chronic diffuse infiltrative lung disease: clinical, roentgenographic, and physiological correlations in 502 patients. Ann Thorac Surg 1980;30(5):411–26.

56. Yu RC, Chu C, Buluwela L, et al. Clonal proliferation of Langerhans cells in Langerhans cell histiocytosis. Lancet 1994;343(8900):767–8.

57. Willman CL, Busque L, Griffith BB, et al. Langerhans'-cell histiocytosis (histiocytosis X)–a clonal proliferative disease. N Engl J Med 1994;331(3):154–60.

58. Dacic S, Trusky C, Bakker A, et al. Genotypic analysis of pulmonary Langerhans cell histiocytosis. Hum Pathol 2003;34(12):1345–9.

59. Vassallo R, Ryu JH, Schroeder DR, et al. Clinical outcomes of pulmonary Langerhans'-cell histiocytosis in adults. N Engl J Med 2002;346(7):484–90.

60. Abbott GF, Rosado-de-Christenson ML, Franks TJ, et al. From the archives of the AFIP: pulmonary Langerhans cell histiocytosis. Radiographics 2004;24(3):821–41.

61. Kambouchner M, Basset F, Marchal J, et al. Three-dimensional characterization of pathologic lesions in pulmonary langerhans cell histiocytosis. Am J Respir Crit Care Med 2002;166(11):1483–90.

62. Allen TC. Pulmonary Langerhans cell histiocytosis and other pulmonary histiocytic diseases: a review. Arch Pathol Lab Med 2008;132(7):1171–81.

63. Wallace WA, Gillooly M, Lamb D. Intra-alveolar macrophage numbers in current smokers and non-smokers: a morphometric study of tissue sections. Thorax 1992;47(6):437–40.

64. Mehta H, Nazzal K, Sadikot RT. Cigarette smoking and innate immunity. Inflamm Res 2008;57(11):497–503.

65. Fraig M, Shreesha U, Savici D, et al. Respiratory bronchiolitis: a clinicopathologic study in current smokers, ex-smokers, and never-smokers. Am J Surg Pathol 2002;26(5):647–53.

66. Vassallo R, Jensen EA, Colby TV, et al. The overlap between respiratory bronchiolitis and desquamative interstitial pneumonia in pulmonary Langerhans cell histiocytosis: high-resolution CT, histologic, and functional correlations. Chest 2003;124(4):1199–205.

67. Churg A, Muller NL, Wright JL. Respiratory bronchiolitis/interstitial lung disease: fibrosis, pulmonary function, and evolving concepts. Arch Pathol Lab Med 2010;134(1):27–32.

68. Attili AK, Kazerooni EA, Gross BH, et al. Smoking-related interstitial lung disease: radiologic-clinical-pathologic correlation. Radiographics 2008;28(5):1383–96 [discussion: 1396–8].

69. Lauweryns JM, Baert JH. Alveolar clearance and the role of the pulmonary lymphatics. Am Rev Respir Dis 1977;115(4):625–83.

70. Lacasse Y, Selman M, Costabel U, et al. Clinical diagnosis of hypersensitivity pneumonitis. Am J Respir Crit Care Med 2003;168(8):952–8.

71. Sieminska A, Kuziemski K. Respiratory bronchiolitis-interstitial lung disease. Orphanet J Rare Dis 2014;9:106.

72. Yousem SA. Respiratory bronchiolitis-associated interstitial lung disease with fibrosis is a lesion distinct from fibrotic nonspecific interstitial pneumonia: a proposal. Mod Pathol 2006;19(11):1474–9.

73. Wells AU, Nicholson AG, Hansell DM. Challenges in pulmonary fibrosis. 4: smoking-induced diffuse interstitial lung diseases. Thorax 2007;62(10):904–10.

74. Heyneman LE, Ward S, Lynch DA, et al. Respiratory bronchiolitis, respiratory bronchiolitis-associated interstitial lung disease, and desquamative interstitial pneumonia: different entities or part of the spectrum of the same disease process? AJR Am J Roentgenol 1999;173(6):1617–22.

75. Craig PJ, Wells AU, Doffman S, et al. Desquamative interstitial pneumonia, respiratory bronchiolitis and their relationship to smoking. Histopathology 2004;45(3):275–82.

76. Ryu JH, Myers JL, Capizzi SA, et al. Desquamative interstitial pneumonia and respiratory bronchiolitis-associated interstitial lung disease. Chest 2005;127(1):178–84.

77. Sverzellati N, Lynch DA, Hansell DM, et al. American Thoracic Society-European Respiratory Society Classification of the Idiopathic Interstitial Pneumonias: Advances in Knowledge since 2002. Radiographics 2015;35(7):1849–71.

78. Kligerman SJ, Henry T, Lin CT, et al. Mosaic attenuation: etiology, methods of differentiation, and pitfalls. Radiographics 2015;35(5):1360–80.

79. Hartman TE, Primack SL, Swensen SJ, et al. Desquamative interstitial pneumonia: thin-section CT findings in 22 patients. Radiology 1993;187(3):787–90.

80. Tazelaar HD, Wright JL, Churg A. Desquamative interstitial pneumonia. Histopathology 2011;58(4):509–16.

81. Auerbach O, Stout AP, Hammond EC, et al. Smoking habits and age in relation to pulmonary changes. Rupture of alveolar septums, fibrosis and thickening of walls of small arteries and arterioles. N Engl J Med 1963;269:1045–54.

82. Franks TJ, Galvin JR. Smoking-related "interstitial" lung disease. Arch Pathol Lab Med 2015;139(8):974–7.

83. Katzenstein AL. Smoking-related interstitial fibrosis (SRIF), pathogenesis and treatment of usual interstitial pneumonia (UIP), and transbronchial biopsy in UIP. Mod Pathol 2012;25(Suppl 1):S68–78.

84. Katzenstein AL, Mukhopadhyay S, Zanardi C, et al. Clinically occult interstitial fibrosis in smokers: classification and significance of a surprisingly common finding in lobectomy specimens. Hum Pathol 2010;41(3):316–25.

85. Watanabe Y, Kawabata Y, Kanauchi T, et al. Multiple, thin-walled cysts are one of the HRCT features of

airspace enlargement with fibrosis. Eur J Radiol 2015;84(5):986–92.

86. Raghu G, Collard HR, Egan JJ, et al. An official ATS/ERS/JRS/ALAT statement: idiopathic pulmonary fibrosis: evidence-based guidelines for diagnosis and management. Am J Respir Crit Care Med 2011;183(6):788–824.

87. Cottin V, Cordier JF. The syndrome of combined pulmonary fibrosis and emphysema. Chest 2009; 136(1):1–2.

Current Update on Interstitial Lung Disease of Infancy
New Classification System, Diagnostic Evaluation, Imaging Algorithms, Imaging Findings, and Prognosis

Paul G. Thacker, MD[a],*, Sara O. Vargas, MD[b],
Martha P. Fishman, MD[c], Alicia M. Casey, MD[c],
Edward Y. Lee, MD, MPH[d]

KEYWORDS

- Interstitial lung disease • High-resolution computed tomography
- Neuroendocrine cell hyperplasia of infancy • Pulmonary interstitial glycogenosis
- Surfactant dysfunction disorder • Bronchopulmonary dysplasia

KEY POINTS

- Childhood interstitial lung disease (chILD) encompasses a spectrum of diffuse childhood lung diseases presenting with at least 3 of 4 criteria: (1) respiratory symptoms, (2) hypoxemia, (3) respiratory signs, (4) diffuse abnormalities on chest radiographs or computed tomography (CT).
- Imaging in chILD primarily relies on CT with whole lung volumetric CT for the initial evaluation and with high-resolution CT for the follow-up evaluation.
- Imaging findings of chILD are typically nonspecific for a particular diagnosis with the exception of neuroendocrine cell hyperplasia of infancy in the appropriate clinical context.
- Imaging of diagnostic quality is paramount for demonstrating the nature and distribution of lung disease as well to help exclude mimickers of interstitial lung disease.

INTRODUCTION

Childhood interstitial lung disease (chILD) represents a heterogeneous group of diffuse lung diseases (DLDs), many of which can result in significant morbidity and mortality in affected pediatric patients. Although many of the encompassed diseases are rare, collectively they are not. Diseases within the chILD spectrum typically involve more than just the pulmonary interstitium, affecting also the airways, airspaces, alveolar epithelium, vasculature, pleura, and pleural spaces. Thus, some investigators have argued that these diseases are more accurately

[a] Department of Radiology and Radiological Science, Medical University of South Carolina, MSC 322, 96 Jonathan Lucas Street, Charleston, SC 29425, USA; [b] Department of Pathology, Boston Children's Hospital, Harvard Medical School, 300 Longwood Avenue, Boston, MA 02115, USA; [c] Pulmonary Division, Department of Medicine, Boston Children's Hospital, Harvard Medical School, 300 Longwood Avenue, Boston, MA 02115, USA; [d] Division of Thoracic Imaging, Department of Radiology, Boston Children's Hospital, Harvard Medical School, 300 Longwood Avenue, Boston, MA 02115, USA
* Corresponding author.
E-mail address: thackerp@musc.edu

Radiol Clin N Am 54 (2016) 1065–1076
http://dx.doi.org/10.1016/j.rcl.2016.05.012
0033-8389/16/$ – see front matter © 2016 Elsevier Inc. All rights reserved.

categorized under the term pediatric DLDs.[1,2] Nevertheless, for this up-to-date review, we use the more common term chILD, acknowledging the exceptions to this term.

The precise incidence of chILD is currently difficult to determine, as the definition of diseases included under the chILD umbrella is evolving, and many cases are either misdiagnosed or underreported. The incidence of pediatric DLD has been projected to range from 0.13 to 16.2 cases per 100,000 children per year[3] based on 3 studies, all of which used different case definitions.[3–6]

Categorization of ILD in children differs significantly from the classification developed for adults by the American Thoracic Society/European Respiratory Society International Multidisciplinary Consensus on Idiopathic Interstitial Pneumonias.[7] In comparison with adult interstitial lung disease, diseases within the chILD classification system have unique clinical, pathologic, genetic, and sometimes radiologic findings. Multicenter studies analyzing lung biopsies in children presenting with chILD syndrome have taken the view that the pathology encompasses many different diseases involving multiple lung compartments, some with a known genetic basis, some with perturbation of lung growth and development, and some arising due to interactions among genetics, environment, and development. Genetic diseases are more likely to present in childhood, sometimes with extrapulmonary syndromic manifestations, which can be a clue to classification. Fibrosis has a much more prominent role in adult ILD in comparison with chILD.[1]

Contemporary classification of chILD is based on the classification scheme published by the chILD Research Network (chILDRN) (Box 1).[8] American Thoracic Society guidelines for pediatric DLD recommend that this classification be used routinely to categorize patients with chILD.[9] The chILDRN scheme categorizes chILD into 2 broad types: those that are more prevalent in infancy and those that are not specific to infancy. As is discernable from the category nomenclature, the first group represents disorders most often occurring in infancy, but that can occur in older children and even adults. The second category has conditions that develop largely in older children and adults, but can manifest in infants.[9]

The chILD classification scheme divides disorders primarily affecting infants into 5 groups, as follows: (1) diffuse developmental disorders, (2) growth abnormalities, (3) structural pulmonary changes with chromosomal abnormalities, (4) specific conditions of undefined etiology, and (5) surfactant dysfunction mutations and related disorders. An advantage of this classification

---

Box 1
Childhood interstitial lung disease classification scheme: disorders more prevalent in infancy

Diffuse developmental disorders

- Acinar dysplasia
- Congenital alveolar dysplasia
- Alveolar-capillary dysplasia with pulmonary vein misalignment

Alveolar growth abnormalities

- Prenatal disorders
  - Pulmonary hypoplasia
- Chronic neonatal lung disease
  - Prematurity-related chronic lung disease
  - Term infants with acquired chronic lung disease
- Chromosomal anomaly associated pulmonary structural changes
  - Trisomy 21
  - Other
- Congenital heart disease associated pulmonary structural changes
- Surfactant dysfunction disorders
  - SPFTB mutations
  - SPFTC mutations
  - ABCA3 mutation
  - Congenital granulocyte-macrophage colony-stimulating factor receptor deficiency
  - Lysinuric protein intolerance

Specific conditions of unknown or poorly understood etiology

- Neuroendocrine cell hyperplasia of infancy
- Pulmonary interstitial glycogenosis

Modified from Deutsch GH, Young LR, Deterding RR, et al. Diffuse lung disease in young children: application of a novel classification scheme. Am J Respir Crit Care Med 2007;176:1120–8; and Lee EY, Cleveland RH, Langston C. Imaging in pediatric pulmonology. New York: Springer; 2012; with permission of the American Thoracic Society.

---

scheme is that it firmly separates the classification ILD in pediatric patients from that in adults. A limitation of the scheme is that, in reality, many individual children present with DLD showing elements of more than 1 of the these categories.

The purpose of this review article was to provide an up to date, comprehensive review of chILD occurring in the neonatal and infant periods. The article is structured to present first the clinical presentation of chILD. We then discuss the diagnostic evaluation, including nonimaging and imaging evaluation, as well as present a diagnostic algorithm. Last, we discuss each disease in more depth, including specific imaging findings and prognosis.

CLINICAL PRESENTATION

The most consistent clinical presentation in those affected by chILD is tachypnea, which occurs in 75% to 93% of cases.[9–12] Cough, failure to thrive, and/or crackles are also common clinical presentations.[8,10,12] However, affected patients may present only with mild wheezing or have normal breath sounds. Profound respiratory failure may occur in the neonatal period, whereas a more insidious course can be seen in older children presenting with failure to thrive or intolerance to exercise.[1]

The term "chILD syndrome" has been developed in an attempt to identify a specific phenotype requiring a rapid diagnostic evaluation.[1,9] Before the moniker can be applied, certain forms of DLD, such as asthma, primary ciliary dyskinesia, cystic fibrosis, infection, and recurrent aspiration, must be excluded (Fig. 1). Once these and other common causes of DLD have been excluded, chILD syndrome is assumed to exist has at least 3 of the following 4 findings: (1) respiratory symptoms (eg, rapid and/or difficult breathing, exercise intolerance, cough), (2) respiratory signs (eg, retractions, resting tachypnea, respiratory failure, digital clubbing, retractions, or failure to thrive), (3) hypoxemia, and (4) diffuse abnormalities on computed tomography (CT) or chest radiography (CXR).[1,9] This definition of chILD syndrome is sensitive for disease presence. However, the specificity of chILD syndrome for underlying chILD disease has not been fully evaluated.[9]

DIAGNOSTIC EVALUATION
Nonimaging Evaluation

Nonradiologic diagnostic testing in chILD includes echocardiography, pulmonary function tests (PFTs), genetic testing, bronchoscopy with bronchoalveolar lavage, and lung biopsy.

The utility of echocardiography is twofold. First, both congenital heart disease and pulmonary vascular disease can coexist with or mimic chILD.[6] Second, in patients with isolated chILD, echocardiography can help in the evaluation of concurrent pulmonary hypertension, a finding that is associated with a worse prognosis.[9,13] The use of echocardiography has been strongly recommended for the evaluation of chILD.[9]

Neonatal and infant PFTs are performed using the raised-volume rapid thoracic compression method with standard procedures, as well as normal values for fractional lung volumes, bronchodilator responsiveness, and forced flows.[9,14–17] Both restrictive and obstructive abnormalities may be seen in chILD. PFT findings are not specific for a particular chILD diagnosis and are combined with other tests, such as high-resolution CT (HRCT) in both the initial diagnostic evaluation as well as the assessment of therapeutic response and disease progression.[9]

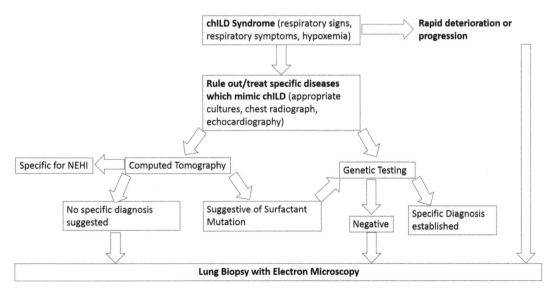

Fig. 1. Diagnostic algorithm for infants and neonates with suspected ILD.

Genetic testing is strongly recommended in the nonimaging workup of chILD, as many single-gene disorders that can result in chILD have been identified.[9,18–20] The phenotypic expression of these disorders has considerable overlap, which often necessitates analysis of a panel of genes. Prioritization of which genes to analyze depends on the patient's age at presentation, extrapulmonary manifestations, mode of inheritance, and other factors.[9] Although full description of each genetic abnormality is beyond the scope of this review article, where applicable, the exact gene mutation is discussed under the specific chILD entity in the following sections. For further discussion of genetic testing in chILD, the authors refer the reader to Ref.[8] as well as its corresponding supplemental material.[9]

Imaging Evaluation

Generally, the first radiologic imaging test used in chILD evaluation is a conventional CXR. Rarely are these radiographs normal, although the abnormalities found are often not specific.[1,9,21,22] CXRs are particularly useful in detecting and/or excluding alternative diagnoses which may mimic chILD. Nevertheless, a normal CXR does not exclude chILD, and advanced cross-sectional imaging is often still necessary; the current imaging test of choice is CT.

In chILD evaluation, the goal of CT is to provide sufficient image quality to aid in refining the differential diagnosis, guide additional diagnostic testing, and, in certain cases, to make or confirm a specific diagnosis.[1] The emphasis on "sufficient image quality" cannot be overstated. That most of these diseases occur during the first year of life confounds these aims, as obtaining high-quality images in this age group is difficult because of small body size, rapid respiratory rate, motion, and inability to comply with breath-holding instructions. Anesthesia is often used to address some of these issues. However, anesthesia-associated atelectasis can obscure underlying lung findings. If anesthesia is necessary, alveolar recruitment measures and positive-pressure ventilation techniques have been shown to decrease associated atelectasis.[23,24] In a study of 42 children using a CT scanning protocol of intubation, lung-recruitment, and controlled ventilation, Newman and colleagues[23] demonstrated a significant difference in terms of image quality and atelectasis amount in those patients who had lung-recruitment versus standard controls.

In terms of normal lung attenuation at CT, in comparison with adults, children have relatively higher contrast between the aerated lung components and the nonaerated pulmonary interstitium. Thus, HRCT technique can be used with very low radiation dosages, estimated at roughly 10 to 15 CXRs. A common misconception is that chest CTs performed on contemporary multidetector CT (MDCT) scanners are "high resolution." This stems from the fact that such scanners can now either scan or reconstruct images at subcentimeter levels, which one could argue is very high spatial resolution. However, in this review, we refer to HRCT in its traditional sense; that is, axial noncontiguous imaging. This is in contrast to volumetric MDCT of the entire lungs. Both techniques have advantages and disadvantages.

HRCT offers a lower total dose than volumetric MDCT because only a sample of the lung is actually imaged. However, HRCT of infants, neonates, and small children is more susceptible to motion artifact, risks missing areas of disease involvement, cannot be adequately reconstructed into multiplanar reformations, and is technically more demanding with limited reproducibility from one scan to another.[1,25,26] Traditionally, inspiratory HRCT is performed at 10-mm intervals in children and 5-mm to 7-mm intervals for infants and neonates. Expiratory HRCT images are then acquired at double the inspiratory interval. The utility of expiratory images lies in their increased sensitivity to air-trapping from underlying small airways diseases and large airway collapse, such as tracheobronchomalacia.[1]

In contract, MDCT uses contiguous axial images encompassing the entire lung. A higher radiation dose compared with HRCT is required. However, the limitations of HRCT in terms of missed pathology and reproducibility are negated by acquiring imaging of the entire lung. MDCT is technically easier to perform with multiplanar reformations readily available. Additional expiratory images may be used to evaluate air-trapping. Alternatively, some institutions use a hybrid approach, acquiring MDCT of the entire lung in inspiration and noncontiguous expiratory images in an effort to decrease the total dose. In the end, the choice of scanning technique depends on scanner type as well as the presence of local expertise. However, it should be noted that the American Thoracic Society in its most recent official guidelines recommend that children with suspected chILD have CT imaging performed at centers with pediatric chest CT expertise.[9]

Currently, MR imaging is not recommended for imaging children with chILD, as there is little evidence evaluating its use for this clinical indication outside of a few recently published articles on MR imaging and bronchopulmonary dysplasia/chronic lung disease of prematurity.[9,27] However, in the future, particularly with increased availability of advanced scanning techniques, such as 0 echo time imaging, MR imaging may become a viable option to CT for chILD imaging. MR imaging has already been shown to be nearly equivalent to CT and CXR for pneumonia and moderate to severe changes of cystic fibrosis.[28,29] Additionally, evidence of the utility of MR imaging for quantifying disease severity in bronchopulmonary dysplasia has recently emerged.[27] With more evidence and improved imaging techniques for evaluating the lung parenchyma, MR imaging may serve as a nonionizing radiation–using alternative to CT for chILD evaluation.

SPECTRUM OF IMAGING FINDINGS

Communication of imaging findings in chILD should closely follow the standard lexicon as put forth by the Fleischner Society in their glossary of terms for thoracic imaging.[30] Using this lexicon, the predominant findings in chILD consist of varying combinations of air-trapping, ground-glass opacities, consolidations, nodules, cysts, and linear/reticular opacities.[2] As can be ascertained, these imaging findings are nonspecific and can be seen in a host of infectious, inflammatory, genetic, neoplastic, and idiopathic processes. To complicate evaluation even further, the lung parenchyma of young children is relatively high in attenuation compared with older individuals. This appearance results from the smaller alveolar diameter, leading to a higher ratio of alveolar septal tissue to intra-alveolar air. To the unwary observer, this can simulate diffuse ground-glass opacity, leading to inaccurate interpretation as a pathologic process when in fact this is a normal finding.[1,31]

Another key difference in young children is that the normal bronchoarterial ratio is less than 0.75. This is in contrast to adults, in whom bronchiectasis is not typically considered until the bronchoarterial ratio is greater than 1.[1] Thus, using the adult criteria can lead to underestimation of airway disease.

Diffuse Developmental Disorders

Diffuse developmental disorders are postulated to occur during the early stages of in utero lung development and are classified into 3 entities: (1) acinar dysplasia (Fig. 2), (2) congenital alveolar dysplasia (CAD), and (3) alveolar-capillary dysplasia with misalignment of the pulmonary veins (ACD/MPV) (Fig. 3).[1,2,32] All are associated with profound impairment of alveolar gas exchange. Acinar dysplasia is characterized by a complete lack of alveolar development. Affected lungs show only airwaylike structures, with nearly all reported cases occurring in female infants (see Fig. 2B).[33] CAD is not well characterized, described by MacMahan[34–36] in 1947 and 1948 as heavy lungs, excess of interalveolar richly vascularized mesenchyme, and a paucity of alveoli with increased variation in size. It was described subsequently by only one other group, who used the term for a group of patients with alveolar septal thickening by interstitial cells (resembling pulmonary interstitial glycogenosis [PIG]) and variably thickened pulmonary arteries.[37] In contrast to acinar dysplasia, infants with CAD can be adequately supported with mechanical ventilation. Last, ACD/MPV combines both vascular changes and abnormal development of the pulmonary lobule and is associated with underlying genetic

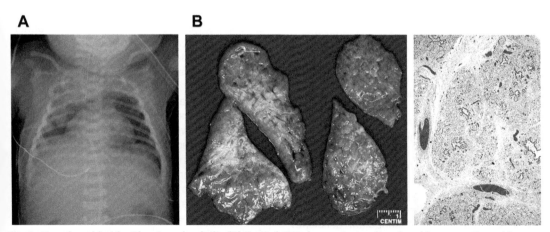

A **B**

Fig. 2. One-day-old girl with acinar dysplasia. (*A*) Frontal CXR demonstrates disordered lung aeration with asymmetrically hyperinflated left lower lung and focal atelectasis in both upper lungs. (*B*) Grossly, the lungs were small and showed small lobules with prominent interlobular septa (*left*). Microscopically, there was virtually no alveolar development (*right*) (H&E).

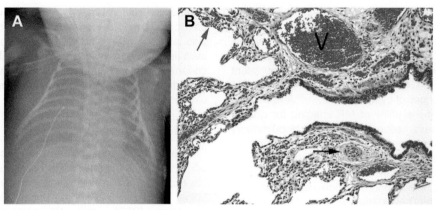

Fig. 3. Four-day-old boy with ACD/MPV. (*A*) Frontal CXR shows asymmetric diffuse granular opacities, right greater than left. (*B*) A large pulmonary vein (*V*) runs along with the bronchovascular bundle. Alveolar septa (*green arrow*) show excess myxoid mesenchyme, and accompanying pulmonary hypertensive remodeling (*black arrow*) is present (H&E).

anomalies; for example, forkhead box (FOX)F1 gene mutation and 16q24.1 microdeletions.[2,32] In ACD/MPV, large venous structures referred to as "misaligned pulmonary veins" run adjacent to the bronchovascular bundles. The alveolar septa are thickened by excess mesenchymal cells and myxoid extracellular matrix, and the capillaries lack close apposition to the alveolar basement membranes (see **Fig. 3**B). There is typically accompanying pulmonary arterial hypertensive change (medial hypertrophy of the pulmonary arterioles), as well as prominent regional or diffuse lymphangiectasis. Also, more than 80% of patients with ACD/MPV have extrapulmonary anomalies, including gastrointestinal (malrotation and alimentary tract atresias), cardiac (aortic coarctation and hypoplastic left heart syndrome), absent or hypoplastic gallbladder, and genitourinary anomalies.[1,32]

Diffuse developmental disorders typically present in a term infant with severe pulmonary hypertension and profound respiratory failure within the first 48 hours of birth.[38] Death typically occurs early in infancy unless lungs are only partially involved or if the patient receives a lung transplant.

Given their rapidly fatal clinical progression, knowledge of the imaging characteristics of diffuse developmental disorders is limited. Imaging is usually restricted to CXRs, which initially maybe normal. On subsequent imaging, lungs become progressively and diffusely hazy, similar to what is seen in surfactant deficiency of prematurity and surfactant deficiency disorders. Sequelae of barotrauma, including pneumothorax and pneumomediastinum commonly develop.[1,32,38–40]

Alveolar Growth Abnormalities

Representing approximately 43% of all cases of chILD in those younger than age 2, alveolar growth abnormalities are the most common cause of DLD in infancy.[32] These include structural pulmonary changes due to chromosomal abnormalities; pulmonary hypoplasia resulting from prenatal conditions such as congenital diaphragmatic hernia, congenital lung masses, oligohydramnios, or neuromuscular conditions; structural pulmonary changes in congenital heart disease; and alveolar simplification of unknown etiology. Bronchopulmonary dysplasia/chronic lung disease of prematurity is generally considered a separate diagnosis.[1,32]

Patient presentation varies widely and is dependent on the underlying cause. However, patients with alveolar growth abnormalities generally have some degree of respiratory distress during the first month of life. Depending on the degree of alveolar development and the amount of alveolar abnormality, these symptoms may improve over time as new alveoli develop or progressively worsen if normal alveoli fail to grow over time or there is ongoing injury.

The imaging appearance in patients with alveolar growth abnormalities is variable and largely dependent on which of the underlying etiology is causing the alveolar growth abnormality. Findings can range from near normal to markedly abnormal with coarse perilobular opacities, ground-glass opacities, cystic lucencies, and disordered aeration. In patients with trisomy 21, airspaces are enlarged and reduced in number ("simplified"), most prominently in the subpleural region where they may form radiologically appreciable cysts in up to 36% of cases (**Fig. 4**).[41] One disorder that may mimic bronchopulmonary dysplasia but is

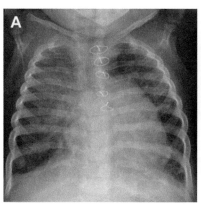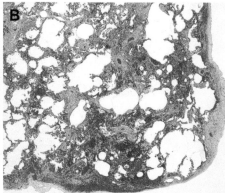

Fig. 4. Sixteen-month-old boy with trisomy 21. (*A*) Frontal CXR demonstrates scattered perihilar interstitial opacities with coarse bibasilar reticular interstitial opacities and patchy bibasilar atelectasis. Additionally, there is cardiomegaly and postoperative changes of a sternotomy in this child with trisomy 21–related alveolar growth abnormalities and congenital heart disease. (*B*) Lung biopsy sample shows grossly enlarged airspaces ("alveolar simplification"), most prominent subpleurally (H&E). (In the background is vasculopathy related to superimposed congenital heart disease.)

distinctly different in etiology is filamin A (*FLNA*) mutation, which is an X-linked gene disorder characterized by hyperlucent lungs, hyperinflation, and pulmonary vascular attenuation affecting all lung lobes.[8,32,42,43] In addition to pulmonary abnormalities, *FLNA* mutation is also associated with cardiovascular anomalies, skeletal dysplasia, airway malacia, Ehlers-Danlos variants, and periventricular nodular gray matter heterotopia.[32,42]

Surfactant Dysfunction Disorders and Related Abnormalities

The third category of chILD includes different genetic abnormalities that impact surfactant function. The most common mutation to affect surfactant function involves the gene for adenosine triphosphate binding cassette transporter protein A3 (*ABCA3*) and has autosomal-recessive inheritance. Other genetic disorders resulting in surfactant dysfunction arise from autosomal-recessive mutations in *SFTPB*, the gene for surfactant protein B (SpB), from autosomal-dominant mutations in *SFTPC*, the gene for surfactant protein C (SpC), from haploinsufficiency in *NKX2.1*, the gene for thyroid transcription factor 1 (TTF1), and from autosomal-recessive mutations in *CSF2RA* or *CSF2RB*, the genes encoding granulocyte-macrophage colony-stimulating factor receptor subunits (GM-CSF-R).[1,32] Collectively, these disorders represent the most common known genetic cause of respiratory distress syndrome in term infants.[1,32]

Depending on the age at presentation, clinical and imaging findings can be quite variable. Patients with *SFTPB* mutations typically present very early after birth with severe respiratory failure. Chest radiographs resemble surfactant deficiency of prematurity with diffuse, hazy, granular opacities and decreased lung volumes. However, the clinical course differs from surfactant deficiency of prematurity in that patients with SpB mutation are unresponsive to exogenous surfactant and extracorporeal membrane oxygenation. Generally, affected patients die within a few months of life unless they receive lung transplantation. If the specific mutation allows some SpB production, milder cases with longer patient survival can occur.

ABCA3 and *SFTPC* mutations have a much more variable clinical and imaging progression compared with SpB mutations, ranging from severe respiratory distress syndrome occurring immediately after birth to presentation later during infancy or childhood. There are even reports of delayed presentation into adulthood.[44–47] *ABCA3* gene mutations, for example, have a variable prognosis depending on the specific genotype.[8,48] Children typically present with variable levels of hypoxemia, tachypnea, cough, and failure to thrive. CXR findings in infants demonstrate patchy or diffuse hazy interstitial opacities (**Fig. 5**).[32] CT findings typically include areas of ground-glass opacity, septal thickening, patchy consolidation, and often small cystic lucencies (see **Fig. 5B**). When significant pulmonary alveolar proteinosis is present, this can result in the appearance of "crazy-paving."[2,32] Affected older children typically have progressively decreasing ground-glass opacity on imaging with increasing cystic changes and septal thickening with age. Pectus excavatum has been reported as a musculoskeletal sequela in

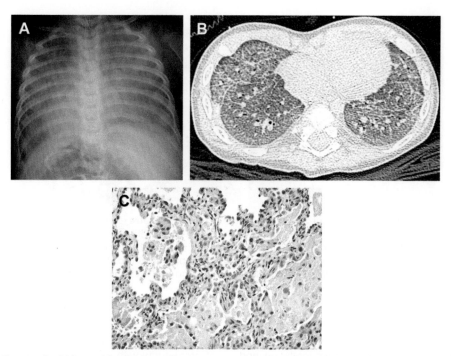

Fig. 5. Eight-month-old boy with ABCA3 surfactant gene mutation. (*A*) Frontal CXR shows situs inversus totalis with diffuse but asymmetric ground-glass opacity and asymmetric lung aeration. (*B*) Corresponding unenhanced CT image demonstrates scattered areas of septal thickening with diffuse ground-glass opacity giving patchy areas of "crazy-paving" in this patient with ABCA3 mutation. (*C*) Mutation in the surfactant gene *ABCA3* accounted for the triad of intra-alveolar proteinaceous material, intra-alveolar macrophages, and prominent type 2 pneumocyte hyperplasia (H&E).

older children and is thought to be related to changes to the developing chest wall by chronic restrictive lung disease.[32,44] Notably, imaging findings do not always correlate with changes in lung function and, thus, need to be interpreted in clinical context.[1] Histologically, the most prominent findings in genetic surfactant protein deficiencies include alveolar proteinosis, increased numbers of intra-alveolar macrophages, and type 2 pneumocyte hyperplasia, in variable proportions (see **Fig. 5**C); fibrosis may be a late sequela.

Although knowledge of other genes in which mutations affect surfactant, for example, *NKX2.1*, *CSF2RA*, and *CSF2RB*, has continually expanded over the past several years, reports of the clinical presentation and imaging findings remain relatively limited. Patients with GM-CSF-Rα mutation present with a combination of failure to thrive and tachypnea with nonspecific diffuse pulmonary opacities on CXR and crazy-paving on CT, related to impaired alveolar macrophage function leading to pulmonary alveolar proteinosis.[1] Patients with *NKX2.1* mutation often have a unique constellation of findings with maldevelopment of the basal ganglia and thyroid in addition to respiratory abnormalities. This has led to the classic name

"brain-lung-thyroid syndrome" with hypotonia, chorea, congenital hypothyroidism, and DLD. Pulmonary symptoms range from a mild asthmalike presentation to severe neonatal respiratory distress.[32] CT findings can be similar to findings seen in other surfactant protein dysfunction, but because TTF-1 is a regulator of early lung growth, findings consistent with growth disorders also can be observed.[32] Notably, an inherited *NKX2.1* was recently described in a family demonstrating classic radiologic and histologic features of "neuroendocrine hyperplasia of infancy."[49,50] *NKX2.1* mutations can present with isolated pulmonary disease and do not consistently present with the classic "triad," so this should be considered in the differential diagnosis even for infants with isolated lung disease.[50]

Last, *SLC747* mutations result in lysinuric protein intolerance and affect a wide range of organs. However, in children, the only life-threatening complication results from pulmonary involvement with acute progressive respiratory failure from pulmonary hemorrhage and pulmonary alveolar proteinosis. Depending on the age at presentation and the disease stage, CXR and CT appearance varies widely from subtle septal thickening, subpleural cysts, and nodules on CT during early stages to diffuse airspace opacities.[1,32]

Given the underlying defect and nonspecific imaging findings, surfactant dysfunction disorders are typically diagnosed by genetic testing, although rarely conclusive, in combination with lung biopsy.[32,51]

Disorders of Poorly Understood or Unknown Etiology

The final chILD category includes 2 relatively common entities that are unique to infants: PIG, previously termed infantile cellular interstitial pneumonitis, and neuroendocrine cell hyperplasia of infancy (NEHI).

Pulmonary interstitial glycogenosis

PIG can affect both full-term and premature infants and is characterized histologically by pulmonary interstitial expansion by immature mesenchymal cells containing finely vacuolated cytoplasm (Fig. 6).[1,8,32] It can be divided into 2 forms: diffuse and patchy, both of which may accompany many different diseases associated with infant respiratory distress. Nearly all patients with PIG present at birth with hypoxemia, most with mild symptoms.[8,32] Clinical outcome is dependent on the presence and severity of any associated alveolar growth abnormalities or other superimposed

pulmonary disease.[2,8] In those with more severe symptoms, corticosteroids may be beneficial.

Imaging characteristics of PIG vary broadly and are dependent on the presence of associated alveolar growth abnormalities.[2] In the diffuse form and in the absence of any growth abnormality, CXR findings include nonspecific hyperinflation and diffuse interstitial opacities.[32] CT findings include ground-glass opacities, interlobular septal thickening, architectural distortion, and hyperlucent areas.[2,32] Patients with patchy PIG, particularly in the presence on an underlying growth disorder, may demonstrate multifocal areas of cystic change which vary in size. Additionally, CT findings of patchy PIG are similar to the diffuse form, although more limited in scope, and include diffuse ground-glass opacities, reticular interstitial opacities, and interlobular septal thickening.[1,32,52,53]

Neuroendocrine cell hyperplasia of infancy

Originally called persistent tachypnea of infancy, NEHI is a disorder of unknown etiology typically affecting term infants within the first 3 months of life.[32] Initially, patients are asymptomatic. When clinical symptoms develop, sometimes following a minor viral respiratory infection, patients present with a mixture of hypoxemia, failure to thrive, persistent tachypnea, wheezing, and crackles.[1,32]

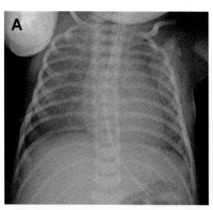
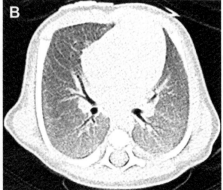
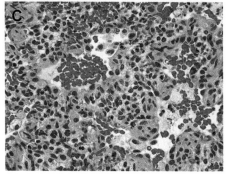

Fig. 6. Twenty-three-day-old girl with PIG. (A) Frontal CXR demonstrates diffuse granular opacities. (B) Unenhanced CT image shows diffuse ground-glass opacity most marked posteriorly. (C) PIG was a major component of the disease observed in the lung biopsy and likely pathogenic biallelic mutations in the ABCA3 gene. Interstitial cells with vacuolated cytoplasm markedly expand the alveolar septa (H&E).

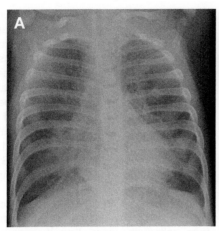
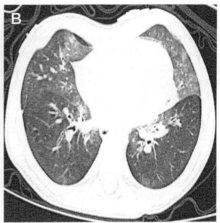

Fig. 7. 9 month old boy with NEHI. (*A*) Front radiograph of the chest demonstrates patchy interstitial and alveolar opacities in a perimediastinal distribution, greatest in the lingula and right middle lobe. (*B*) Corresponding axial, non-contrast enhanced CT image demonstrates patchy groundglass opacities, predominantly in the perimediastinal right middle lobe and lingula in the classic distribution of NEHI.

Characteristically, the clinical presentation is out of proportion to the minor, nonspecific histologic changes seen on lung biopsy specimens.[8,47] PFTs demonstrate marked air-trapping with decreased forced expiratory volume, elevated residual volume, and an elevated total lung capacity.[32]

On CXRs and CT, infants with NEHI typically manifest with hyperinflation and geographic ground-glass opacities in the paramediastinal lungs, particularly in the right middle lobe and the lingula. The presence of these findings on HRCT has been found to have a specificity of 100% when interpreted by experienced radiologists familiar with the disorder.[54] The same study found the sensitivity to be 78%, leading to the conclusion that HRCT cannot definitively exclude NEHI as a possible diagnosis.

Histologic diagnosis of NEHI is determined by an increased number of bombesin-immunopositive pulmonary neuroendocrine cells, the only consistent histologic abnormality.[8] Expanded bronchus-associated lymphoid tissue or subtle airway injury resembling postviral changes also may be seen (**Fig. 7**). Nevertheless, with a CT diagnostic specificity of nearly 100%, lung biopsy may be unnecessary in those who present with characteristic imaging findings and classic symptomatology.[32] Familial cases of NEHI have been described, suggesting a possible genetic etiology.[49,55]

Despite significant pulmonary symptomatology, patients with NEHI typically do not develop respiratory failure.[8] However, even with the relative lack of histologic changes on lung biopsy, patients often require supplemental oxygen and demonstrate persistent hyperinflation on imaging well into childhood.[2,56]

SUMMARY

Despite their rarity, childhood interstitial lung diseases are an important cause of morbidity and mortality in infants and young children. Many have nonspecific imaging findings, and, thus, a definitive diagnosis cannot be made on imaging alone. For the interpreting radiologist, obtaining appropriate and adequate imaging is paramount. Furthermore, familiarity with these diseases and their classification is important, as the treating physician may be unfamiliar, or at least not considering, these rare diseases in their differential diagnosis.

REFERENCES

1. Lee EY, Cleveland RH, Langston C. Imaging in pediatric pulmonology. New York: Springer; 2012.
2. Zucker EJ, Lee EY. Radiology illustrated: pediatric radiology. New York: Springer; 2014.
3. Hime NJ, Zurynski Y, Fitzgerald D, et al. Childhood interstitial lung disease: a systematic review. Pediatr Pulmonol 2015;50(12):1383–92.
4. Griese M, Haug M, Brasch F, et al. Incidence and classification of pediatric diffuse parenchymal lung diseases in Germany. Orphanet J Rare Dis 2009;4:26.
5. Kornum JB, Christensen S, Grijota M, et al. The incidence of interstitial lung disease 1995-2005: a Danish nationwide population-based study. BMC Pulm Med 2008;8:24.
6. Dinwiddie R, Sharief N, Crawford O. Idiopathic interstitial pneumonitis in children: a national survey in

the United Kingdom and Ireland. Pediatr Pulmonol 2002;34:23–9.

7. American Thoracic Society, European Respiratory Society. American Thoracic Society/European Respiratory Society International Multidisciplinary Consensus Classification of the Idiopathic Interstitial Pneumonias. This joint statement of the American Thoracic Society (ATS), and the European Respiratory Society (ERS) was adopted by the ATS board of directors, June 2001 and by the ERS Executive Committee, June 2001. Am J Respir Crit Care Med 2002;165:277–304.

8. Deutsch GH, Young LR, Deterding RR, et al. Diffuse lung disease in young children: application of a novel classification scheme. Am J Respir Crit Care Med 2007;176:1120–8.

9. Kurland G, Deterding RR, Hagood JS, et al. An official American Thoracic Society clinical practice guideline: classification, evaluation, and management of childhood interstitial lung disease in infancy. Am J Respir Crit Care Med 2013;188:376–94.

10. Clement A, Force ERST. Task force on chronic interstitial lung disease in immunocompetent children. Eur Respir J 2004;24:686–97.

11. Fan LL, Kozinetz CA, Deterding RR, et al. Evaluation of a diagnostic approach to pediatric interstitial lung disease. Pediatrics 1998;101:82–5.

12. Fan LL, Mullen AL, Brugman SM, et al. Clinical spectrum of chronic interstitial lung disease in children. J Pediatr 1992;121:867–72.

13. Fan LL, Kozinetz CA. Factors influencing survival in children with chronic interstitial lung disease. Am J Respir Crit Care Med 1997;156:939–42.

14. Castile R, Filbrun D, Flucke R, et al. Adult-type pulmonary function tests in infants without respiratory disease. Pediatr Pulmonol 2000;30:215–27.

15. Feher A, Castile R, Kisling J, et al. Flow limitation in normal infants: a new method for forced expiratory maneuvers from raised lung volumes. J Appl Physiol (1985) 1996;80:2019–25.

16. Goldstein AB, Castile RG, Davis SD, et al. Bronchodilator responsiveness in normal infants and young children. Am J Respir Crit Care Med 2001;164:447–54.

17. Jones M, Castile R, Davis S, et al. Forced expiratory flows and volumes in infants. Normative data and lung growth. Am J Respir Crit Care Med 2000;161:353–9.

18. Nogee LM. Genetic mechanisms of surfactant deficiency. Biol Neonate 2004;85:314–8.

19. Wert SE, Whitsett JA, Nogee LM. Genetic disorders of surfactant dysfunction. Pediatr Dev Pathol 2009;12:253–74.

20. Whitsett JA, Wert SE, Xu Y. Genetic disorders of surfactant homeostasis. Biol Neonate 2005;87:283–7.

21. Copley SJ, Coren M, Nicholson AG, et al. Diagnostic accuracy of thin-section CT and chest radiography of pediatric interstitial lung disease. AJR Am J Roentgenol 2000;174:549–54.

22. Owens C. Radiology of diffuse interstitial pulmonary disease in children. Eur Radiol 2004;14(Suppl 4):L2–12.

23. Newman B, Krane EJ, Gawande R, et al. Chest CT in children: anesthesia and atelectasis. Pediatr Radiol 2014;44:164–72.

24. Halter JM, Steinberg JM, Schiller HJ, et al. Positive end-expiratory pressure after a recruitment maneuver prevents both alveolar collapse and recruitment/derecruitment. Am J Respir Crit Care Med 2003;167:1620–6.

25. Studler U, Gluecker T, Bongartz G, et al. Image quality from high-resolution CT of the lung: comparison of axial scans and of sections reconstructed from volumetric data acquired using MDCT. AJR Am J Roentgenol 2005;185:602–7.

26. Vikgren J, Johnsson AA, Flinck A, et al. High-resolution computed tomography with 16-row MDCT: a comparison regarding visibility and motion artifacts of dose-modulated thin slices and "step and shoot" images. Acta Radiol 2008;49:755–60.

27. Walkup LL, Tkach JA, Higano NS, et al. Quantitative magnetic resonance imaging of bronchopulmonary dysplasia in the NICU environment. Am J Respir Crit Care Med 2015;192(10):1215–22.

28. Yikilmaz A, Koc A, Coskun A, et al. Evaluation of pneumonia in children: comparison of MRI with fast imaging sequences at 1.5T with chest radiographs. Acta Radiol 2011;52:914–9.

29. Sileo C, Corvol H, Boelle PY, et al. HRCT and MRI of the lung in children with cystic fibrosis: comparison of different scoring systems. J Cyst Fibros 2014;13:198–204.

30. Hansell DM, Bankier AA, MacMahon H, et al. Fleischner Society: glossary of terms for thoracic imaging. Radiology 2008;246:697–722.

31. Hansell DM. Thin-section CT of the lungs: the Hinterland of normal. Radiology 2010;256:695–711.

32. Lee EY. Interstitial lung disease in infants: new classification system, imaging technique, clinical presentation and imaging findings. Pediatr Radiol 2013;43:3–13 [quiz p: 128–9].

33. Langston C, Dishop MK. Diffuse lung disease in infancy: a proposed classification applied to 259 diagnostic biopsies. Pediatr Dev Pathol 2009;12:421–37.

34. MacMahan MH. Congenital alveolar dysplasia of the lungs. Bull New Engl Med Cent 1947;9:48.

35. MacMahan MH. Congenital alveolar dysplasia; a developmental anomaly involving pulmonary alveoli. Pediatrics 1948;2:43–57.

36. MacMahan MH. Congenital alveolar dysplasia of the lungs. Am J Pathol 1948;24:919–31.

37. Galambos C, Vargas SO, Arnold J, et al. Congenital alveolar dysplasia [abstract]. Mod Pathol 2003;16:3P.

38. Gillespie LM, Fenton AC, Wright C. Acinar dysplasia: a rare cause of neonatal respiratory failure. Acta Paediatr 2004;93:712–3.

39. Newman B, Yunis E. Primary alveolar capillary dysplasia. Pediatr Radiol 1990;21:20–2.

40. Hugosson CO, Salama HM, Al-Dayel F, et al. Primary alveolar capillary dysplasia (acinar dysplasia) and surfactant protein B deficiency: a clinical, radiological and pathological study. Pediatr Radiol 2005; 35:311–6.

41. Biko DM, Schwartz M, Anupindi SA, et al. Subpleural lung cysts in Down syndrome: prevalence and association with coexisting diagnoses. Pediatr Radiol 2008;38:280–4.

42. Lord A, Shapiro AJ, Saint-Martin C, et al. Filamin A mutation may be associated with diffuse lung disease mimicking bronchopulmonary dysplasia in premature newborns. Respir Care 2014;59: e171-7.

43. Lucaya J, Garcia-Pena P, Herrera L, et al. Expiratory chest CT in children. AJR Am J Roentgenol 2000; 174:235–41.

44. Doan ML, Guillerman RP, Dishop MK, et al. Clinical, radiological and pathological features of ABCA3 mutations in children. Thorax 2008;63: 366–73.

45. Guillot L, Epaud R, Thouvenin G, et al. New surfactant protein C gene mutations associated with diffuse lung disease. J Med Genet 2009;46: 490–4.

46. Thouvenin G, Abou Taam R, Flamein F, et al. Characteristics of disorders associated with genetic mutations of surfactant protein C. Arch Dis Child 2010; 95:449–54.

47. Fan LL, Deterding RR, Langston C. Pediatric interstitial lung disease revisited. Pediatr Pulmonol 2004; 38:369–78.

48. Wambach JA, Casey AM, Fishman MP, et al. Genotype-phenotype correlations for infants and children with ABCA3 deficiency. Am J Respir Crit Care Med 2014;189:1538–43.

49. Young LR, Deutsch GH, Bokulic RE, et al. A mutation in TTF1/NKX2.1 is associated with familial neuroendocrine cell hyperplasia of infancy. Chest 2013; 144:1199–206.

50. Hamvas A, Deterding RR, Wert SE, et al. Heterogeneous pulmonary phenotypes associated with mutations in the thyroid transcription factor gene NKX2-1. Chest 2013;144:794–804.

51. Gower WA, Nogee LM. Surfactant dysfunction. Paediatr Respir Rev 2011;12:223–9.

52. Lanfranchi M, Allbery SM, Wheelock L, et al. Pulmonary interstitial glycogenosis. Pediatr Radiol 2010; 40:361–5.

53. Castillo M, Vade A, Lim-Dunham JE, et al. Pulmonary interstitial glycogenosis in the setting of lung growth abnormality: radiographic and pathologic correlation. Pediatr Radiol 2010;40:1562–5.

54. Brody AS, Guillerman RP, Hay TC, et al. Neuroendocrine cell hyperplasia of infancy: diagnosis with high-resolution CT. AJR Am J Roentgenol 2010; 194:238–44.

55. Popler J, Gower WA, Mogayzel PJ Jr, et al. Familial neuroendocrine cell hyperplasia of infancy. Pediatr Pulmonol 2010;45:749–55.

56. Deterding RR. Infants and young children with children's interstitial lung disease. Pediatr Allergy Immunol Pulmonol 2010;23:25–31.

Imaging of Occupational Lung Disease

Jay Champlin, MD*, Rachael Edwards, MD, Sudhakar Pipavath, MBBS

KEYWORDS

- Occupational lung disease • Occupational lung diseases • Pneumoconiosis • Pneumoconioses
- Imaging • Radiology • Radiograph • Computed tomography

KEY POINTS

- In general, high-resolution computed tomography is more sensitive and specific than radiography for the detection of occupational lung diseases.
- Imaging findings are often nonspecific and must be interpreted with a multidisciplinary approach in the context of occupational history.
- Although often thought of as a static topic, occupational lung diseases are changing with evolving understanding of old diseases and new and emerging diseases.

OVERVIEW

Occupational lung disease refers to a variety of disorders that affect the lungs following inhalation of dusts or chemical antigens in a vocational setting. Despite the safety standards established by health organizations, occupational lung disease represents one of the most common work-related illnesses. Occupational lung diseases are responsible for approximately 70% of all deaths from occupational diseases.[1]

Pneumoconisosis is a subset of occupational lung diseases and is defined as a pulmonary disease caused by inhalation of inorganic mineral dust. Pneumoconioses may be further subdivided clinicopathologically into nonfibrotic and fibrotic subtypes.[2] The nonfibrotic subtype, resulting from inert dusts (iron, tin, barium), involves an accumulation of dust-containing macrophages and may lead to radiographic abnormalities. However, substantial fibrosis and functional impairment do not occur. In contrast, the fibrotic subtype, as seen in silicosis, coal worker's pneumoconiosis (CWP), asbestosis, berylliosis, and talcosis, results in focal or diffuse fibrosis and manifests as substantial radiographic abnormalities as well as functional impairment.

IMAGING IN OCCUPATIONAL LUNG DISEASE

Since 1930, the International Labor Organization (ILO), with support from the National Institute for Occupational Safety and Health (NIOSH), has provided a classification system, which is used worldwide to objectively classify the changes associated with pneumoconiosis based on posteroanterior chest radiographs. This system was revised in 2000 and, following widespread adaptation of digital radiography, extended from analog radiography to include digital radiography in 2011.[3,4]

Chest radiographs are relatively low radiation dose, inexpensive, and widely available. Thus, it is not surprising that radiography remains the first-line imaging examination for both occupational-exposure surveillance programs and the workup of suspected occupational lung diseases. However, high-resolution computed tomography (HRCT) is more sensitive and specific than radiography for the evaluation of occupational lung disease,

Dr J. Champlin and Dr R. Edwards have no financial relationships to disclose. Dr S. Pipavath is a consultant and expert advisor for Boehringer Ingelheim and expert reader for Imbio.
Department of Radiology, 1959 Northeast Pacific Street, RR 215, Box 357115, Seattle, WA 98195, USA
* Corresponding author.
E-mail address: jaychamp@uw.edu

radiologic.theclinics.com

particularly during the early stages.[5–11] HRCT is used to further characterize radiographic abnormalities and for evaluation of symptomatic patients. Given the increased sensitivity and specificity of HRCT, the use of HRCT in screening and surveillance programs has been suggested, and multiple classification schemes for evaluating the HRCT findings of occupational lung diseases similar to the ILO system for radiographs have been developed.[12,13]

No such system has of yet been adopted, mainly because of concerns over radiation exposure and cost. However, the recent adoption of lung cancer screening programs using low-dose computed tomography (CT) as well as studies showing adequate pleural and parenchymal detail in asbestos-exposed patients screened for lung cancer with low-dose HRCT suggests that low-dose HRCT may be a viable future one-stop screening option.[14,15]

The American College of Radiology has developed evidence-based guidelines regarding the imaging of occupational lung diseases, providing direction regarding the 3 classic mineral pneumoconioses: silicosis, CWP, and asbestosis.[16] These guidelines assert the increased sensitivity of CT relative to radiography and note a limited role for MR imaging and PET/CT.

A final note should be made regarding interpretation of imaging findings in occupational lung diseases. With relatively few exceptions, most imaging findings found on radiography and HRCT overlap with other diffuse lung diseases. As such, establishing the diagnosis is often a multidisciplinary endeavor requiring integration of occupational history, physical examination, laboratory testing, pulmonary function testing (PFT), imaging findings, and when the diagnosis is uncertain, pathologic evaluation of bronchoalveolar lavage (BAL) fluid and/or transbronchial or surgical lung biopsy.

Coal Mine Dust Lung Disease

Inhalation of coal mine dust places coal miners at risk for developing a variety of disorders, including chronic obstructive pulmonary disease (COPD), silicosis, CWP, mixed dust pneumoconiosis, and the relatively recently recognized dust-related diffuse fibrosis (DDF). The term coal mine dust lung disease (CMDLD) is now being used to reference this spectrum of diseases.

SILICOSIS

Silicosis is caused by inhalation of inorganic crystalline silicon dioxide (silica) dust. Crystalline silica occurs naturally in rocks and sand. Despite

occupational exposure limits in many countries, silicosis remains a common pneumoconiosis worldwide, with recent reports highlighting the risks of new construction materials, quartz conglomerates, and artificial stone products.[17–19] In addition, hydraulic fracturing or "fracking," in which large quantities of pressurized sand, water, and other chemicals are injected into fracture sites during the process of natural gas extraction exposes workers to silica as well as other volatile organic compounds. A recent study conducted by NIOSH researchers found that among 11 sites tested over 5 states, full-shift samples exceeded the permissible exposure limits for silica, in some cases by 10 times the occupational health criteria.[20] Additional potential avenues of exposure include mining, tunneling, drilling, quarrying, stonecutting, concrete manufacturing, polishing, masonry, brick lining, sandblasting, glass manufacturing, foundry work, pottery, ceramic and porcelain manufacturing, boiler scaling, vitreous enameling, and even clothing production (from sandblasting denim).[20–23]

There are multiple identified clinical forms of silicosis, including simple, complicated, accelerated, and acute. Simple silicosis occurs after 10 to 20 years of low- to moderate-level exposure.[24] Following inhalation, macrophages engulf silica, resulting in cytokine release, fibroblast proliferation, and formation of silicotic nodules with concentric layers of collagen and silica-laden macrophages as well as lymphoid cells, which become acellular and hyalinized.[25] Simple silicosis typically causes no symptoms or respiratory impairment.

Radiographic findings include small, well-circumscribed nodules (1–10 mm but typically 2–5 mm) favoring the upper posterior lungs. Nodules can calcify, often diffusely. Pseudoplaques occasionally form because of clustering of subpleural nodules. Mediastinal and hilar lymphadenopathy with or without calcification may be present. Additional findings include pleural thickening and pleural effusions.[26]

HRCT findings include multiple small well-defined nodules, often seen in a centrilobular and perilymphatic distribution (Fig. 1). Nodules may be diffuse in distribution or favor the upper lobes. CT can also demonstrate pseudoplaques, pleural thickening, and pleural effusions.[26] Additional CT findings include hilar and/or mediastinal lymphadenopathy, which may calcify.[27] Lymphadenopathy may be the first manifestation following lower levels of silica exposure, preceding the development of parenchymal findings.[23] Subsequent exposure and lymph node damage may interfere with lymph drainage and increase the propensity for parenchymal disease.[28] Eggshell

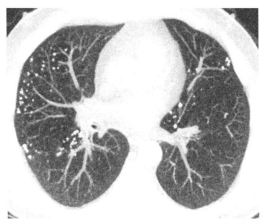

Fig. 1. Axial maximum intensity projection (MIP) reconstruction depicts numerous upper lobe predominant calcified nodules in a centrilobular distribution in setting of simple silicosis.

calcification can be seen as in sarcoidosis, amyloidosis, chronic beryllium disease (CBD), and mycobacterial infection. Although there are some similarities between simple silicosis and sarcoidosis, there are many distinguishing factors (Box 1).

Complicated silicosis, also known as progressive massive fibrosis (PMF), results when silica in periphery of the silicotic nodules incites further fibrotic response.[29] Unlike simple silicosis, PMF is usually debilitating with progressive dyspnea and respiratory and functional impairment. On radiographs, PMF is characterized by large opacities greater than 1 cm, which develop in the periphery of the mid and upper lungs (usually in the apical and posterior segments of upper lobes) and migrate toward the hila with resulting paracicatricial emphysema (Fig. 2A).[30] These large opacities, also known as conglomerate masses, occur because of conglomeration of small nodules and are often bilateral, usually symmetric, and tend

---

Box 1
Distinguishing features of simple silicosis and early stage sarcoidosis

- Occupational history
- Clustering of nodules around perihilar regions and bronchi is more common in sarcoidosis
- Nodular septa, fissural thickening, and reticular opacities are not found in silicosis

Data from Ooi C, Arakawa H. Silicosis. Imaging of occupational and environmental disorders of the chest. Berlin: Springer-Verlag Berlin Heidelberg, 2006.

---

to have irregular margins with a lateral border paralleling the pleura. They may calcify or cavitate, with cavitation suggesting ischemic necrosis or superimposed tuberculosis (TB). The damage caused by inhaled silica to alveolar macrophages and impaired cell-mediated immunity results in increased risk for TB.

HRCT better demonstrates the coalescent nodular margin of large opacities as well as the background profusion of small nodules. The profusion of small nodules decreases as they coalesce into larger opacities (Fig. 2B). These findings may be difficult to distinguish from the conglomerate masses that form in advanced sarcoidosis simulating PMF (Box 2, Fig. 3). In addition, CT also better demonstrates surrounding paracicatricial emphysema (Fig. 4). Interestingly, silica has been shown to be a risk factor for the development of emphysema independent of smoking.[31,32] CT scoring of emphysema and extent of air trapping have been shown to correlate with PFTs.[33,34] In addition to these findings, patients may also develop diffuse fibrosis in a nonspecific interstitial pneumonia or usual interstitial pneumonia (UIP) pattern.[35,36]

Silica is a known carcinogen and increases risk for lung cancer.[37] Large opacities/conglomerate masses in complicated silicosis may resemble cancer. Distinguishing large opacities in this setting from lung cancer can be difficult on CT. However, identifying conglomerate masses in complicated silicosis is often possible based on slow progression and symmetry, but in challenging cases, MR imaging can be helpful. Large opacities of PMF demonstrate low signal intensity on T2-weighted imaging (T2WI), whereas lung cancer typically has increased signal intensity on T2WI.[38] Contrary to one's expectation, PET is not helpful because intense FDG uptake can occur in both lung cancer and PMF.[39]

Accelerated silicosis occurs following short but intense exposure (4–10 years). Clinical presentation and radiographic findings are similar to complicated silicosis; however, patients are more likely to progress, even following exposure removal.

Acute silicosis or silicoproteinosis is a rare condition seen in individuals with heavy exposure to silica in enclosed spaces with little or no protection. This high-level inhalation results in proliferation of type II pneumocytes and exuberant surfactant production.[40,41] Acute silicosis has been reported following exposure times as short as several months up to 8 years.[42] Patients often present with constitutional symptoms and rapidly progressive dyspnea, often resulting in respiratory failure and death, frequently due to cor

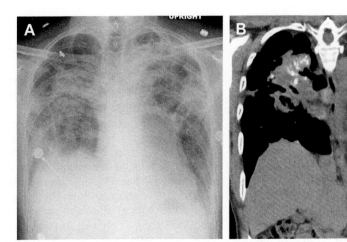

Fig. 2. PMF as a result of silicosis. Chest radiograph (*A*) demonstrates large opacities with a peripheral and upper long predominance with volume loss and distortion of the hila. Correlative coronal CT image (*B*) with upper lobe predominant mass like consolidation with calcifications.

pulmonale.[41,42] Imaging findings are similar to pulmonary alveolar proteinosis. Radiographically, ground-glass opacities (GGO) and consolidation with air bronchograms in a perihilar distribution are seen.[43] On HRCT, interlobular septal thickening and "crazy-paving" may be seen with numerous bilateral centrilobular nodules, multifocal GGO, and consolidation (**Fig. 5**).[44]

COAL WORKER'S PNEUMOCONIOSIS

CWP results from inorganic coal dust inhalation, primarily in miners exposed to coal mine dust. Following the introduction of the Federal Coal Mine Health and Safety Act of 1969, which reduced the allowable dust levels in mines, the incidence of CWP in the United States decreased from 11.2% from 1970 to 1974 to 2% from 1995 to 1999. In 2007, however, the Centers for Disease Control and Prevention reported multiple cases of rapidly progressing pneumoconiosis among underground coal miners who began working after the implementation of these federally mandated prevention measures.[45] Adding to the concern is the fact that the incidence of CWP has been increasing in recent years, particularly in smaller mines with fewer than 50 employees.[46,47]

CWP can occur in those with exposure to washed coal dust as well as mixed dust containing coal, kaolin, mica, and silica in various proportions.[2] Development of disease depends on several factors, including level and duration of exposure, mine size and configuration, coal type, coal rank (hardness of coal), proportion of other mineral dust contamination, mining methods, and personal protective measures used.[48,49]

The relationship between coal and silica in the development of CWP and progression is complex, and although studies have shown that silica is not required, the fact that exposure to both minerals is often simultaneous suggests that silica often likely contributes.[50–53] The nearly identical imaging appearance of silicosis and CWP further complicates the matter, and distinguishing between the 2 based on imaging is not usually possible. Fortunately, the histologic findings of CWP and silicosis differ with CWP characterized by coal macules, which are aggregates of coal dust–laden macrophages entangled with collagen lacking the hyalinization and laminated collagen typically seen in silicotic nodules.[49]

As with silicosis, there are simple and complicated forms of CWP. Simple CWP generally requires at least 20 years of coal dust exposure

---

Box 2

Distinguishing features of complicated silicosis and conglomerate masses of late-stage sarcoidosis

- Occupational history
- Conglomerate masses of sarcoidosis form near hila instead of at periphery
- Conglomerate masses in complicated silicosis may calcify or cavitate, an uncommon finding in sarcoidosis
- No surrounding lung distortion or paracicatricial emphysema

Data from Pipavath S, Godwin JD. Imaging of interstitial lung disease. Clin Chest Med 2004;25(2):455–65, v–vi.

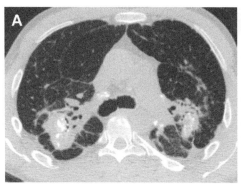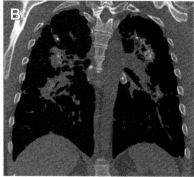

Fig. 3. (*A*, *B*) PMF as a result of sarcoidosis. CT axial (*A*) and coronal (*B*) images show upper lobe predominant masslike consolidation with calcifications in combination with calcified mediastinal lymph nodes.

with shorter exposures more likely to cause chronic bronchitis. Patients with CWP may be asymptomatic or gradually develop dyspnea and decline in PFTs.

Radiographic findings of simple CWP include small nodules or reticulonodular opacities (**Fig. 6**). Compared with silicotic nodules, the nodules of CWP may be smaller and less distinct. The nodules may calcify in up to 20% of patients and are typically central in location.[54] Nodules are often seen in a mid and upper lung–predominant distribution. However, when extensive, all lobes may be involved.[55] As with silicosis, subpleural nodules may coalesce, resembling pleural plaques (pseudoplaques). Lymph node calcification is not as common as in silicosis (up to one-third), and eggshell calcification is uncommon.[5,56]

HRCT will typically show nodules in a centrilobular or perilymphatic/subpleural pattern (**Fig. 7**).[2,57] These nodules tend to favor the apical and posterior segments of the upper lobes and superior segments of the lower lobes. A right, upper-lobe preponderance has been described because of local differences in lymphatic clearance.[5] Subpleural nodules may coalesce into pseudoplaques.[57] Mediastinal or hilar lymphadenopathy can be seen in up to 30% of patients.[5]

PMF may occur in the setting of CWP, but is less common than in silicosis and tends to develop in patients with long exposure times.[58] It is hypothesized that this difference is due to decreased fibrogenicity of coal relative to silica. The large opacities in CWP are made of mineral dust, calcium salts, and proteinaceous material and can be distinguished from those seen in silicosis by the presence of coal dust and absence of silicotic nodules.

On imaging, PMF is characterized by one or more large opacities 1 cm or larger that typically begin peripherally with round or lentiform shape and a lateral border paralleling the chest wall. Paracicatricial emphysema often develops as the large opacities enlarge and migrate toward the hila. Like silicosis, the process is accompanied by a decrease in small nodule profusion. Similarly, the large opacities can calcify or cavitate, due to either infection or ischemia, and patients may report coughing up black sputum (melanoptysis). As with silicosis, cavitation should alert to the possibility of mycobacterial infection, because there is an increased risk of TB. Coal mining is associated with an increased incidence of lung cancer.[59,60] Thus, similar to silicosis, it is important to distinguish large opacities of PMF from lung cancer. In

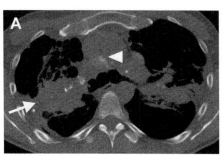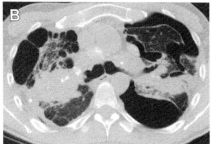

Fig. 4. (*A*, *B*) Axial CT images of PMF with upper lobe masslike consolidation containing calcification (*arrow*) in the background of emphysema and bullae. Calcified mediastinal lymph nodes (*arrowhead*) are seen additionally.

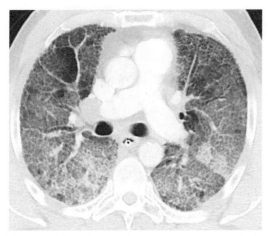

Fig. 5. Axial CT image demonstrating acute silicosis in a patient who presented with dyspnea following sand blasting without respiratory protection. Classic, although not specific, imaging pattern of GGO with superimposed interlobular septal thickening ("crazy-paving").

addition, coal dust exposure has been found to be a risk factor, independent of smoking, for development of emphysema and COPD.[61]

In 1953, Caplan[62] described a characteristic radiographic pattern in coal miners afflicted with rheumatoid arthritis that was distinct from simple CWP or PMF. It consisted of multiple, well-defined nodules ranging from 0.5 cm to several centimeters scattered throughout the lung but with a peripheral preponderance and often seen in clusters.[62] This disease has subsequently been referred to as Caplan syndrome or rheumatoid pneumoconiosis. Nodule onset is typically sudden, with the clinical course ranging from regression to progression. Histologically,

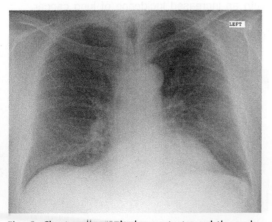

Fig. 6. Chest radiograph demonstrates subtle nodularity most pronounced in the upper lobes.

rheumatoid nodules are distinct from typical nodules of PMF in that they are inflammatory and consist of central necrosis surrounded by a collagenous layer containing polymorphonuclear leukocytes and a few macrophages.[63] Since the initial description by Caplan, it has been recognized that these same nodules can also occur following asbestos, silica, aluminum, carbon, and dolomite exposure.

DUST-RELATED DIFFUSE FIBROSIS

DDF is a recently recognized phenomenon shown on autopsy series to occur in 15% to 20% of coal miners.[64] DDF may be mistaken for idiopathic pulmonary fibrosis (IPF) without careful occupational history; however, the distinction is important, because DDF is associated with longer survival than IPF.[64,65] On histologic analysis, there have been reports of fibrosis with areas of anthracotic nodules and pigment and inflammation.[66] Separate reports have described bridging fibrosis connecting macular, nodular, or PMF lesions of CWP or silicosis, often with pigmented interlobular septal thickening.[64,65] On HRCT, diffuse interlobular septal thickening is seen.[66]

MIXED-DUST PNEUMOCONIOSIS

Mixed-dust pneumoconiosis (MDP) is a generic term for pneumoconiosis caused by simultaneous exposure to silica and less fibrogenic dusts, such as coal or iron. Several types of MDP have been described, including silicosiderosis. In the setting of CMDLD, MDP refers to disease caused by inhalation of silica and coal dust. A pathologic definition for MDP has been proposed as a pneumoconiosis with dust macules or mixed-dust fibrotic nodules with or without silicotic nodules in an individual with history of exposure to mixed dust.[67] Although studies have described the imaging findings of MDP from a variety of causes, the findings seen in CMDLD have yet to be widely published.[57,68]

ASBESTOS-RELATED THORACIC DISEASE

Asbestos is a generic term applied to several naturally occurring, fibrous silicate minerals united in their heat-resistant properties. Exposure to asbestos historically occurred through a variety of occupations including insulation and textile manufacturing, construction, shipbuilding and shipyard trades, and brake manufacture and repair. Although global consumption of asbestos has decreased and asbestos-related diseases have plateaued in most of the developed world, consumption is increasing in many developing

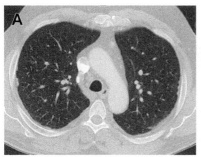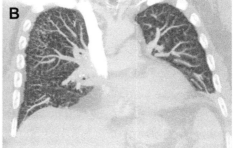

Fig. 7. Axial (A) and coronal MIP (B) CT from the same patient demonstrate centrilobular and perilymphatic nodules.

countries.[69] Furthermore, despite decreased domestic use, asbestos exposure continues to be of concern in industrial maintenance and repair and during the course of renovations and demolitions. In addition, the long latency from exposure to disease manifestation results in asbestos-related conditions being a perpetual dilemma.

There are 2 main groups of asbestos based on physical characteristics of the fibers: serpentines and amphiboles. Chrysotile, the sole asbestiform mineral in the serpentine group, is curly, flexible, and easily decomposable. These fibers, which account for greater than 90% of the asbestos used in the United States, do not penetrate deeply into the lung and are relatively chemically stable. Amphiboles fibers, including amosite, crocidolite, and tremolitie, are stiff, straight, needlelike, and more fibrogenic and carcinogenic.[70]

There are a variety of pulmonary and extrapulmonary sequelae related to asbestos exposure. Pulmonary processes range from benign pleural (pleural effusion, pleural plaques, and diffuse pleural thickening [DPT]) and parenchymal diseases (asbestosis, rounded atelectasis), to malignancies (lung carcinoma and mesothelioma). Extrapulmonary manifestations include peritoneal mesothelioma, gastrointestinal carcinoma, renal carcinoma, leukemia, and head and neck carcinoma.[71]

Pleural plaque is the most commonly recognized manifestation following asbestos exposure, developing in up to 80% of exposed workers.[29] Plaques generally develop 20 to 30 years following initial exposure. They do not typically cause symptoms or substantial functional impairment but serve as a biomarker of asbestos exposure.[72] Importantly, pleural plaques do not undergo malignant degeneration and are not precursor lesions of mesothelioma. Histologically, pleural plaques are composed of generally acellular bundles of collagen in an undulating "basket-weave" pattern, which may contain asbestos fibers but no asbestos bodies.

Radiographically, plaques are best seen in profile as focal areas of pleural thickening, typically along the posterolateral chest wall between the sixth through tenth ribs and along the dome of diaphragm, with sparing of the apices and costophrenic sulci (Fig. 8A).[73] En face lesions may have the appearance of a holly leaf (Fig. 9A). Plaques can be mistaken for extrapleural fat, although symmetry and smooth margins with extension over the apices and into fissures are typical of extrapleural fat.

HRCT is more sensitive than radiography for the detection of pleural plaques.[57] CT will show focal, irregular areas of pleural thickening, which almost always affect the parietal pleura and only rarely affect the visceral pleura and interlobar fissures. Plaques are usually bilateral but can be unilateral in up to 36% of patients.[74] Diaphragmatic lesions may be best appreciated on coronal or sagittal reformats (Fig. 8B). The lesions typically involve the mid chest and can calcify over time (Fig. 9B). CT can easily distinguish plaques from extrapleural fat.

DPT is usually the sequelae of prior asbestos-related pleural effusion and occurs in 22% to 25% of those exposed to asbestos.[29,75] Chronic inflammation results in fusion of the visceral and parietal layers and is often accompanied by rounded atelectasis. Although there are many causes of DPT (pleurisy, parapneumonic effusion or empyema, hemothorax, connective tissue disease, or previous instrumentation), bilateral pleural thickening is usually the result of asbestos exposure, particularly when pleural plaques are identified. Unlike pleural plaques, DPT can cause functional impairment.

Although various radiological definitions exist, McLoud and colleagues[76] define DPT as smooth, continuous thickening over at least one-fourth of the chest wall. On HRCT, Lynch and colleagues[71] define DPT as continuous thickening greater than 3 mm, which is greater than 5 cm wide and greater

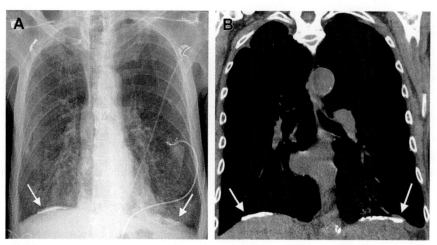

Fig. 8. Chest radiograph (*A*) demonstrating calcified pleural plaque in profile (*arrows*) along the diaphragm with correlative CT coronal reconstruction (*B*).

than 8 cm in craniocaudal extent; however, less extensive thickening may be physiologically significant, and a less strict definition may be useful. There are no specific imaging features of pleural thickening itself; however, the presence of pleural plaques is suggestive of asbestos-related DPT. DPT is generally less than 10 mm thick, and thickness greater than 10 mm, nodularity, and circumferential or mediastinal pleural involvement should raise the possibility of malignant pleural disease.

Benign pleural effusions are probably the earliest manifestation following asbestos exposure and usually develop within 7 to 10 years of initial exposure or anytime thereafter. Effusions are exudative, often blood tinged, and can be unilateral or bilateral.[77] They are seen in 3% to 7% of exposed patients; however, because effusions are often subclinical, these figures are likely underestimated.[78] When symptomatic, patients may present with mild chest pain, fever, and leukocytosis.

Effusions often spontaneously resolve but can lead to DPT. Histologic analysis may reveal nonspecific inflammation and fibrosis with rare asbestos bodies or fibers, which may be better demonstrated by electron microscopy.

HRCT may show features of exudative effusion with or without parietal pleural thickening (**Fig. 10**). The presence of pleural plaques is suggestive of asbestos-related pleural effusion. Patients can have multiple recurrences, with increases in DPT after each episode. Substantial pain or long-lasting effusion should raise the possibility of mesothelioma, which has been shown to arise from an apparent benign but persistent pleural effusion.[77]

Mesothelioma is a rare, progressive neoplasm of the mesothelium. It most often arises from pleura, less frequently from the peritoneum or pericardium. Patients with the pleural form of the disease may present with persistent or recurrent unilateral pleural effusion. Radiographic

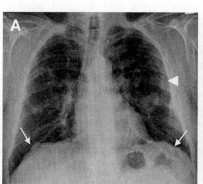
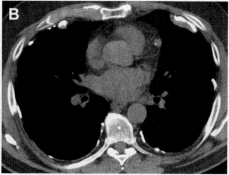

Fig. 9. Chest radiograph (*A*) depicting calcified pleural plaque both in profile (*arrows*) and en face (*arrowhead*) with correlative axial CT image (*B*).

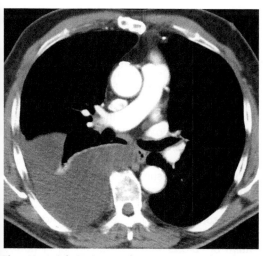

Fig. 10. Axial CT image demonstrates right pleural effusion, a sequela of asbestos exposure.

findings include large unilateral pleural effusion, multiple pleural soft tissue lesions, often in the setting of pleural plaques. HRCT findings suggestive of malignancy include nodular and circumferential pleural thickening greater than 10 mm, mediastinal or fissural involvement, or invasion of the chest wall, diaphragm, or mediastinum (Fig. 11).[79]

Asbestosis is interstitial fibrosis resulting from exposure to asbestos. There is a dose-response relationship with cases typically seen following high levels of exposure for long periods of time, usually at least 20 years after initial exposure. Asbestos-related fibrosis begins around the respiratory bronchioles in the periphery of the lower lobes where asbestos fibers accumulate and can progress to diffuse interstitial fibrosis and honeycombing with loss of alveolar architecture. Asbestos bodies are typically seen on BAL or tissue specimens.[80] Patients present with symptoms and progressive decline in vital capacity and diffusion capacity.

Radiography typically shows basal predominant reticular opacities consistent with fibrosis. The HRCT findings of asbestosis are often indistinguishable from a UIP pattern of fibrosis with reticulation, traction bronchiectasis and bronchiolectasis, and honeycombing, typically basal predominant.[81,82] Early in the disease, HRCT may also show subpleural dotlike opacities and branching structures, which may coalesce into subpleural curvilinear lines and small subpleural irregular nodules.[83] Additional HRCT findings include parenchymal bands, patchy subpleural GGO, small cystic spaces, and areas of hypoattenuation.[71,83] Interestingly, in one study, many of the early findings seen in asbestosis, including subpleural dotlike or branching opacities as well as subpleural curvilinear lines mosaic attenuation, and parenchymal bands, were reported to be more common in asbestosis and visible intralobular bronchioles, traction bronchiectasis, bronchiolectasis within consolidations, and honeycombing more common in IPF (Box 3).[82] In another study, fibrosis seen in asbestosis was actually more often basal and subpleural than that seen in biopsy-proven UIP; however, when a logistic regression model was applied adjusting for age, sex, and extent of fibrosis, no CT feature,

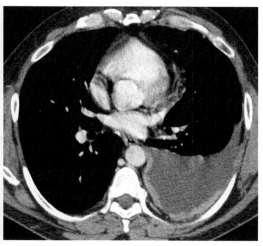

Fig. 11. Axial CT image depicts mesothelioma with left-sided nodularity along the pleura and a left-sided pleural effusion.

Box 3
Distinguishing features of asbestosis and idiopathic pulmonary fibrosis

- Pleural plaques may serve as a marker for asbestos exposure
- Digital clubbing is less common with asbestosis than IPF
- Slower progression of fibrosis in asbestosis
- Subpleural dotlike or branching opacities, subpleural curvilinear lines, mosaic attenuation, and parenchymal bands were reported to be more common in asbestosis and visible intralobular bronchioles, traction bronchiectasis and bronchiolectasis, and honeycombing more common in IPF

Data from Copley SJ. Asbestosis. In: De Vuyst P, Gevenois PA, editors. Imaging of occupational and environmental disorders of the chest. Berlin: Springer; 2006. p. 207–21.

including distribution of disease, varied between asbestosis and UIP groups.[84] Often in the setting of fibrosis, the only feature suggesting the diagnosis of asbestosis is the presence of concomitant pleural plaques; however, this is not infallible, because not all patients with asbestosis will have pleural plaques and not all fibrosis in the presence of pleural plaques is asbestosis.[81] Importantly, the risk of death from asbestosis increases with increasing severity of fibrosis on imaging.[85] In mild cases, prone imaging can help distinguish mild posterior fibrosis from dependent atelectasis.

Asbestos is a known carcinogen, and the incidence of lung carcinoma is increased among those exposed to asbestos. In smokers, the risk is greatly increased due to the synergistic effect between asbestos and cigarette smoke.[86,87] Fortunately, smoking cessation can decrease lung cancer risk back to levels seen in exposed nonsmokers.[87]

Rounded atelectasis is nonspecific and can occur in a variety of conditions that cause pleural thickening. It occurs when visceral pleural fibrosis invaginates, resulting in atelectasis. Rounded atelectasis is the most common cause of masslike opacity of patients with asbestosis. Given the increased incidence of lung carcinoma in patients with asbestos exposure, correct identification of a mass as rounded atelectasis can prevent unnecessary biopsy or resection. Findings of rounded atelectasis on HRCT include rounded masslike opacity in lung periphery adjacent to thickened pleura with associated volume loss and distortion of bronchi and vessels leading to the mass ("comet-tail" sign).[88,89] PET may be helpful to distinguish rounded atelectasis from lung carcinoma, because rounded atelectasis is not usually FDG avid.[90,91]

OTHER PNEUMOCONIOSES
Siderosis

Siderosis is an inert dust pneumoconiosis caused by inhalation of inorganic iron dust. It has also been called arc welder's pneumoconiosis because of its prevalence among electric arc or oxyacetylene welders exposed to iron oxide fumes from consumable electrodes during the welding process. Other occupational exposures associated with siderosis include mining and processing of iron ores, steel mill and foundry workers, and silver polishers.

Following inhalation, macrophages ingest iron oxide and aggregate along perivascular and peribronchial lymphatics.[2] Although patients may present with cough and dyspnea, siderosis is generally not associated with fibrosis or functional impairment.[2,75,92] When both iron oxide and silica are inhaled together, however, silicosiderosis (a mixed dust pneumoconiosis) can develop, which, unlike siderosis, is often associated with fibrosis and disability.[2]

On radiography, siderosis generally appears as micronodules concentrated in the middle thirds of the lungs in the perihilar regions.[92] The nodules are typically less dense than those seen in silicosis and may be accompanied by diffuse, fine reticulonodular opacities. Unlike most pneumoconiosis, the radiographic abnormalities may resolve following removal from exposure.[93] HRCT findings include diffuse, poorly defined centrilobular nodules and branching linear structures or extensive GGO without zonal predominance.[57,92,94,95] Additional reported findings include emphysema or a UIP pattern of fibrosis with honeycombing, or rarely, conglomerate masses with high attenuation.[92]

Talcosis

Occupational talcosis is caused by inhalation of talc, a hydrated magnesium silicate used in the manufacture and processing of leather, paper, rubber, plastics, paint, cosmetic, textiles, and ceramics. Pulmonary talcosis can also occur following illicit intravenous drug injection of oral medications in which talc is used as a filler and lubricant. Histologically, talc incites nonnecrotizing granulomatous inflammation that may progress to pulmonary fibrosis.[2]

Radiographic findings of occupational talcosis include small nodules, large opacities, a diffuse reticular pattern, and lymphadenopathy.[57,96] HRCT findings include small centrilobular and subpleural nodules, septal and subpleural lines, GGO, and lobular low-attenuation areas due to air trapping.[57,96,97] Some investigators have reported no zonal predominance, whereas others have reported that findings are most severe in the upper and mid lungs with relative sparing of the bases.[96,97] Large opacities may be irregular, round, or crescent-shaped and often contain foci of high attenuation, reflecting talc deposition.[96] Rarely, honeycombing can be seen.[96] Noncalcified pleural plaques and enlarged lymph nodes with focal areas of high attenuation have also been reported.[57,96]

It is worth noting that the HRCT findings of talcosis resulting from intravenous drug abuse differ somewhat from inhalational talcosis occurring in the occupational setting and include diffuse small nodules, confluent perihilar conglomerate masses with increased attenuation, diffuse GGO, and lower lobe panacinar emphysema.[98,99] The imaging features of talcosis and other common and uncommon occupational lung disease can be found in Table 1.

Table 1
Imaging features of common and uncommon occupational thoracic disease

Disease	Imaging Findings
Simple silicosis	Radiographs: small, well-circumscribed nodules favoring the upper posterior lungs, which may calcify HRCT: small, well-defined centrilobular and perilymphatic nodules, upper lobe predominance, pseudoplaques, hilar, or mediastinal lymphadenopathy with or without calcification
Complicated silicosis	Radiographs: large, often bilateral, usually symmetric opacities (usually >1 cm) in the periphery of the mid/upper lungs; central distribution of the opacities from migration toward the hila. These opacities may calcify or cavitate and demonstrate paracicatricial emphysema HRCT: small nodules, conglomerate masses (large opacities), coalescent nodular margin of large conglomerate masses, emphysema. Findings that are present but may not help in distinguishing from other diseases include mosaic attenuation and air trapping, and paracicatricial emphysema
Silicoproteinosis	Radiographs: GGO and/or consolidations in a perihilar distribution (similar to any alveolar filling process, not a specific imaging pattern) HRCT: interlobular septal thickening and "crazy-paving" pattern (may not always be present), centrilobular nodules, multifocal patchy GGO, and consolidation. Exposure history is key in making an accurate diagnosis
Simple CWP	Radiographs: small nodules often seen in a mid and upper lung predominant distribution, which may calcify. Pseudoplaques, quite often very similar to simple silicosis HRCT: nodules ranging from 2 to 12 mm in centrilobular and perilymphatic distribution favoring the apical and posterior segments of the upper lobes and superior segments of the lower lobes, pseudoplaques, mediastinal, or hilar lymphadenopathy that may calcify
Complicated CWP	Imaging: similar to complicated silicosis
Asbestosis	Radiographs: predominant reticular opacities in a basal distribution HRCT: subpleural dotlike opacities and branching structures, which may coalesce into subpleural curvilinear lines and small pleural-based irregular nodules (early findings), interlobular septal and intralobular interstitial thickening, traction bronchiectasis and bronchiolectasis, and honeycombing, often with a basal predominance. Other findings such as parenchymal bands, subpleural GGO, small cystic spaces, and areas of hypoattenuation (mosaic attenuation). None of the findings are specific for asbestosis. Exposure history and asbestos-related pleural plaques are helpful in suggesting this possibility
Siderosis	Radiographs: micronodules concentrated in the middle third of the lungs. Diffuse fine reticulonodular opacities HRCT: diffuse, ill-defined centrilobular nodules, extensive GGO without zonal predominance, emphysema, fibrosis, honeycombing, conglomerate masses with high attenuation. Exposure history or histologic confirmation is often required for accurate diagnosis
Talcosis	Radiographs: small nodules, large opacities, lymphadenopathy HRCT: small centrilobular and subpleural nodules, GGO, and lobular low-attenuation areas due to air trapping, possibly with upper and mid lung predominance. Irregular, round, or crescent-shaped large opacities similar to conglomerate masses, often of high attenuation due to talc deposition, noncalcified pleural plaques, and enlarged lymph nodes with focal areas of high attenuation

IMMUNE-MEDIATED OCCUPATIONAL LUNG DISEASES
Hypersensitivity Pneumonitis

Hypersensitivity pneumonitis (HP) is an immunologically mediated diffuse granulomatous lung disease of the pulmonary interstitium and terminal airways. It develops in susceptible individuals following sensitization and repeated exposure to and inhalation of certain antigenic organic and low-molecular-weight inorganic particles. The pathogenesis is related to a combination of type III and type IV hypersensitivity reactions.

A variety of microbes, animal antigens, and inorganic compounds have been associated with the development of HP, and new agents and occupational exposures are routinely being identified.[100] Known antigens include isocyanates (paint sprays) (which are also a common cause of occupational asthma), plastic vapors (plastics and packing plants), nontuberculous mycobacteria (microbially contaminated metal working fluid), *Aspergillus* and thermophilic *Actinomyces* (agriculture), and avian proteins (bird breeders); however, the causative antigen is not identified in up to 38% of cases of histologically confirmed cases of HP.[101] A short description of general imaging features seen in HP and other immune-mediated occupational lung diseases can be found in **Table 2**, and findings of more newly described occupational lung diseases found in **Table 3**.

Beryllium

Beryllium is a lightweight metal used in a variety of industries, ranging from aerospace, defense, nuclear power and weapons, electronics, metal manufacturing, dentistry, ceramics, and recreational equipment. Clinically, acute and chronic forms of lung injury related to beryllium exposure have been recognized when exposed to dust, fumes, or aerosols of beryllium or its salts.

Acute beryllium disease (ABD) is a chemical pneumonitis resembling acute respiratory distress syndrome. The disease may be self-limited or fatal. Imaging often reveals diffuse airspace opacities occurring 1 to 3 weeks following high levels of exposure.[102] Fortunately, since adoption of OSHA standards in 1949 and resulting improved industrial control measures, ABD is no longer seen in the United States.

CBD is a multisystem granulomatous disease, which develops in up to 15% of exposed workers.[103–105] It is the result of a beryllium-specific lymphocyte-mediated delayed-type hypersensitivity response in which inhalation leads to activation of CD4+ T lymphocytes, which migrate to the lungs, causing an inflammatory response with macrophage accumulation and noncaseating, epithelioid granulomata formation.[106,107] There is no clear dose-response relationship, because CBD can occur after short-term low-level exposure, or may

---

Table 2
Imaging features of other common occupational lung diseases

Disease	Diagnostic Imaging Features
HP	Radiographs: small nodules, reticulonodular pattern, or air space opacities, often with relative sparing of the bases and loss of lung volume when chronic HRCT: small poorly defined GGO attenuation centrilobular nodules (helps in diagnosis), patchy or diffuse GGO, mosaic attenuation, and air trapping. Headcheese pattern when appreciated is a useful clue, as is relative sparing of the bases. Reticulation, architectural distortion, and traction bronchiectasis may be seen in chronic HP
Chronic berylliosis	Radiographs: can be normal; when abnormal, small nodules and reticulation, typically in a mid and upper lung predominant distribution (early). Reticulation, architectural distortion, honeycombing, and masslike lesions due to coalescence of small nodules, and lymphadenopathy HRCT: nodules in a perilymphatic distribution, aggregate nodules forming pseudoplaques. Reticulation, architectural distortion, and honeycombing may also be seen
Hard metal lung	Radiographs: bilateral GGO, small nodules, reticulation, lymphadenopathy, small cystic spaces HRCT: mosaic attenuation and air trapping, small centrilobular nodules, bilateral GGO, consolidation, reticulation, traction bronchiectasis, possibly with a lower lobe predominance, honeycombing

Table 3
Newer occupational lung diseases

Disease	Inciting Agent	Clinical	Imaging
Flock worker's lung	Due to inhalation of flock, an ultrafine nylon fiber used in the production of some fabrics First recognized at a Canadian plant in 1995[140]	Histologic findings: lymphocytic bronchiolitis and peribronchiolitis with lymphoid hyperplasia represented by lymphoid aggregates[141] Cough and dyspnea, which typically improves following cessation of exposure	Radiographs: normal or diffuse reticulonodular infiltrates and patchy consolidations[141] HRCT: patchy GGO and consolidations or diffuse micronodules, reticulation, traction bronchiectasis, and peripheral honeycombing can also be seen[141,142]
Flavor worker's lung	Due to exposure to the ketone diacetyl (2,3-butanedione) used in artificial butter flavoring of microwave popcorn First reported in 2002 among 8 (later 9) workers at a microwave popcorn plant in Missouri[143–145]	Histologic findings: constrictive bronchiolitis characterized by concentric fibrosis of the submucosa and peribronchial tissues of the terminal and respiratory bronchioles, with advanced lesions often demonstrating airway obliteration[29,75] Progressive dyspnea and obstructive lung disease	Radiographs: normal or hyperinflation HRCT: bronchial wall thickening with findings of small airways diseases, including mosaic attenuation and air trapping on expiratory imaging, bronchiectasis, upper lobe volume loss, and subpleural nodularity suggestive of fibrosis[145]
Indium	Due to exposure to indium-tin oxide, which is used in manufacture of transparent conductive coatings for LCD and plasma TVs[146] First reported in 2003 in a 27-y-old Japanese man who worked in indium target production[147] Subsequent studies have identified substantial interstitial disease on HRCT in up to 21% of indium workers[148]	Histologic findings: intra-alveolar exudates typical of alveolar proteinosis, cholesterol clefts, and granulomas and fibrosis[149] Cough, dyspnea, and sputum production	Radiographs: findings simulating pulmonary alveolar proteinosis with diffuse GGO, and fibrosis with fine reticulonodular opacities[147,148] HRCT: "crazy-paving" pattern with GGO superimposed on interlobular septal thickening in a geographic distribution, fine reticulation or interstitial fibrosis, and traction bronchiectasis, and bronchiolectasis.[148,150] Centrilobular and perilymphatic nodules have also been reported, as have emphysema, subpleural blebs, and increased propensity toward developing pneumothorax[147,149]

never develop despite long-term high-level exposure.[102,105,108]

CBD and sarcoidosis may be clinically, histologically, and radiographically indistinguishable. In fact, one study showed that upon re-evaluation, 40% (34/80) of patients diagnosed with sarcoidosis actually had CBD.[109] Definitive diagnosis can be established through establishing evidence of immune sensitization to beryllium through beryllium-specific lymphocyte proliferation test performed on blood or BAL fluid and in vivo patch testing (known as BeS), which can distinguish CBD from sarcoidosis.[103,110]

Although the lung is the primary organ involved, there are a variety of extrapulmonic manifestations, including skin lesions, granulomatous hepatitis, hypercalcemia, and renal stones.[111] In addition, beryllium exposure is thought to be a risk factor for the development of lung carcinoma.[112]

Patients may remain asymptomatic or present with fever, anorexia, weight loss, dry cough, chest pain, dyspnea on exertion, fatigue, and night sweats. PFTs may show restrictive or obstructive patterns or evidence of abnormal gas exchange.[102,104] CBD may be self-limited or respond to steroids or progress to fibrosis and respiratory failure.[113,114]

CBD may be nearly radiographically indistinguishable from sarcoidosis (Box 4). During the early course of the disease, radiographs may be normal or show multiple small nodules and reticulation, typically in a mid and upper lung predominant distribution.[115,116] As the disease progresses, reticulation, honeycombing, and masslike lesions formed by coalescence of small nodules may be present.[116] Hilar and mediastinal lymphadenopathy may also be seen.[116] HRCT usually shows septal lines, bronchial wall thickening, and well-defined perilymphatic nodules.[115] Other findings include patchy GGO, honeycombing, bronchiectasis, and aggregate nodules forming pseudoplaques.[115] Hilar and mediastinal lymphadenopathy is less common than in sarcoidosis, present in only 25% to 32% of patients.[115] Eggshell calcification may be present as in silicosis or sarcoidosis.[117,118] Late in the disease, upper lobe or diffuse fibrosis may develop.[119] Overall, the constellation of findings may resemble those seen in HP.[115,120,121]

Hard Metal Disease

Hard metal disease (HMD), also known as hard metal pneumoconiosis, was previously called giant cell pneumonia (GIP) and classified as an interstitial lung disease. HMD is usually caused by inhalation of hard metals, alloys composed primarily of cobalt and tungsten carbide, which may contain other metals in small proportions.[122] Cobalt is thought to be the main contributor to pulmonary toxicity, because the disease has been documented in diamond polishers working with high-speed cobalt-diamond polishing disks that did not contain hard metal.[123] Hard metals are widely used in several industries because of their great strength, heat resistance, and resistance to oxidation.[122] Occupational exposure can occur in the aircraft, automobile, and electrical industries, in the production of cutting, drilling, and grinding tools, as well as in polishing.[122]

Histopathologically, HMD usually manifests as GIP, although desquamative interstitial pneumonia and UIP can occasionally be seen.[124,125] GIP is characterized by the presence of bizarre multinucleated giant cells (MGC), which have engulfed other host cells, often macrophages or neutrophils (cannibalistic MGCs).[125] Areas of fibroblastic foci mixed with mature collagen may be present, making it difficult to distinguish it from UIP.[125] In addition, interstitial paucicellular granulomata similar to those seen in HP may also be present, but more well-developed granulomata reminiscent of sarcoidosis are rarely detected.[125–127]

Analysis of BAL fluid typically reveals an increased number of cells, MGCs, and increased inflammatory cells and can avoid biopsy in the appropriate clinical and occupational setting.[128] Detection of tungsten and cobalt on scanning electron microscopy and energy-dispersive spectroscopy can be diagnostic and is helpful when light microscopy findings are inconclusive.

Reported radiographic findings include bilateral GGO, small nodules, and reticulation, often with lymphadenopathy and small cystic spaces in advanced disease.[2,93,129] The earliest findings seen on HRCT are those of constrictive bronchiolitis as manifested by mosaic attenuation with air trapping on expiratory imaging. Subsequently, small centrilobular nodules, bilateral GGO or consolidation, reticulation, and traction bronchiectasis can develop either without zonal predominance or with a lower lobe predominance (Fig. 12).[57,130,131] Honeycombing is a late

---

Box 4
Distinguishing features of chronic berylliosis and sarcoidosis

- Occupational history
- Beryllium sensitivity
- Extrathoracic manifestations are rare in berylliosis

Data from Lynch DA, Gamsu G, Ray CS, et al. Asbestos-related focal lung masses: manifestations on conventional and high-resolution CT scans. Radiology 1988;169(3):603–7; and Lynch DA. Beryllium-related diseases. In: De Vuyst P, Gevenois PA, editors. Imaging of occupational and environmental disorders of the chest. Berlin: Springer; 2006. p. 249–56.

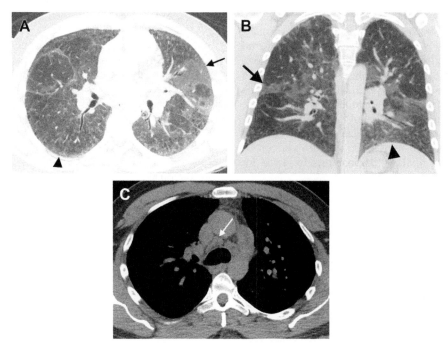

Fig. 12. Axial (*A*) and coronal CT (*B*) images in patient with HMD depicting both GGO (*black arrow*) and reticulation (*black arrowhead*). (*C*) Axial CT image of the same patient demonstrating mediastinal lymphadenopathy (*white arrow*).

finding, typically with a peripheral and basilar predominance.[57,131]

Occupational Asthma

Work-related asthma is an encompassing term that describes both work-exacerbated asthma and occupational asthma. Work-exacerbated asthma is pre-existing or concurrent asthma made worse by nonspecific vocational stimuli. In contrast, occupational asthma is asthma caused by exposure to airborne dusts, gases, vapors, or fumes in the workplace.

Occupational asthma is the most common form of occupational lung disease, responsible for 15% to 17% of new-onset asthma in adults.[132–135] Hundreds of inciting agents have been identified, of both high and low molecular weight, including animal and plant proteins, cleaning agents, reactive chemicals (isocyanates [also a cause of HP], anhydrides, reactive dyes glues), flour, and latex.[132] As a result, occupational asthma has been reported among several occupations ranging from agriculture, individuals exposed to cleaning products and spray paints, hairdressers, bakers, and nurses.[132] These lists are constantly growing as new agents and occupations are routinely being identified.[100]

There are 2 types of occupational asthma, immunologic and nonimmunologic, which can be distinguished by the presence or absence of a latency period. Immunologic occupational asthma is the result of an immunoglobulin E–mediated hypersensitivity reaction and can only develop after a latent period of exposure necessary to induce sensitization.[136] This type is incited by most high-molecular-weight and some low-molecular-weight compounds. Nonimmunologic occupational asthma, also known as irritant-induced asthma, occurs following exposure to very high levels of irritants and does not require a latent period.[137,138] The pathophysiology of nonimmunologic occupational asthma is not fully elucidated. However, it has been suggested that this type may result from direct injury to and desquamation of the bronchial epithelium.[139] This type is incited by some other low-molecular-weight compounds.

Radiographic features include hyperinflation and bronchial wall thickening with peribronchial cuffing. HRCT may demonstrate bronchial wall thickening, mosaic attenuation, expiratory air trapping, and small foci of atelectasis.

Newer Occupational Lung Diseases

In summary, occupational lung diseases encompass many pulmonary diseases caused by inhalation of dusts or chemical antigens in the workplace. Occupational lung diseases remain a large cause of morbidity and mortality, particularly in developing countries. Although radiography remains the initial imaging modality used in screening and evaluating symptomatic workers, HRCT has higher sensitivity and specificity, and low-dose HRCT may promise to be a viable screening option in the future. Despite imaging advances, a large proportion of the imaging findings seen in occupational lung diseases is nonspecific and a multidisciplinary approach with a focus on history of occupational exposure is essential for accurate diagnosis.

REFERENCES

1. Weston A. Work-related lung diseases. IARC Sci Publ 2011;163:387–405.

2. Chong S, Lee KS, Chung MJ, et al. Pneumoconiosis: comparison of imaging and pathologic findings. Radiographics 2006;26(1):59–77.

3. Hering KG, Jacobsen M, Bosch-Galetke E, et al. Further development of the International Pneumoconiosis Classification–from ILO 1980 to ILO 2000 and to ILO 2000/German Federal Republic version. Pneumologie 2003;57(10):576–84 [in German].

4. Henry DA. International Labor Office Classification System in the age of imaging: relevant or redundant. J Thorac Imaging 2002;17(3):179–88.

5. Remy-Jardin M, Degreef JM, Beuscart R, et al. Coal worker's pneumoconiosis: CT assessment in exposed workers and correlation with radiographic findings. Radiology 1990;177(2):363–71.

6. Akira M, Higashihara T, Yokoyama K, et al. Radiographic type p pneumoconiosis: high-resolution CT. Radiology 1989;171(1):117–23.

7. Gevenois PA, Pichot E, Dargent F, et al. Low grade coal worker's pneumoconiosis. Comparison of CT and chest radiography. Acta Radiol 1994;35(4):351–6.

8. Sun J, Weng D, Jin C, et al. The value of high resolution computed tomography in the diagnostics of small opacities and complications of silicosis in mine machinery manufacturing workers, compared to radiography. J Occup Health 2008;50(5):400–5.

9. Savranlar A, Altin R, Mahmutyazicioğlu K, et al. Comparison of chest radiography and high-resolution computed tomography findings in early and low-grade coal worker's pneumoconiosis. Eur J Radiol 2004;51(2):175–80.

10. Spyratos D, Chloros D, Haidich B, et al. Chest imaging and lung function impairment after long-term occupational exposure to low concentrations of chrysotile. Arch Environ Occup Health 2012; 67(2):84–90.

11. Muravov OI, Kaye WE, Lewin M, et al. The usefulness of computed tomography in detecting asbestos-related pleural abnormalities in people who had indeterminate chest radiographs: the Libby, MT, experience. Int J Hyg Environ Health 2005; 208(1–2):87–99.

12. Suganuma N, Kusaka Y, Hering KG, et al. Reliability of the proposed international classification of high-resolution computed tomography for occupational and environmental respiratory diseases. J Occup Health 2009;51(3):210–22.

13. Hering KG, Tuengerthal S, Kraus T. Standardized CT/HRCT-classification of the German Federal Republic for work and environmental related thoracic diseases. Radiologe 2004;44(5):500–11 [in German].

14. Carrillo MC, Alturkistany S, Roberts H, et al. Low-dose computed tomography (LDCT) in workers previously exposed to asbestos: detection of parenchymal lung disease. J Comput Assist Tomogr 2013; 37(4):626–30.

15. Remy-Jardin M, Sobaszek A, Duhamel A, et al. Asbestos-related pleuropulmonary diseases: evaluation with low-dose four-detector row spiral CT. Radiology 2004;233(1):182–90.

16. Bacchus L, Shah RD, Chung JH, et al. ACR appropriateness criteria review ACR Appropriateness Criteria® occupational lung diseases. J Thorac Imaging 2016;31(1):W1–3.

17. Pérez-Alonso A, Córdoba-Doña JA, Millares-Lorenzo JL, et al. Outbreak of silicosis in Spanish quartz conglomerate workers. Int J Occup Environ Health 2014;20(1):26–32.

18. Moitra S, Puri R, Paul D, et al. Global perspectives of emerging occupational and environmental lung diseases. Curr Opin Pulm Med 2015;21(2):114–20.

19. Kramer MR, Blanc PD, Fireman E, et al. Artificial stone silicosis [corrected]: disease resurgence among artificial stone workers. Chest 2012;142(2): 419–24.

20. Esswein EJ, Breitenstein M, Snawder J, et al. Occupational exposures to respirable crystalline silica during hydraulic fracturing. J Occup Environ Hyg 2013;10(7):347–56.

21. Bang KM, Attfield MD, Wood JM, et al. National trends in silicosis mortality in the United States, 1981-2004. Am J Ind Med 2008;51(9):633–9.

22. Akgun M, Mirici A, Ucar EY, et al. Silicosis in Turkish denim sandblasters. Occup Med (Lond) 2006; 56(8):554–8.

23. Laney AS, Weissman DN. The classic pneumoconioses: new epidemiological and laboratory observations. Clin Chest Med 2012;33(4):745–58.

24. Rom WN, Markowitz SB. Environmental and occupational medicine. Philadelphia (PA): Lippincott Williams & Wilkins; 2007.

25. Fujimura N. Pathology and pathophysiology of pneumoconiosis. Curr Opin Pulm Med 2000;6(2): 140–4.

26. Arakawa H, Honma K, Saito Y, et al. Pleural disease in silicosis: pleural thickening, effusion, and invagination. Radiology 2005;236(2):685–93.

27. Ooi CGC, Khong PL, Cheng RSY, et al. The relationship between mediastinal lymph node attenuation with parenchymal lung parameters in silicosis. Int J Tuberc Lung Dis 2003;7(12):1199–206.

28. Cox-Ganser JM, Burchfiel CM, Fekedulegn D, et al. Silicosis in lymph nodes: the canary in the miner? J Occup Environ Med 2009;51(2):164–9.

29. Ahuja J, Kanne JP, Meyer CA. Occupational lung disease. Semin Roentgenol 2015;50(1):40–51.

30. Ferreira AS, Moreira VB, Ricardo HMV, et al. Progressive massive fibrosis in silica-exposed workers. High-resolution computed tomography findings. J Bras Pneumol 2006;32(6):523–8.

31. Cowie RL, Hay M, Thomas RG. Association of silicosis, lung dysfunction, and emphysema in gold miners. Thorax 1993;48(7):746–9.

32. Bégin R, Filion R, Ostiguy G. Emphysema in silica- and asbestos-exposed workers seeking compensation. A CT scan study. Chest 1995; 108(3):647–55.

33. Gevenois PA, Sergent G, De Maertelaer V, et al. Micronodules and emphysema in coal mine dust or silica exposure: relation with lung function. Eur Respir J 1998;12(5):1020–4.

34. Arakawa H, Gevenois PA, Saito Y, et al. Silicosis: expiratory thin-section CT assessment of airway obstruction. Radiology 2005;236(3):1059–66.

35. Arakawa H, Fujimoto K, Honma K, et al. Progression from near-normal to end-stage lungs in chronic interstitial pneumonia related to silica exposure: long-term CT observations. AJR Am J Roentgenol 2008; 191(4):1040–5.

36. Arakawa H, Johkoh T, Honma K, et al. Chronic interstitial pneumonia in silicosis and mix-dust pneumoconiosis: its prevalence and comparison of CT findings with idiopathic pulmonary fibrosis. Chest 2007;131(6):1870–6.

37. Steenland K, Ward E. Silica: a lung carcinogen. CA Cancer J Clin 2014;64(1):63–9.

38. Matsumoto S, Miyake H, Oga M, et al. Diagnosis of lung cancer in a patient with pneumoconiosis and progressive massive fibrosis using MRI. Eur Radiol 1998;8(4):615–7.

39. O'Connell M, Kennedy M. Progressive massive fibrosis secondary to pulmonary silicosis appearance on F-18 fluorodeoxyglucose PET/CT. Clin Nucl Med 2004;29(11):754–5.

40. Dumontet C, Biron F, Vitrey D, et al. Acute silicosis due to inhalation of a domestic product. Am Rev Respir Dis 1991;143(4 Pt 1):880–2.

41. Goodman GB, Kaplan PD, Stachura I, et al. Acute silicosis responding to corticosteroid therapy. Chest 1992;101(2):366–70.

42. Marchiori E, Souza CA, Barbassa TG, et al. Silicoproteinosis: high-resolution CT findings in 13 patients. AJR Am J Roentgenol 2007;189(6): 1402–6.

43. Dee P, Suratt P, Winn W. The radiographic findings in acute silicosis. Radiology 1978;126(2):359–63.

44. Marchiori E, Ferreira A, Müller NL. Silicoproteinosis: high-resolution CT and histologic findings. J Thorac Imaging 2001;16(2):127–9.

45. Centers for Disease Control and Prevention (CDC). Advanced pneumoconiosis among working underground coal miners–Eastern Kentucky and Southwestern Virginia, 2006. MMWR Morb Mortal Wkly Rep 2007;56(26):652–5.

46. Centers for Disease Control and Prevention (CDC). Pneumoconiosis and advanced occupational lung disease among surface coal miners–16 states, 2010-2011. MMWR Morb Mortal Wkly Rep 2012; 61(23):431–4.

47. Laney AS, Attfield MD. Coal workers' pneumoconiosis and progressive massive fibrosis are increasingly more prevalent among workers in small underground coal mines in the United States. Occup Environ Med 2010;67(6):428–31.

48. Antao VCDS, Petsonk EL, Sokolow LZ, et al. Rapidly progressive coal workers' pneumoconiosis in the United States: geographic clustering and other factors. Occup Environ Med 2005;62(10):670–4.

49. Vallyathan V, Brower PS, Green FH, et al. Radiographic and pathologic correlation of coal workers' pneumoconiosis. Am J Respir Crit Care Med 1996; 154(3):741–8.

50. Hurley JF, Burns J, Copland L, et al. Coalworkers' simple pneumoconiosis and exposure to dust at 10 British coalmines. Br J Ind Med 1982;39(2):120–7.

51. Nagelschmidt G, Rivers D, King EJ, et al. Dust and collagen content of lungs of coal-workers with progressive massive fibrosis. Br J Ind Med 1963;20(3): 181–91.

52. Naeye RL, Dellinger WS. Coal workers' pneumoconiosis. Correlation of roentgenographic and postmortem findings. JAMA 1972;220(2):223–7.

53. Morgan WK, Lapp NL. Respiratory disease in coal miners. Am Rev Respir Dis 1976;113(4):531–59.

54. Young RC, Rachal RE, Carr PG, et al. Patterns of coal workers' pneumoconiosis in Appalachian former coal miners. J Natl Med Assoc 1992;84(1):41–8.

55. Laney AS, Petsonk EL. Small pneumoconiotic opacities on U.S. coal worker surveillance chest radiographs are not predominantly in the upper lung zones. Am J Ind Med 2012;55(9):793–8.

56. Green FH, Laqueur WA. Coal workers' pneumoconiosis. Pathol Annu 1980;15(Pt 2):333–410.

57. Akira M. Imaging of occupational and environmental lung diseases. Clin Chest Med 2008;29(1):117–31, vi.

58. Williams JL, Moller GA. Solitary mass in the lungs of coal miners. Am J Roentgenol Radium Ther Nucl Med 1973;117(4):765–70.

59. Hosgood HD, Chapman RS, Wei H, et al. Coal mining is associated with lung cancer risk in Xuanwei, China. Am J Ind Med 2012;55(1):5–10.

60. Taeger D, Pesch B, Kendzia B, et al. Lung cancer among coal miners, ore miners and quarrymen: smoking-adjusted risk estimates from the synergy pooled analysis of case-control studies. Scand J Work Environ Health 2015;41(5):467–77.

61. Santo Tomas LH. Emphysema and chronic obstructive pulmonary disease in coal miners. Curr Opin Pulm Med 2011;17(2):123–5.

62. Caplan A. Certain unusual radiological appearances in the chest of coal-miners suffering from rheumatoid arthritis. Thorax 1953;8(1):29–37.

63. Gough J, Rivers D, Seal RME. Pathological studies of modified pneumoconiosis in coal-miners with rheumatoid arthritis (Caplan's syndrome). Thorax 1955;10(1):9–18.

64. Petsonk EL, Rose C, Cohen R. Coal mine dust lung disease. New lessons from old exposure. Am J Respir Crit Care Med 2013;187(11):1178–85.

65. McConnochie K, Green FHY, Vallyathan V, et al. Interstitial fibrosis in coal workers—experience in Wales and West Virginia. Ann Occup Hyg 1988; 32(inhaled particles VI):553–60.

66. Thrumurthy SG, Kearney S, Sissons M, et al. Diffuse interlobular septal thickening in a coal miner. Thorax 2010;65(1):82–4.

67. Honma K, Abraham JL, Chiyotani K, et al. Proposed criteria for mixed-dust pneumoconiosis: definition, descriptions, and guidelines for pathologic diagnosis and clinical correlation. Hum Pathol 2004;35:1515–23.

68. Shida H, Chiyotani K, Honma K, et al. Radiologic and pathologic characteristics of mixed dust pneumoconiosis. Radiographics 1996;16(3):483–98.

69. Stayner L, Welch LS, Lemen R. The worldwide pandemic of asbestos-related diseases. Annu Rev Public Health 2013;34(1):205–16.

70. Peacock C, Copley SJ, Hansell DM. Asbestos-related benign pleural disease. Clin Radiol 2000; 55(6):422–32.

71. Lynch DA, Gamsu G, Aberle DR. Conventional and high resolution computed tomography in the diagnosis of asbestos-related diseases. Radiographics 1989;9(3):523–51.

72. Copley SJ, Wells AU, Rubens MB, et al. Functional consequences of pleural disease evaluated with chest radiography and CT. Radiology 2001; 220(1):237–43.

73. Kim JS, Lynch DA. Imaging of nonmalignant occupational lung disease. J Thorac Imaging 2002; 17(4):238.

74. Gevenois PA, De Maertelaer V, Madani A, et al. Asbestosis, pleural plaques and diffuse pleural thickening: three distinct benign responses to asbestos exposure. Eur Respir J 1998;11(5):1021–7.

75. Seaman DM, Meyer CA, Kanne JP. Occupational and environmental lung disease. Clin Chest Med 2015;36(2):249–68, viii–ix.

76. McLoud TC, Woods BO, Carrington CB, et al. Diffuse pleural thickening in an asbestos-exposed population: prevalence and causes. AJR Am J Roentgenol 1985;144(1):9–18.

77. Gaensler EA, Kaplan AI. Asbestos pleural effusion. Ann Intern Med 1971;74(2):178–91.

78. Epler GR, McLoud TC, Gaensler EA. Prevalence and incidence of benign asbestos pleural effusion in a working population. JAMA 1982;247(5):617–22.

79. Leung AN, Müller NL, Miller RR. CT in differential diagnosis of diffuse pleural disease. AJR Am J Roentgenol 1990;154(3):487–92.

80. Vathesatogkit P, Harkin TJ, Addrizzo-Harris DJ, et al. Clinical correlation of asbestos bodies in BAL fluid. Chest 2004;126(3):966–71.

81. Primack SL, Hartman TE, Hansell DM, et al. End-stage lung disease: CT findings in 61 patients. Radiology 1993;189(3):681–6.

82. Akira M, Yamamoto S, Inoue Y, et al. High-resolution CT of asbestosis and idiopathic pulmonary fibrosis. AJR Am J Roentgenol 2003;181(1):163–9.

83. Akira M, Yokoyama K, Yamamoto S, et al. Early asbestosis: evaluation with high-resolution CT. Radiology 1991;178(2):409–16.

84. Copley SJ, Wells AU, Sivakumaran P, et al. Asbestosis and idiopathic pulmonary fibrosis: comparison of thin-section CT features. Radiology 2003; 229(3):731–6.

85. Markowitz SB, Morabia A, Lilis R, et al. Clinical predictors of mortality from asbestosis in the North American Insulator Cohort, 1981 to 1991. Am J Respir Crit Care Med 1997;156(1):101–8.

86. Erren TC, Jacobsen M, Piekarski C. Synergy between asbestos and smoking on lung: cancer risks. Epidemiology 1999;10(4):405.

87. Markowitz SB, Levin SM, Miller A, et al. Asbestos, asbestosis, smoking, and lung cancer. New findings from the North American insulator cohort. Am J Respir Crit Care Med 2013;188(1):90–6.

88. Lynch DA, Gamsu G, Ray CS, et al. Asbestos-related focal lung masses: manifestations on conventional and high-resolution CT scans. Radiology 1988;169(3):603–7.

89. Batra P, Brown K, Hayashi K, et al. Rounded atelectasis. J Thorac Imaging 1996;11(3):187.

90. Gilkeson RC, Adler LP. Rounded atelectasis. Evaluation with (18)PET scan. Clin Positron Imaging 1998;1(4):229–32.

91. McAdams HP, Erasums JJ, Patz EF, et al. Evaluation of patients with round atelectasis using 2-[18F]-fluoro-2-deoxy-D-glucose PET. J Comput Assist Tomogr 1998;22(4):601–4.

92. Akira M. Uncommon pneumoconioses: CT and pathologic findings. Radiology 1995;197(2):403–9.

93. Kim KI, Kim CW, Lee MK, et al. Imaging of occupational lung disease. Radiographics 2001;21(6): 1371–91.

94. Kim KI, Choi SJ, Sohn HS, et al. High-resolution CT findings of Welders' pneumoconiosis. J Korean Radiol Soc 1996;34(3):367–71.

95. Han D, Goo JM, Im JG, et al. Thin-section CT findings of arc-welders' pneumoconiosis. Korean J Radiol 2000;1(2):79–83.

96. Akira M, Kozuka T, Yamamoto S, et al. Inhalational talc pneumoconiosis: radiographic and CT findings in 14 patients. AJR Am J Roentgenol 2007;188(2):326–33.

97. Marchiori E, Souza Júnior AS, Müller NL. Inhalational pulmonary talcosis: high-resolution CT findings in 3 patients. J Thorac Imaging 2004;19(1):41–4.

98. Padley SP, Adler BD, Staples CA, et al. Pulmonary talcosis: CT findings in three cases. Radiology 1993;186(1):125–7.

99. Ward S, Heyneman LE, Reittner P, et al. Talcosis associated with IV abuse of oral medications: CT findings. AJR Am J Roentgenol 2000;174(3):789–93.

100. Fishwick D. New occupational and environmental causes of asthma and extrinsic allergic alveolitis. Clin Chest Med 2012;33(4):605–16.

101. Vourlekis JS, Schwarz MI, Cherniack RM, et al. The effect of pulmonary fibrosis on survival in patients with hypersensitivity pneumonitis. Am J Med 2004;116(10):662–8.

102. Mayer AS, Hamzeh N, Maier LA. Sarcoidosis and chronic beryllium disease: similarities and differences. Semin Respir Crit Care Med 2014;35(3):316–29.

103. Kreiss K, Wasserman S, Mroz MM, et al. Beryllium disease screening in the ceramics industry. Blood lymphocyte test performance and exposure-disease relations. J Occup Med 1993;35(3):267–74.

104. Sprince NL, Kanarek DJ, Weber AL, et al. Reversible respiratory disease in beryllium workers. Am Rev Respir Dis 1978;117(6):1011–7.

105. Kreiss K, Mroz MM, Zhen B, et al. Epidemiology of beryllium sensitization and disease in nuclear workers. Am Rev Respir Dis 1993;148(4 Pt 1):985–91.

106. Fontenot AP, Newman LS, Kotzin BL. Chronic beryllium disease: T cell recognition of a metal presented by HLA-DP. Clin Immunol 2001;100(1):4–14.

107. Fontenot AP, Canavera SJ, Gharavi L, et al. Target organ localization of memory CD4(+) T cells in patients with chronic beryllium disease. J Clin Invest 2002;110(10):1473–82.

108. Richeldi L, Kreiss K, Mroz MM, et al. Interaction of genetic and exposure factors in the prevalence of berylliosis. Am J Ind Med 1997;32(4):337–40.

109. Müller-Quernheim J, Gaede KI, Fireman E, et al. Diagnoses of chronic beryllium disease within cohorts of sarcoidosis patients. Eur Respir J 2006;27(6):1190–5.

110. Santo Tomas LH. Beryllium hypersensitivity and chronic beryllium lung disease. Curr Opin Pulm Med 2009;15(2):165–9.

111. Stoeckle JD, Hardy HL, Weber AL. Chronic beryllium disease. Long-term follow-up of sixty cases and selective review of the literature. Am J Med 1969;46(4):545–61.

112. Steenland K, Ward E. Lung cancer incidence among patients with beryllium disease: a cohort mortality study. J Natl Cancer Inst 1991;83(19):1380–5.

113. Freiman DG, Hardy HL. Beryllium disease. The relation of pulmonary pathology to clinical course and prognosis based on a study of 130 cases from the U.S. beryllium case registry. Hum Pathol 1970;1(1):25–44.

114. Sood A, Beckett WS, Cullen MR. Variable response to long-term corticosteroid therapy in chronic beryllium disease. Chest 2004;126(6):2000–7.

115. Newman LS, Buschman DL, Newell JD, et al. Beryllium disease: assessment with CT. Radiology 1994;190(3):835–40.

116. Maier LA. Clinical approach to chronic beryllium disease and other nonpneumoconiotic interstitial lung diseases. J Thorac Imaging 2002;17(4):273–84.

117. Lynch DA. Beryllium-related diseases. In: De Vuyst P, Gevenois PA, editors. Imaging of occupational and environmental disorders of the chest. Berlin: Springer; 2006. p. 249–56.

118. Flors L, Domingo ML, Leiva-Salinas C, et al. Uncommon occupational lung diseases: high-resolution CT findings. AJR Am J Roentgenol 2010;194(1):W20–6.

119. Harris KM, McConnochie K, Adams H. The computed tomographic appearances in chronic berylliosis. Clin Radiol 1993;47(1):26–31.

120. Naccache J-M, Marchand-Adam S, Kambouchner M, et al. Ground-glass computed tomography pattern in chronic beryllium disease: pathologic substratum and evolution. J Comput Assist Tomogr 2003;27(4):496–500.

121. Daniloff EM, Lynch DA, Bartelson BB, et al. Observer variation and relationship of computed tomography to severity of beryllium disease. Am J Respir Crit Care Med 1997;155(6):2047–56.

122. Kelleher P, Pacheco K, Newman LS. Inorganic dust pneumonias: the metal-related parenchymal disorders. Environ Health Perspect 2000;108(Suppl 4):685–96.

123. Demedts M, Gheysens B, Nagels J, et al. Cobalt lung in diamond polishers. Am Rev Respir Dis 1984;130(1):130–5.

124. Coates EO, Watson JH. Pathology of the lung in tungsten carbide workers using light and electron microscopy. J Occup Med 1973;15(3):280–6.

125. Naqvi AH, Hunt A, Burnett BR, et al. Pathologic spectrum and lung dust burden in giant cell interstitial pneumonia (hard metal disease/cobalt pneumonitis): review of 100 cases. Arch Environ Occup Health 2008;63(2):51–70.

126. Newman LS. Metals that cause sarcoidosis. Semin Respir Infect 1998;13(3):212–20.

127. Satoh-Kamachi A, Munakata M, Kusaka Y, et al. A case of sarcoidosis that developed three years after the onset of hard metal asthma. Am J Ind Med 1998;33(4):379–83.

128. Forni A. Bronchoalveolar lavage in the diagnosis of hard metal disease. Sci Total Environ 1994; 150(1–3):69–76.

129. Pipavath SNJ, Godwin JD, Kanne JP. Occupational lung disease: a radiologic review. Semin Roentgenol 2010;45(1):43–52.

130. Dunlop P, Müller NL, Wilson J, et al. Hard metal lung disease: high resolution CT and histologic correlation of the initial findings and demonstration of interval improvement. J Thorac Imaging 2005;20(4):301–4.

131. Choi JW, Lee KS, Chung MP, et al. Giant cell interstitial pneumonia: high-resolution CT and pathologic findings in four adult patients. AJR Am J Roentgenol 2005;184(1):268–72.

132. Kogevinas M, Zock J-P, Jarvis D, et al. Exposure to substances in the workplace and new-onset asthma: an international prospective population-based study (ECRHS-II). Lancet 2007;370(9584): 336–41.

133. Blanc PD, Toren K. How much adult asthma can be attributed to occupational factors? Am J Med 1999; 107(6):580–7.

134. Balmes J, Becklake M, Blanc P, et al. American Thoracic Society Statement: occupational contribution to the burden of airway disease. Am J Respir Crit Care Med 2003;167(5):787–97.

135. Torén K, Blanc PD. Asthma caused by occupational exposures is common—a systematic analysis of estimates of the population-attributable fraction. BMC Pulm Med 2009;9(1):7.

136. Maestrelli P, Boschetto P, Fabbri LM, et al. Mechanisms of occupational asthma. J Allergy Clin Immunol 2009;123(3):531–42 [quiz: 543–4].

137. Tarlo SM, Broder I. Irritant-induced occupational asthma. Chest 1989;96(2):297–300.

138. Brooks SM, Weiss MA, Bernstein IL. Reactive airways dysfunction syndrome (RADS). Persistent asthma syndrome after high level irritant exposures. Chest 1985;88(3):376–84.

139. Lemière C, Malo JL, Boutet M. Reactive airways dysfunction syndrome due to chlorine: sequential bronchial biopsies and functional assessment. Eur Respir J 1997;10(1):241–4.

140. Lougheed MD, Roos JO, Waddell WR, et al. Desquamative interstitial pneumonitis and diffuse alveolar damage in textile workers. Potential role of mycotoxins. Chest 1995;108(5):1196–200.

141. Kern DG, Crausman RS, Durand KT, et al. Flock worker's lung: chronic interstitial lung disease in the nylon flocking industry. Ann Intern Med 1998; 129(4):261–72.

142. Weiland DA, Lynch DA, Jensen SP, et al. Thin-section CT findings in flock worker's lung, a work-related interstitial lung disease. Radiology 2003; 227(1):222–31.

143. Parmet AJ, Essen Von S. Rapidly progressive, fixed airway obstructive disease in popcorn workers: a new occupational pulmonary illness? J Occup Environ Med 2002;44(3):216.

144. Kreiss K, Gomaa A, Kullman G, et al. Clinical bronchiolitis obliterans in workers at a microwave-popcorn plant. N Engl J Med 2002;347(5):330–8.

145. Akpinar-Elci M, Travis WD, Lynch DA, et al. Bronchiolitis obliterans syndrome in popcorn production plant workers. Eur Respir J 2004;24(2): 298–302.

146. Larici AR, Mereu M, Franchi P. Imaging in occupational and environmental lung disease. Curr Opin Pulm Med 2014;20(2):205–11.

147. Homma T, Ueno T, Sekizawa K, et al. Interstitial pneumonia developed in a worker dealing with particles containing indium-tin oxide. J Occup Health 2003;45(3):137–9.

148. Chonan T, Taguchi O, Omae K. Interstitial pulmonary disorders in indium-processing workers. Eur Respir J 2007;29(2):317–24.

149. Cummings KJ, Nakano M, Omae K, et al. Indium lung disease. Chest 2012;141(6):1512–21.

150. Sauler M, Gulati M. Newly recognized occupational and environmental causes of chronic terminal airways and parenchymal lung disease. Clin Chest Med 2012;33(4):667–80.

Pulmonary Vasculitis
Spectrum of Imaging Appearances

Shamseldeen Mahmoud, MD[a], Subha Ghosh, MD[a], Carol Farver, MD[b], Jason Lempel, MD[a], Joseph Azok, MD[a], Rahul D. Renapurkar, MD[a,c],*

KEYWORDS

• Pulmonary vasculitis • Computed tomography • Imaging

KEY POINTS

- Vasculitis can be broadly classified into small vessel, medium vessel, and large vessel vasculitis, depending on the size of the predominantly affected vessel.
- Pulmonary involvement in vasculitis is uncommon, and is most commonly seen with small vessel vasculitis.
- Granulomatosis with polyangiitis is the most common anti-neutrophil cytoplasm antibody–associated vasculitis and can manifest with lung and airway findings.

 Video content accompanies this article at http://www.radiologic.theclinics.com.

INTRODUCTION

The term "vasculitis" refers to disorders characterized by inflammation of blood vessel walls.[1] "Vasculopathy," on the other hand, is generally used to describe any disease that affects the blood vessels[2] and can be used to describe various pathologies, such as degenerative, embolic, metabolic, and inflammatory processes. The term "vasculopathy" can be used in place of "vasculitis" before a diagnosis is pathologically proven. Primary vasculitides are rare disorders with an annual incidence of approximately 20 to 100 cases per million and a prevalence of 150 to 450 cases per million.[3–7]

All vasculitides are characterized by the presence of leukocytes and fibrinoid necrosis in the blood vessel wall, with consequent compromise of vessel integrity and hemorrhage. There is also narrowing of the blood vessel lumen, which leads to downstream tissue ischemia and necrosis. Depending on the size and type of blood vessel that is predominantly affected, the disorder can be classified as large, medium, or small vessel vasculitis (LVV, MVV, or SVV, respectively). Vasculitides can also be broadly classified as infectious or noninfectious. This article focuses on noninfectious vasculitis, conditions in which direct pathogens are not involved. However, in some cases of noninfectious vasculitis, pathogens are indirectly involved in the pathogenesis of the disease. For example, cryoglobulinemic vasculitis (CV) is caused by an autoimmune response initiated by hepatitis C virus infection.[8]

Clinical features of each disease depend on the site, size, and type of vessel involved and by the relative amounts of inflammation, vessel destruction, and tissue necrosis. Evaluation of patients with suspected vasculitis can be challenging, as these patients present with nonspecific signs and symptoms. The clinical presentation of systemic vasculitis mimics and overlaps that of infections, connective tissue diseases, and malignancies.

Disclosures: None.
[a] Section of Thoracic Imaging, Imaging Institute, Cleveland Clinic, 9500 Euclid Avenue, Cleveland, OH 44195, USA; [b] Department of Pathology, Cleveland Clinic, 9500 Euclid Avenue, Cleveland, OH 44195, USA; [c] Section of Cardiovascular Imaging, Imaging Institute, Cleveland Clinic, 9500 Euclid Avenue, Cleveland, OH 44195, USA
* Corresponding author. Thoracic Imaging, L10, Imaging Institute, Cleveland Clinic, Cleveland, OH 44195.
E-mail address: renapur@ccf.org

Radiol Clin N Am 54 (2016) 1097–1118
http://dx.doi.org/10.1016/j.rcl.2016.05.007
0033-8389/16/$ – see front matter © 2016 Elsevier Inc. All rights reserved.

Additionally, in patients with known vasculitis, clinical deterioration can pose a diagnostic challenge; this can be caused by disease activity, drug complication, superimposed infection, or a combination of all 3. Hence, the diagnosis and management of these cases requires a high index of suspicion, and the clinician often must rely on a multidisciplinary approach to reach a conclusion.

In this article, we review the classification and salient radiological findings of different vasculitides and discuss their common differential diagnoses. We also emphasize the clinicoradiologic approach to diagnosing pulmonary vasculitis.

HISTORICAL BACKGROUND AND EVOLUTION OF CLASSIFICATION SYSTEMS

Since the first classification system was proposed by Zeek[9] in 1952, the nomenclature and classification of pulmonary vasculitis have undergone several revisions and modifications. Most of the early revisions were built on these existing criteria and introduced additional parameters, such as size of the vessel, histologic features, and whether the vasculitis was primary or secondary. These modifications were fueled by better understanding of the disease processes and their respective molecular pathogenesis. Some of these early classification systems are summarized in **Table 1**.[9–14] Other efforts have included the American College of Rheumatology (ACR) criteria (1990)[15–20] and nomenclature from the Chapel Hill Consensus Conferences (CHCC) (1994 and 2012).[8,21]

Most clinical trials and studies have relied on the ACR-proposed criteria.[15–20] The CHCC 1994 nomenclature is also frequently used in studies. However, this nomenclature is often mistakenly used as a classification system, which was not the primary intention of the authors.[22] The authors' goals for the CHCC 1994 nomenclature were to reach a consensus on names for the most common forms of vasculitis and to construct a specific definition for each.[21] The CCHC 1994 nomenclature was revised in 2012, with the addition of new definitions and modification of existing definitions when appropriate (**Box 1**).[8] For example, the CHCC 2012 introduced definitions of dominant vessel size affected in each vasculitis category; however, it also stated that any size vessel could be affected in each category. Large vessels include the aorta and its major branches (with analogous veins). The medium-sized vessels include the main visceral arteries (eg, renal, hepatic, coronary, mesenteric) with their corresponding veins. The small vessels include the intraparenchymal arteries, arterioles, capillaries, venules, and veins.

Despite these efforts, the current definitions and classifications still do not meet all of the criteria of a reliable classification system, such as naturalness, exhaustiveness, and disjointedness, and these classification proposals remain a work in progress.[23] The most recent global endeavor, entitled "Diagnostic and Classification Criteria in Vasculitis Study (DCVAS)," plans to recruit patients with known vasculitis until December 2017.[24]

Table 1	
Summary of historical classification criteria for vasculitis	

Author(s)/Date	Key Points
Zeek,[9] 1952	First classification system; has served as the basis for all subsequent classification systems Five groups were described based on review of existing literature: hypersensitivity angiitis (variant of polyarteritis nodosa; also called leukocytoclastic vasculitis), granulomatous allergic angiitis (recognizable as eosinophilic granulomatosis with polyangiitis), rheumatic arteritis, periarteritis nodosa (polyarteritis nodosa), and temporal arteritis (giant cell arteritis)
Alarçon Segovia and Brown,[10] 1964	Granulomatosis with polyangiitis and immunoglobulin A vasculitis added
De Shazo,[11] 1975	A few subgroups added
Gilliam and Smiley,[12] 1976	Better appreciation of the degree of overlap in the size of vessels involved for vasculitis subgroups
Fauci et al,[13] 1978	Kawasaki disease added
Lie,[14] 1994	Subdivisions into primary or secondary forms, as well as predominant vessel size involvement

---

Box 1
Names for vasculitides adopted by the 2012 International Chapel Hill Consensus Conference on the nomenclature of vasculitides

Large vessel vasculitis
Takayasu arteritis
Giant cell arteritis

Medium vessel vasculitis
Polyarteritis nodosa
Kawasaki disease

Small vessel vasculitis
Antineutrophil cytoplasmic antibody-associated vasculitis
   Microscopic polyangiitis
   Granulomatosis with polyangiitis
   Eosinophilic granulomatosis with polyangiitis
Immune complex small vessel vasculitis
   Anti-glomerular basement membrane disease
   Cryoglobulinemic vasculitis
   Immunoglobulin A vasculitis
   Hypocomplementemic urticarial vasculitis (anti-C1q vasculitis)

Variable vessel vasculitis
Behçet disease
Cogan syndrome

Single-organ vasculitis
Cutaneous leukocytoclastic angiitis
Cutaneous arteritis
Primary central nervous system vasculitis
Isolated aortitis
Others

Vasculitis associated with systemic disease
Lupus vasculitis
Rheumatoid vasculitis
Sarcoid vasculitis
Others

Vasculitis associated with probable etiology
Hepatitis C virus–associated cryoglobulinemic vasculitis
Hepatitis B virus–associated vasculitis
Syphilis-associated aortitis
Drug-associated immune complex vasculitis
Drug-associated antineutrophil cytoplasmic antibody-associated vasculitis
Cancer-associated vasculitis
Others

From Jennette JC, Falk RJ, Bacon PA, et al. 2012 revised International Chapel Hill Consensus Conference nomenclature of vasculitides. Arthritis Rheum 2013;65(1):1–11; with permission.

PULMONARY VASCULITIS

Pulmonary vasculitis is usually a facet of systemic vasculitis, except in the rare instances in which it presents as an isolated or single-organ vasculitis.[25–27] The term "pulmonary vasculitis" can be used to describe inflammation of vessel walls (of any size) involving the lower respiratory tract; however, it commonly refers to vasculitides with increased involvement of the respiratory system, specifically the anti-neutrophil cytoplasm antibody (ANCA)-associated vasculitides. Lung involvement in systemic vasculitis can present via 3 major pathologic mechanisms:

1. Necrosis of pulmonary parenchyma with inflammatory cell infiltration,
2. Stenosis of the tracheobronchial tree as a result of inflammation, and
3. Pulmonary capillaritis resulting in diffuse alveolar hemorrhage (DAH).

Most vasculitides involve the capillaries; involvement of other vessels, such as large pulmonary and bronchial arteries and pulmonary veins, is relatively rare.[28] In most cases, pulmonary vasculitis is primary or idiopathic.

In our discussion, we use the most current nomenclature scheme from CHCC 2012 (see Box 1); using the size of the involved vessel to classify vasculitides allows us to systematically discuss clinical and imaging findings. Thoracic involvement is most common with LVV, such as Takayasu arteritis (TAK), Behçet disease, and with ANCA-associated SVV, such as granulomatosis with polyangiitis (GPA), eosinophilic GPA (EGPA), and microscopic polyangiitis (MPA).

Large Vessel Vasculitis

The 2 main diseases involving the large vessels are TAK and giant cell arteritis (GCA). CHCC 2012 defines LVV as vasculitis that involves the aorta and its major branches more often than other vasculitides; however, any size artery may be affected. This definition does not state that LVV predominantly affects large vessels, because the number of medium and small vessels affected is often greater than the number of involved large arteries.

Although both TAK and GCA are often characterized by granulomatous inflammation, there are some distinct differences between these 2 entities. TAK predominantly involves the aorta and its major branches, whereas GCA has a predilection for branches of the carotid and vertebral arteries and often involves the temporal arteries. Another major discriminator between TAK and GCA is the age of the patient; TAK almost exclusively occurs in patients younger than 40 years, whereas GCA is usually seen in patients older than 50 years and is often associated with polymyalgia rheumatica.[8]

Takayasu arteritis

Named after Dr Mikito Takayasu, an ophthalmologist from Japan, TAK is an LVV that predominantly affects the aorta and its branches.[29,30] It is also known as pulseless disease, occlusive thromboaortopathy, and Martorell syndrome.[31] Classically described in young women from Eastern Asia, it is now increasingly recognized worldwide and in both sexes, although the clinical manifestations may vary among populations. The female-to-male ratio appears to decline from Eastern Asia toward the West.[29] TAK is a chronic inflammatory disease of unknown etiology and is characterized by granulomatous inflammation of medium and large arteries.[32] This vessel inflammation leads to wall thickening, fibrotic stenosis, and vessel thrombosis. Typically, the vessel involvement is segmental and patchy.[29]

The classic presentation of TAK is characterized by 3 stages: (1) a systemic or prepulseless phase, (2) a vascular phase, and (3) a quiescent "burnt-out" phase. This classic sequential presentation is uncommon in clinical practice, however. In the vascular phase, vascular medial necrosis may lead to aneurysm formation.[33] Constitutional symptoms, low-grade fever, and arthralgias are often early manifestations of disease, whereas characteristic late symptoms include variable pulses of the extremities and claudication of affected vascular territories. Renovascular hypertension, pulmonary hypertension, and ischemia of affected organs also can occur.[28] Although symptomatic pulmonary involvement is relatively uncommon in TAK, studies have shown involvement of the large and medium pulmonary arteries in roughly 50% of patients with this condition.[34] Progressive medial defects of the arteries and ingrowth of granulation tissues with intimal thickening and subendothelial smooth muscle proliferation can lead to stenosis and occlusion of pulmonary arteries and pulmonary hypertension. The ACR criteria for the diagnosis of TAK include

- Disease onset at age 40 years or younger
- Claudication of an extremity
- Decreased brachial artery pulse
- Greater than 10 mm Hg difference in systolic blood pressure between arms
- A bruit over the subclavian arteries or the aorta
- Arteriographic evidence of narrowing or occlusion of the entire aorta, its primary

branches, or large arteries in the proximal upper or lower extremities

The presence of 3 or more of these 6 criteria is considered diagnostic, with a sensitivity of 90.5% and a specificity of 97.8%.[15]

Chest radiography is often performed as a baseline investigation, but this modality is nonspecific and the results are often unremarkable. Superior mediastinal widening may sometimes be seen because of ascending aortic or proximal aortic branch vessel dilation. In suspected early disease, vascular ultrasound can be considered, although this modality does not allow comprehensive vascular evaluation.

Cross-sectional imaging techniques, such as computed tomography (CT) and magnetic resonance (MR) imaging allow detailed evaluation of the aortic and pulmonary vasculature and are the tests of choice for TAK. Both CT and MR imaging offer excellent depiction of smooth wall thickening of the involved aorta, which may show enhancement (Fig. 1).[35,36] MR imaging is preferred over CT as it avoids radiation exposure in this younger patient population.[35] The wall enhancement is related to disease activity and can be shown with both CT and MR imaging.[37] In later stages, areas of luminal irregularities, stenosis, and occlusion are seen; there may be associated aneurysmal dilation. Imaging also may show changes in pulmonary arteries that are not suspected clinically. Often seen are areas of segmental and subsegmental arterial stenoses or occlusions (see Fig. 1).[38] As with the aorta, there is associated wall thickening that may enhance. In late stages, wall calcification and stenosis/occlusion can develop; unilateral occlusion of pulmonary arteries has been described.[38] In chronic cases, collaterals can develop depending on the location and severity of stenotic lesions. For instance, bronchial artery collateralization has been noted with pulmonary artery involvement. With pulmonary involvement, the lungs may show focal areas of oligemia and hypoperfusion secondary to stenotic lesions (see Fig. 1, Video 1).[39] Nonspecific peripheral fibrotic changes also have been reported.[28]

Angiography in TAK demonstrates changes similar to those seen with CT or MR imaging, although assessment of the vessel wall with this modality is suboptimal.[38] PET with 18-fluorodeoxyglucose (FDG) can show FDG uptake in actively inflamed vessels[40]; this information can be valuable for monitoring disease activity.

Giant cell arteritis

GCA is the most common systemic vasculitis in individuals aged older than 50 years, with an incidence of 3.5 per 100,000 per year.[41] The incidence is higher in Scandinavian populations, and women are affected approximately 2 to 6 times more often than men.[42] Familial clustering has been reported.[43] After the age of 50, the incidence of GCA increases with age.[42] GCA is an LVV or MVV predominantly involving the aorta and its branches, most notably the temporal artery. The frequency of aortic aneurysm in patients with GCA is higher than in the general population, although the exact risk is not known. In one

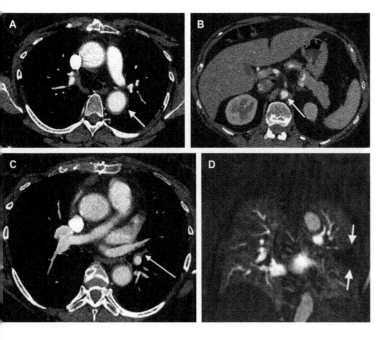

Fig. 1. A 38-year-old woman with TAK. (*A* and *B*) Contrast-enhanced CT of the chest shows circumferential thickening of walls of the descending thoracic and upper abdominal aorta (*arrows*). The aorta is narrowed in caliber at the level of the origin of the celiac axis (*arrow*). (*C*) CT image at the level of left atrial appendage shows occlusion of the lingular branch of the left pulmonary artery (*arrow*). (*D*) Corresponding coronal MR angiography image in the same patient shows a perfusion defect in the lingula secondary to occlusion of the lingular branch (*arrows*).

retrospective study, patients with GCA were 17 times more likely to develop thoracic aortic aneurysms and 2.4 times more likely to develop abdominal aortic aneurysms than age-matched and sex-matched patients without GCA. The thoracic aorta is more often involved than the abdominal aorta. Aortic dissection also can occur, with studies showing an incidence of up to 6%.[44] The exact etiology of this condition is unknown, although both humoral and cellular immune mechanisms and infection may be involved.[45,46] GCA is characterized by granulomatous inflammation of blood vessel walls, as observed in 60% of temporal artery biopsy specimens. The intracranial vessels are uncommonly affected. Histologically, the lesions are indistinguishable from those of TAK.[47]

The clinical presentation of GCA tends to be subacute. Constitutional symptoms, such as fever, are seen in approximately half of patients with GCA. Other characteristic findings include headaches, transient vision loss, polymyalgia rheumatic, and jaw claudication. The ACR criteria for diagnosis of GCA include the following:

- Age of onset at 50 years or older (symptoms or signs beginning at ≥50 years)
- New headache (new onset of or new type of localized pain in the head)
- Temporal artery abnormality (tenderness or decreased pulsation)
- Erythrocyte sedimentation rate greater than or equal to 50 mm/h (by the Westergren method)
- Abnormal artery biopsy (vasculitis characterized by predominance of mononuclear cell infiltrates or granulomatous inflammation with multinucleated giant cells)

The presence of 3 or more criteria yields a sensitivity of 93.5% and a specificity of 91.2% for GCA diagnosis.[48]

Respiratory involvement with GCA is uncommon. Upper respiratory tract symptoms, such as nonproductive cough, have been reported in approximately 10% of patients. Thus, GCA should be considered in elderly patients with new-onset throat pain, hoarseness, or cough without any identifiable cause.[49]

The imaging findings of GCA are identical to those of TAK on CT and MR imaging, with findings of arterial wall thickening, stenosis, and thrombosis (**Fig. 2**).[50] In one study of 40 patients with biopsy-proven GCA, evidence of LVV was found on CT angiography in two-thirds of patients, and aortic dilation was found in 15% of patients at the time of diagnosis. In this study, 47% of patients showed involvement of the brachiocephalic trunk, whereas the subclavian arteries and femoral arteries were affected in 42% and 30% of patients, respectively.[51]

Lung findings are often nonspecific, although basal reticulation and bullae have been reported on CT. Pulmonary artery involvement is much less common with GCA than with TAK.[50] FDG-PET can be useful in monitoring disease activity by showing areas of increased uptake in aorta and branch vessels, similar to the use of PET in TAK.[52] However, diagnosing GCA with FDG-PET can be challenging, due to concomitant presence of atherosclerosis in this older patient population.[47] In one study, the utility of FDG-PET in predicting relapses based on previous FDG uptake scoring was found to be limited.[52]

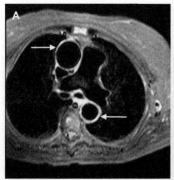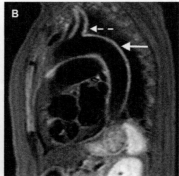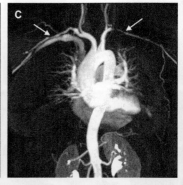

Fig. 2. A 70-year-old man with GCA. (*A*). Axial T2 short-tau inversion recovery (STIR) images of the chest show circumferential thickening of the ascending and descending thoracic aorta (*arrows*). The ascending thoracic aorta is ectatic in caliber. (*B*). Sagittal T2 STIR image shows thickening of the aortic arch branch vessels (*broken arrow*) and the descending thoracic aorta (*arrow*). (*C*). Coronal MR angiography image shows narrowing of the aortic branch vessels. Specifically, both subclavian and axillary arteries are diffusely involved, left greater than right (*arrows*).

Medium Vessel Vasculitis

MVV predominantly affects the medium arteries, such as the main visceral arteries and their branches.[22] The 2 main vasculitides affecting medium-sized vessels are polyarteritis nodosa (PAN) and Kawasaki disease. PAN is a necrotizing-type arteritis that can affect medium or small arteries. An important feature is the absence of ANCA, which is a valuable diagnostic finding to distinguish PAN from MPA.[53] Because MVV does not affect capillaries, PAN does not cause glomerulonephritis or alveolar hemorrhage. Isolated case reports of classic PAN affecting bronchial or bronchiolar arteries have been reported as a cause of lung hemorrhage.[28] However, lung involvement is extremely rare in PAN, and its presence argues against a diagnosis of PAN.[54] Kawasaki disease, formerly called mucocutaneous lymph node syndrome, predominantly affects medium and small arteries. The coronary arteries are often involved, and the aorta and large arteries may be involved.[8] Kawasaki disease usually occurs in children younger than 5 years.[55]

Small Vessel Vasculitis

Larger vessels (>1 mm in external diameter) have elastic laminae in their walls and are referred to as elastic arteries. Smaller vessels (>100 μm to 1 mm in diameter) have a smooth muscle medial layer and are referred to as muscular arteries.[56] The exact point at which pulmonary vessels should be called "small vessels" is debatable, and the definition may be influenced by the spatial resolution of the CT scan. The morphologic differentiation between elastic and muscular arteries is an oversimplification and underestimates the gradual transition of the vessel wall composition from elastic to muscular arteries and further to arterioles.[56] Because of this lack of clear-cut distinction between large and small vessels, true classification of small-vessel disease (such as vasculitis) is arbitrary but generally refers to preferential involvement of smaller pulmonary vessels, such as small intraparenchymal arteries, arterioles, capillaries, and venules. With SVV, medium-sized arterioles and veins also can be affected.

SVV is subdivided into ANCA-associated vasculitis (AAV) and immune complex SVV. These subcategories were introduced in CHCC 2012 to reflect the pathognomonic significance of ANCA positivity in the diagnosis of AAV. The primary difference in these 2 groups is the small number or lack of immune deposits in vessel walls in patients with AAV in contrast to moderate to marked vessel wall immune deposition in patients with immune complex SVV.

Anti-Neutrophil Cytoplasm Antibody–Associated Vasculitis

ANCAs can be distinguished into 2 major categories by indirect immunofluorescence microscopy: cytoplasmic (c-ANCA) and perinuclear (p-ANCA). On enzyme-linked immunosorbent assay testing, c-ANCA nearly always reacts with proteinase 3 (ANCA-PR3), whereas p-ANCA reacts with myeloperoxidase (ANCA-MPO). Patients with AAV also can be ANCA negative. It is unclear whether patients with ANCA-negative AAV have ANCA that cannot be detected with current methods, have ANCA with an as-yet-undiscovered specificity, or have AAV with a pathogenic mechanism that does not involve ANCA at all.[8]

Granulomatosis with polyangiitis

Formerly referred to as Wegener granulomatosis, this entity was renamed GPA in 2011 to better highlight the disease process.[57] GPA, the most common AAV, is most frequently seen in adults but has been reported across all age groups.[58] Both sexes are equally affected. Pathologically, GPA is characterized by necrotizing vasculitis of the small and medium vessels, granulomatous inflammation, and areas of geographic parenchymal necrosis (**Figs. 3** and **4**).[59] Additional histologic variants, such as bronchocentric, eosinophilic, capillaritis, and organizing pneumonia-like patterns also have been described.[60]

The classic clinical triad includes upper airway diseases (such as sinusitis, otitis, ulcerations, and subglottic and bronchial stenosis), lower respiratory tract involvement (clinically presenting as hemoptysis, chest pain, dyspnea, and cough), and glomerulonephritis (presenting as hematuria and azotemia), although patients may not have

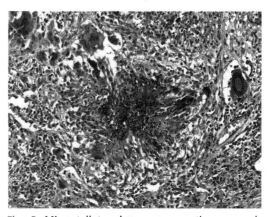

Fig. 3. Microstellate abscess representing an early lesion of GPA (hematoxylin-eosin; original magnification ×200).

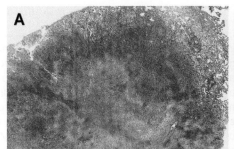
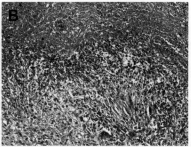

Fig. 4. (A) A necrotizing granulomatous nodule of GPA involving the lung (hematoxylin-eosin; original magnification ×12.5). (B) The palisading histiocytic border of the GPA nodule with characteristic neutrophilic necrosis and giant cells (hematoxylin-eosin; original magnification ×200).

all of these symptoms at the initial presentation. Although 80% to 90% of patients ultimately develop renal disease, as few as 40% have renal involvement at first presentation.[61–63] A total of 85% to 90% of patients with active systemic disease test positive for cytoplasmic ANCA or anti-PR3 compared with only 60% to 65% of patients with organ-limited disease and 40% of patients in remission.[64–67] Advanced age, poor renal function, alveolar hemorrhage, and anti-PR3 positivity are correlated with poor outcomes.[68,69]

Several attempts have been made over the years to define diagnostic criteria for GPA and allow this entity to be distinguished from MPA; these attempts have included the ACR criteria, CCHC nomenclature, and a European Medicines Agency algorithm. However, gaps still exist, and GPA and MPA often cannot be reliably distinguished. Limited expressions of GPA can occur, particularly cases limited to the upper respiratory system or the eye.[70] These patients are included in the GPA category if they are ANCA positive and have clinical and pathologic evidence supporting GPA respiratory tract involvement despite the lack of identifiable evidence of systemic vasculitis.[8]

Imaging findings Chest radiography is often performed as a baseline investigation. Unlike with other vasculitides, chest radiography can be abnormal with GPA and may show findings such as cavitary and noncavitary pulmonary nodules diffuse lung opacities.[71,72] CT is the imaging test of choice, allowing detailed assessment of disease.

Lung findings The most common findings with GPA are nodules and masses of varying sizes, occurring in approximately 90% of patients at the initial presentation (Fig. 5).[73] In one study, nodules or masses were multiple in 85% of patients, and bilateral disease was seen in 67% of patients.[73] Additionally, subpleural nodules were

present in 89% of patients and peribronchovascular nodules were seen in 41% of patients.[73] The nodules can coalesce into larger masses with diameters greater than 10 cm.[35] These nodules frequently cavitate (30%–50%), reflecting their necrotic nature.[73,74] Larger nodules (>2 cm) often cavitate; the cavity is usually thick walled.[35] Secondary infection of the nodules is not uncommon and may be seen as a new air-fluid level in the nodule or mass.[73,74] A CT halo sign manifesting as an area of ground-glass opacity (GGO) surrounding a nodule is seen in 15% of cases (see Fig. 5).[75] A reverse halo appearance also may be seen, likely reflecting an organizing pneumonia reaction in the periphery of focal hemorrhage.[76] There may be evidence of an artery leading into a nodule or mass, known as the feeding vessel sign. Noncavitary nodules may demonstrate central low attenuation on contrast-enhanced CT, likely due to necrosis.[35] GGO and consolidation are other common findings, seen in 25% to 50% of patients (Fig. 6).[73,77] These opacities can be diffuse or patchy and represent either active vasculitis or DAH secondary to capillaritis.[73,77] Centrilobular nodules with tree-in-bud distribution can be seen in approximately 10% of patients; these are likely secondary to inflammatory bronchiolitis (Fig. 7).[73]

Tracheobronchial involvement Airway abnormalities are also common with GPA, with segmental and subsegmental bronchial thickening seen in approximately 70% of patients. Larger airways are involved in 30% of patients. The distribution may be diffuse or focal but classically involves the subglottic region (Fig. 8).[76] Concentric wall thickening leading to airway stenosis is seen in approximately 15% of patients (see Fig. 8; Fig. 9). Postobstructive atelectasis also may occur. Bronchiectasis is less common, occurring in approximately 10% to 20% of patients.[77]

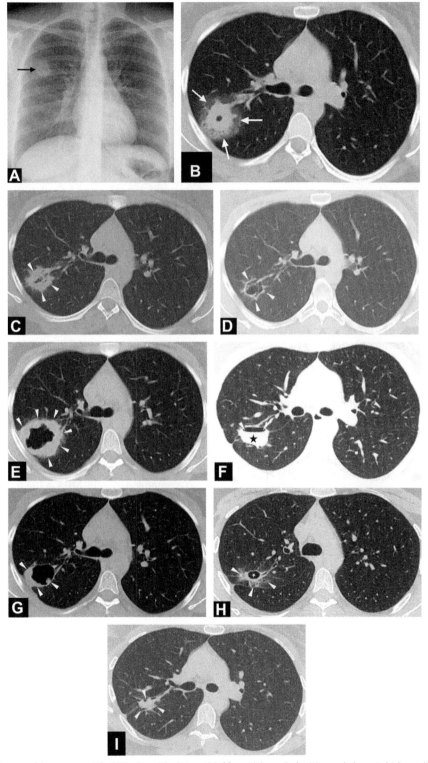

Fig. 5. A 35-year-old woman with GPA, sinusitis, interstitial keratitis, episcleritis, and chronic kidney disease. (A–I). Chest radiographs and serial CT scans showing serial fluctuations of a GPA nodule. (A) Frontal chest radiograph in May 2005 shows a thick-walled cavitary lesion in the right upper lobe (arrow). (B) Axial CT image of the chest shows a 2.6-cm nodule with a small central cavity (arrows). There is surrounding ground-glass halo (CT halo sign). Further images (C–I) show waxing and waning appearance of nodular disease (arrowheads). The nodule shows interval increase in June 2005 (C), decreases in July 2005 (D), followed by recurrent increase in size and wall thickness in October 2005 (E). Subsequently, there is interval development of air-fluid level (asterisk) in December 2005 (F), followed by decrease in size (G) and (H) in 2006, leaving a scar in 2007 after treatment (I).

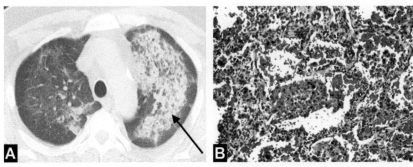

Fig. 6. (*A*) A 45-year-old man with GPA. Axial CT image shows diffuse ground-glass and consolidative opacities, worse on the left, compatible with DAH (*arrow*). (*B*) Capillaritis/DAH in a surgical lung biopsy in another patient with GPA (hematoxylin-eosin; original magnification ×100).

Less frequent findings include interlobular septal thickening, enlarged mediastinal and hilar lymph nodes, and pleural effusions.[72,74] Diffuse lung disease has been reported in patients with AAV, although this finding is more common with MPA than with GPA. Usual interstitial pneumonia pattern is most commonly seen.[78]

Role of imaging in follow-up Patients with GPA are treated with immunosuppressive therapy, and CT is often performed to assess their response to treatment. In patients treated with immunosuppressive therapy, 50% of the nodules and masses resolve without scarring, and 40% diminish significantly with residual scar (see **Fig. 6**). GGO usually resolves.[73,79–81] Lesions involving the airways usually improve with treatment.[69] Relapses are fairly common with GPA; in these cases, CT findings may be similar to or different from the initial presentation.[73]

One of the key features of GPA is the rapid temporal evolution of these nodules and airspace opacities. The other diagnostic challenge is identification of disease relapse. Both relapses and infection are common and may often coexist. In such situations, imaging findings may show a significant overlap; often, a clear-cut differentiation is not possible. For example, centrilobular nodular disease is considered a typical sign of small airway infection but has also been described with GPA (see **Fig. 7**).

Microscopic polyangiitis

MPA is an SVV without any granulomatous inflammation. Characterized by pulmonary capillaritis and glomerulonephritis, MPA is the most common cause of pulmonary-renal syndrome.[82] As with GPA, it is seen across all age groups.[58] Usually, patients present with renal manifestations, with more than 90% of patients demonstrating rapidly progressive glomerulonephritis (RPGN) at presentation. Before the development of RPGN, there is often a protracted prodromal phase of intense constitutional symptoms, such as fever and weight

---

Differential diagnosis:
GPA is often a diagnostic challenge, with imaging findings mimicking those of several other disease processes

Nodular disease (subpleural)

- Infections such as septic thromboembolic disease
- Neoplasms (eg, hematogenous metastases, lymphoma)

Airspace disease

- Several pneumonias (bacterial, fungal)
- Neoplasms, such as adenocarcinoma

Airway disease

- Postintubation stenosis
- Granulomatous disease
- Amyloidosis
- Relapsing polychondritis

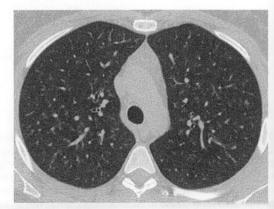

Fig. 7. A 51-year-old woman with GPA showing diffuse centrilobular nodules bilaterally.

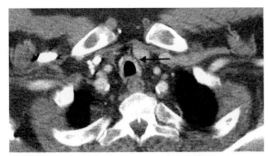

Fig. 8. A 47-year-old woman with GPA with airway involvement. Axial CT image shows circumferential subglottic tracheal wall thickening (*arrow*).

loss. Pulmonary involvement is less common, seen in 30% of patients.[83–85] Gastrointestinal involvement is relatively common; other organs also may be involved, including the peripheral nervous system, in addition to the skin and joints.[84]

The underlying pathology of MPA consists of focal segmental necrotizing vasculitis and mixed inflammatory infiltrates with no evidence of granuloma formation.[8] As noted earlier, it can be difficult or sometimes impossible to differentiate between MPA and GPA; the only difference on pathology specimens is the absence of granuloma formation with MPA, and this finding may be missed because of sampling errors. Among patients with MPA, 50% to 75% are positive for p-ANCA and 35% to 65% are positive for anti-MPO.[83] In 10% to 15% of patients, the c-ANCA is positive.

Imaging findings Radiologically, MPA manifests as DAH secondary to pulmonary capillaritis. On chest radiography, this is seen as diffuse airspace opacities. CT is more definitive in the assessment of lung disease, showing patchy or diffuse GGO

and consolidation (**Fig. 10**). Typically, DAH is more extensive in the perihilar regions, sparing the lung apices and the costophrenic regions.[86] The presence of dense consolidation reflects alveolar blood filling.[86] Interstitial fibrosis and diffuse lung disease may be seen in some patients; this finding is more common with MPA than with GPA.[78] The extent to which repeated alveolar hemorrhage contributes to fibrosis is unclear.

Differential diagnosis
• GPA
• Goodpasture syndrome (presence of anti–glomerular basement membrane [GBM] antibodies)
• Systemic lupus erythematosus (SLE) immune deposits seen on surgical biopsy

Eosinophilic granulomatosis with polyangiitis
Formerly called Churg-Strauss syndrome, EGPA consists of a triad of eosinophilia, asthma, and necrotizing vasculitis. The mean age of onset is relatively late, typically in the third decade. Although this condition is a vasculitic process involving the small and medium vessels, the vasculitis is initially not apparent. The characteristic feature of EGPA is lung involvement, with virtually all patients having asthma.[87] Cardiac involvement is seen in roughly 13% to 47% of patients and is responsible for half of the deaths attributable to EGPA.[60,88] Pulmonary hemorrhage and glomerulonephritis are less commonly seen in EGPA than in the other types of AAV.[89–92] Involvement of other organs, such as the skin, kidneys, gastrointestinal system, and neurologic

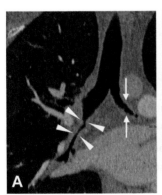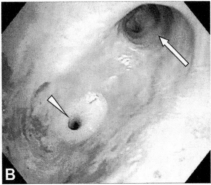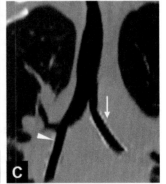

Fig. 9. A 20-year-old woman with GPA. (*A*) Coronal multiplanar reformatted CT image shows long segment stenosis of the bronchus intermedius (*arrowheads*) and moderate stenosis of the left mainstem bronchus (*arrows*). (*B*) Flexible bronchoscopy was done that shows the severe stenosis of the bronchus intermedius (*arrowhead*). The *arrow* points to the origin of the left mainstem bronchus (*C*) Coronal multiplanar reformatted CT image after stenting shows stents in the bronchus intermedius (*arrowhead*) and left mainstem bronchus (*arrow*) with improved patency.

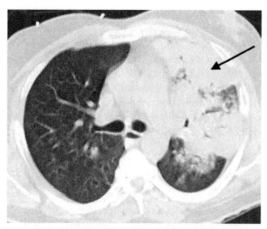

Fig. 10. A 51-year-old man with history of MPA and hemoptysis. Axial CT image shows multifocal consolidation in the left lung compatible with pulmonary hemorrhage (*arrow*).

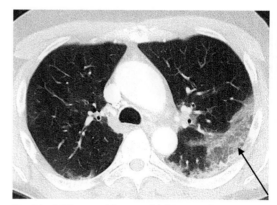

Fig. 11. A 52-year-old man with history of EGPA. Axial CT image shows peripheral GGO in both lungs, largest on the left (*arrow*).

system, is common, with peripheral neuropathy seen in 75% of patients.[89] Histologically, necrotizing SVV is seen along with eosinophilic inflammatory infiltrate and necrotizing granulomas.[93] Lung biopsy may show a spectrum of changes, such as asthmatic bronchitis, eosinophilic pneumonia, extravascular granulomas, or vasculitis.[93] Among patients with EGPA active disease, 35% to 75% will have positive p-ANCA (or anti-MPO).[94] Additionally, 10% of patients will have positive c-ANCA.

Clinically, EGPA has a triphasic presentation. Patients initially present with atopy-sinusitis-asthma, followed by eosinophilia; this is followed by the vasculitis phase. These phases may not be seen in the same order in all patients. The asthmatic phase usually precedes the vasculitic phase by 8 to 10 years.[89] During the second phase, peripheral blood eosinophilia is universal and is associated with eosinophilic infiltration of various organs; the lungs are involved in 40% of patients.[91] The vasculitic phase may be heralded by constitutional symptoms such as fever and weight loss.

Imaging findings An abnormal chest radiograph is noted in approximately 72% of cases of EGPA. Findings include patchy transient consolidation, nonsegmental opacities that may be nodular and cavitary, and diffuse linear opacities.[95–97] These abnormalities tend to be peripheral with no zonal predominance. Pleural effusions are seen in approximately one-third of patients.[91] The most common finding on CT is bilateral areas of GGO or consolidation.[98] These areas are usually lower lobe predominant and peripheral in distribution, although peribronchial and random distribution patterns can also be seen (**Figs. 11** and **12B**).[98,99]

Interlobular septal thickening is seen in approximately half of patients; this thickening may be secondary to cardiogenic pulmonary edema, eosinophilic septal infiltration, or mild fibrosis.[100] Airway involvement is an equally important manifestation of EGPA; in one study, small nodules were seen in 63% of patients, and bronchial wall thickening was seen in 53% of patients (see **Fig. 12**).[100] Small centrilobular nodules correlate to eosinophilic bronchiolitis and peribronchiolar vasculitis, and bronchial wall thickening correlates to eosinophilic and lymphocytic infiltration of the airway wall.[100] Typically, patients with lung opacities respond better to therapy than those with predominant airway involvement.[100] Other imaging findings include enlarged peripheral vessels, noncavitary pulmonary nodules, and linear opacities.[98,99] Unilateral or bilateral pleural effusions are seen in 50% of patients and may be secondary to cardiomyopathy or eosinophilic pleuritis.[101]

Differential diagnosis[60]

Airspace disease
- Simple eosinophilic pneumonia (Loeffler syndrome)
- Chronic eosinophilic pneumonia
- Organizing pneumonia

Airway-predominant pattern
- Subacute hypersensitivity pneumonitis
- MPA
- SLE
- Metastatic calcification
- Infectious bronchiolitis
- Respiratory bronchiolitis

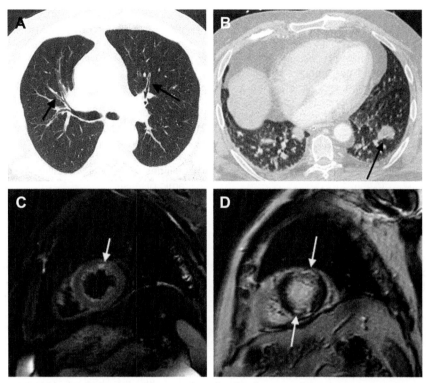

Fig. 12. A 54-year-old man with EGPA and lung and cardiac involvement. (*A*) Axial CT image shows diffuse bronchial wall thickening (*arrows*). (*B*) CT image on the same patient 3 months later shows a new peribronchial nodular opacity in the left lower lobe (*arrow*); these fleeting opacities are typical of EGPA. (*C*) T2 STIR short-axis Cardiac MR image shows increased signal in the distal anterior wall suggestive of myocardial inflammation (*arrow*). (*D*) Corresponding phase-sensitive inversion recovery (PSIR) delayed enhancement MR short-axis image shows mid-myocardial enhancement in the apical anterior and inferior segments consistent with myocarditis (*arrows*).

Immune Complex SVV

Immune complex SVV is characterized by immunoglobulin and/or complement deposition in the visible walls of the small vessels. Glomerulonephritis is frequently seen.

Antiglomerular basement membrane disease

Anti-GBM disease is characterized by circulating antibodies directed against an antigen intrinsic to the GBM.[102] The diagnosis is made via renal biopsy by demonstrating characteristic linear deposition of immunoglobulin G (IgG) on GBM with immunofluorescence microscopy. Goodpasture syndrome is a term used for patients with glomerulonephritis and pulmonary hemorrhage irrespective of the cause, whereas Goodpasture disease is a term used for patients with glomerulonephritis and pulmonary hemorrhage with anti-GBM antibodies. This condition is usually seen in older children and young adults. Glomerulonephritis with basement membrane necrosis and crescent formation occurs as a result of renal involvement, with patients presenting with symptoms of acute

renal failure.[103] Pulmonary involvement is less common, occurring in approximately 40% to 60% of patients; the typical imaging features of DAH are seen in these patients. Rarely, isolated pulmonary involvement can occur.[104] On surgical biopsy, alveolar hemorrhage with pulmonary capillaritis is seen.[104] The variable nature of pulmonary involvement may be the result of restricted access of the circulating antibodies to the alveolar basement membrane; underlying pulmonary injury such as that caused by smoking or cocaine inhalation may predispose patients to pulmonary disease.[105,106]

Immunoglobulin A vasculitis

Formerly known as Henoch-Schönlein purpura, IgA vasculitis is characterized by IgA1-dominant immune deposits within the small vessels. Predominantly a disease of childhood, this condition usually involves the skin, gastrointestinal tract (commonly the small bowel), and joints. Additionally, glomerulonephritis indistinguishable from IgA nephropathy can occur. Symptomatic IgA vasculitis is frequently preceded by an upper respiratory tract or gastrointestinal infection; unidentified chemical and infectious triggers have been postulated as being involved in its pathogenesis.[107] The disease is usually self-limiting in children, although end-stage renal disease can occur in adults.[108] Pulmonary involvement is rare in children but more common in adults. Deposition of anti-GBM IgA to the alveolar basement membrane leads to alveolitis and capillaritis in these patients, and imaging findings related to DAH are seen.[109] Pleural effusions also are seen in cases of IgA vasculitis.[110] Interstitial fibrosis with the usual interstitial pneumonia pattern has also been reported.[109]

Hypocomplementemic urticarial vasculitis

As the name implies, hypocomplementemic urticarial vasculitis or anti-C1 Q vasculitis is an SVV associated with urticaria and hypocomplementemia. Characteristic features include glomerulonephritis, arthritis, ocular inflammation, and obstructive pulmonary disease. The presence of anti-C1q antibodies is a distinctive feature of this condition.[111,112] Pulmonary involvement is reported in 20% of patients, with chronic obstructive pulmonary disease and asthma reported as the most common manifestations. Vasculitis of the lung tissue leads to neutrophilic release of elastase and the development of emphysematous lung disease. Smoking contributes to this disease by helping neutrophil recruitment.[113] Panacinar emphysema with a basilar predominance is commonly seen[113] (**Fig. 13**); pleural effusions have also been reported.[114]

Cryoglobulinemic vasculitis

CV is characterized by deposition of cryoglobulin immune complexes on small vessel walls and subsequent complex activation.[8] A wide variety of organs, such as the kidneys (glomeruli), joints, peripheral joints, and skin are affected in patients with this condition. Pulmonary involvement is

rare, occurring in approximately 2% of patients. The imaging features are related to DAH; the prognosis for patients with this condition is poor.[60,115]

Variable Vessel Vasculitis

As the name implies, variable vessel vasculitis can affect vessels of any size and any type, including arteries, capillaries, and veins. The 2 diseases included in this category are Behçet disease and Cogan syndrome. These are considered primary vasculitides rather than vasculitis associated with systemic disease.[8]

Behçet disease

Behçet disease vasculitis is characterized by recurrent oral and/or genital aphthous ulcers with associated inflammatory lesions involving the skin and the articular, ocular, gastrointestinal, and/or central nervous system. The pathogenesis of this condition is unknown, although a variety of inciting factors, such as genetic and infectious agents, have been postulated.[116] Predominantly seen in young men, this disease is commonly seen along the geographic ancient Silk Road (extending from Eastern Asia to the Mediterranean), with the highest frequency seen in Turkey.[117] Most of the symptoms are attributed to vasculitis, with the classic lesion demonstrating necrotizing leukocytoclastic obliterative perivasculitis and venous thrombosis with lymphocytic infiltration of vessels, irrespective of their size. Thoracic involvement has been reported in 1% to 8% of patients.[118] The common types of vascular lesions are arterial and venous occlusions, aneurysms, and varices.[119] Clinical manifestations include hemoptysis, chest pain, cough, and dyspnea.[120] Behçet disease is the most common cause of pulmonary artery aneurysm.[35] Typically, these aneurysms are fusiform or saccular, often multiple and bilateral, and located in the main or

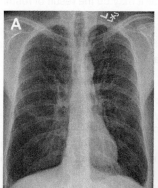 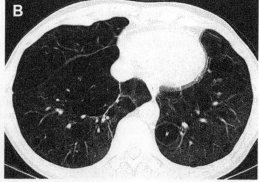

Fig. 13. A 60-year-old man with hypocomplementemic urticarial vasculitis. (*A*) Frontal chest radiograph shows diffuse hyperinflation of the lungs. (*B*) Axial CT image shows lower lobe predominant emphysematous changes in both lungs.

lower lobar pulmonary arteries.[121] Other findings can include superior vena cava (SVC) obstruction, thromboembolism, and pulmonary infarction.[122]

On chest radiographs, hemorrhage or infarction appears as wedge-shaped airspace consolidation in 56% of patients.[123] Infarcts may appear as subpleural nodular opacities in 33% to 83% of patients and may cavitate. These nodules can resolve or rupture in the pleural space.[123,124] Pulmonary artery aneurysms, which can appear as a lung nodule or mass on radiography, may cause hilar enlargement if located centrally. Mediastinal widening may be seen and may be secondary to SVC thrombosis.[123] CT and MR imaging provide better characterization of pulmonary arterial aneurysms. Typically, these aneurysms are partially or totally thrombosed; thrombus formation is an in situ process.[35] There is often wall thickening, likely secondary to periadventitial hematoma (Fig. 14).[121] If untreated, these aneurysms have a high risk of rupture, with a mortality of 30% within 2 years.[120] Perianeurysmal consolidation or GGO is a sign suggestive of impending rupture.[60,121] Approximately 75% of the aneurysms resolve after immunosuppressive therapy, and CT can be used for follow-up in such cases.[125] Pulmonary calcification and thromboemboli can also be seen in patients with Behçet disease, as can thrombosis of the SVC and other mediastinal veins (see Fig. 14).[123] Intracardiac thrombi and endomyocardial fibrosis may occur; these entities are better evaluated with MR imaging.[121] Thickening of the vessel wall can be seen in the aorta and SVC.[35] Mosaic attenuation can occur in the lung due to small vessel disease, and pleural effusions can be seen due to SVC obstruction (chylous) or secondary to pulmonary infarction.[126]

Hughes-Stovin syndrome is an extremely rare disorder characterized by multiple pulmonary aneurysms and deep venous thrombosis without oral or genital ulceration.[127] Typically, large vessels, such as pulmonary and bronchial arteries, are affected, along with systemic veins. This condition is considered to be a limited form or "forme fruste" of Behçet disease, and the imaging findings are similar between the 2.[128]

Vasculitis Associated with Systemic Disease

Vasculitis can be associated with or caused by a systemic disease. Common disease associations include collagen vascular diseases such as rheumatoid arthritis (RA), SLE, and systemic sclerosis, as well as sarcoidosis and relapsing polychondritis. This type of vasculitis is considered a secondary vasculitis, although the differentiation between primary and secondary causes is becoming increasingly blurry as more etiologies for secondary vasculitis are discovered.[8] Typically, small vessels are involved, with evidence of capillaritis.[129]

Although pulmonary involvement in RA is very common,[130] pulmonary vasculitis constitutes a rare finding. RA-related pulmonary vasculitis may be confined to the lungs (isolated vasculitis) or, more commonly, may present in the context of a systemic vasculitic process.[131] Chest radiograph in these patients may be normal or may show signs of pulmonary hypertension and interstitial opacities.[132] Focal and diffuse alveolar opacities and DAH can be seen.[131]

SLE is the most common collagen vascular disease with lung and pleural involvement; lung and pleural involvement is seen in approximately 50% to 70% of patients with SLE.[60] Pulmonary vasculitis is relatively rare but can cause nodules in SLE (Fig. 15); these may cavitate.[133] Asymptomatic DAH is a common autopsy finding in patients with SLE.[134] Although acute DAH is uncommon, it is seen more commonly in SLE

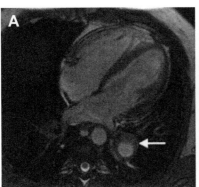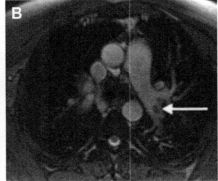

Fig. 14. A 25-year-old-man with Behçet disease. (*A*) Steady-state free precession (SSFP) image shows an aneurysm of the left lower lobar pulmonary artery (*arrow*) with associated wall thickening. (*B*) SSFP image at a higher level shows a pulmonary embolism in the left pulmonary artery (*arrow*).

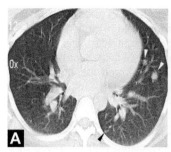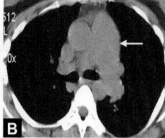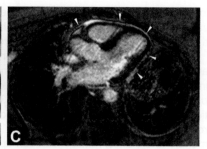

Fig. 15. A 45-year-old woman with SLE. (*A*) Axial CT of the chest shows few scattered pulmonary nodules in the lingula (*white arrowheads*) and left lower lobe (*black arrowhead*). (*B*) Axial image in mediastinal window setting shows dilated pulmonary artery, which can be indicative of pulmonary hypertension (*arrow*). (*C*) PSIR delayed enhancement MR 3-chambered image on the same patient demonstrates circumferential contrast enhancement of the pericardium compatible with pericardial inflammation (*arrowheads*).

than in other connective tissue diseases. In one series, DAH was present in 3.7% of hospital admissions for SLE, and 80% of those patients had pulmonary capillaritis.[135] Patients with DAH often have concomitant findings of congestive heart failure, aspiration, infection, or lupus pneumonitis.[135,136] Chest radiography and CT in these patients show typical findings of patchy or diffuse GGO and consolidation.[137] Necrotizing vasculitis of the arterioles may manifest as centrilobular nodules on CT; this vasculitis may contribute to pulmonary hypertension, which can be seen in 0.5% to 14% of patients with SLE (see **Fig. 15**).[138] Other contributing factors to pulmonary hypertension include recurrent thromboembolism, bland vasculopathy, interstitial fibrosis, and hypoxia.[139] Pulmonary infarcts with cavitating consolidation also can be seen.[128]

Vasculitis Associated with Probable Etiology

These vasculitides include conditions in which there is a probable association with a specific etiology. In such cases, a prefix should be added to specify the underlying disease; for example,

hepatitis C virus–associated CV.[8] Drugs such as propylthiouracil, gemcitabine, diphenylhydantoin, transretinoic acid, and crack cocaine may cause pulmonary capillaritis and lead to DAH (**Fig. 16**).[60] Foreign materials, such as talc, often used as fillers for tablets and capsules, can elicit a perivascular giant cell reaction centered on arterioles; this is seen as diffuse centrilobular nodules on CT.

DIAGNOSTIC CLUES

Although there is no algorithm that can comprehensively allow the systematic classification of vasculitis, radiologists must be aware of clinicoradiologic clues that can help to narrow the differential diagnoses. A diagnostic approach using imaging manifestations correlated with laboratory and clinical findings is shown in **Fig. 17**.

SUMMARY

The diagnosis of vasculitis is often challenging and is complicated by nonspecific and protean clinical findings. Laboratory tests can help to narrow the

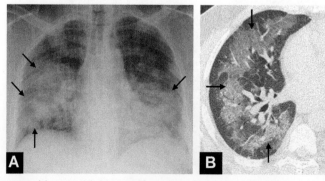

Fig. 16. A 51-year-old man with history of cocaine abuse presented to the emergency department with hemoptysis. (*A*) Chest radiograph and (*B*) CT images show diffuse consolidation and groundglass opacities (*arrows*) in both lungs, compatible with DAH; this was thought to be secondary to crack cocaine.

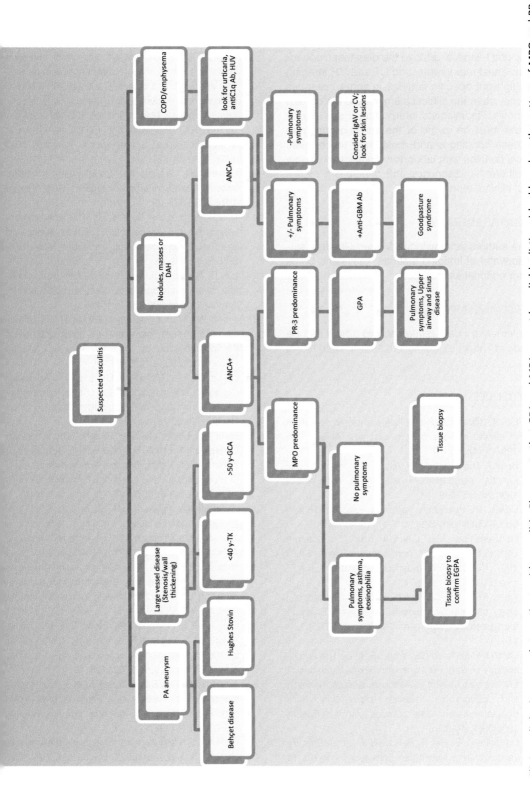

Fig. 17. Clinicoradiologic approach to patients with vasculitis. Please note that GPA and MPA cannot be reliably distinguished based on the pattern of MPO and PR-3 predominance. With EGPA, MPO, and PR-3 positivity is variable, although MPO-ANCA is slightly more common. COPD, chronic obstructive pulmonary disease.

differential diagnoses, although these results show a degree of overlap with other vasculitides and with other disease processes. The unpredictable nature of these disorders, with their potential for flares and relapses, adds to the diagnostic conundrum. Chest radiography and CT and MR imaging can highlight specific findings in some instances that may steer the clinical team toward the correct diagnosis. Radiologists interpreting these examinations must be aware of the imaging spectrum for these conditions and must learn to correlate clinical findings with laboratory findings to narrow the differential diagnoses and generate a meaningful clinical report.

ACKNOWLEDGMENTS

The authors acknowledge Megan Griffiths, scientific writer of Imaging Institute, Cleveland Clinic for her editorial assistance.

SUPPLEMENTARY DATA

Supplementary data related to this article can be found at http://dx.doi.org/10.1016/j.rcl.2016.05.007.

REFERENCES

1. Lie JT. Classification and histopathologic spectrum of central nervous system vasculitis. Neurol Clin 1997;15(4):805–19.
2. Berlit P. The spectrum of vasculopathies in the differential diagnosis of vasculitis. Semin Neurol 1994;14(4):370–9.
3. Brown KK. Pulmonary vasculitis. Proc Am Thorac Soc 2006;3(1):48–57.
4. Gonzalez-Gay MA, Garcia-Porrua C. Systemic vasculitis in adults in northwestern Spain, 1988-1997. Clinical and epidemiologic aspects. Medicine (Baltimore) 1999;78(5):292–308.
5. Watts RA, Lane SE, Bentham G, et al. Epidemiology of systemic vasculitis: a ten-year study in the United Kingdom. Arthritis Rheum 2000;43(2):414–9.
6. Cotch MF, Hoffman GS, Yerg DE, et al. The epidemiology of Wegener's granulomatosis. Estimates of the five-year period prevalence, annual mortality, and geographic disease distribution from population-based data sources. Arthritis Rheum 1996;39(1):87–92.
7. Haugeberg G, Bie R, Bendvold A, et al. Primary vasculitis in a Norwegian community hospital: a retrospective study. Clin Rheumatol 1998;17(5):364–8.
8. Jennette JC, Falk RJ, Bacon PA, et al. 2012 revised International Chapel Hill Consensus Conference nomenclature of vasculitides. Arthritis Rheum 2013;65(1):1–11.
9. Zeek PM. Periarteritis nodosa; a critical review. Am J Clin Pathol 1952;22(8):777–90.
10. Alarcon Segovia D, Brown AL Jr. Classification and etiologic aspects of necrotizing angiitides: an analytic approach to a confused subject with a critical review of the evidence for hypersensitivity in polyarteritis nodosa. Mayo Clin Proc 1964;39:205–22.
11. deShazo RD. The spectrum of systemic vasculitis: a classification to aid diagnosis. Postgrad Med 1975;58(4):78–82.
12. Gilliam JN, Smiley JD. Cutaneous necrotizing vasculitis and related disorders. Ann Allergy 1976;37(5):328–39.
13. Fauci AS, Haynes B, Katz P. The spectrum of vasculitis: clinical, pathologic, immunologic and therapeutic considerations. Ann Intern Med 1978;89(5 Pt 1):660–76.
14. Lie JT. Nomenclature and classification of vasculitis: plus ca change, plus c'est la meme chose. Arthritis Rheum 1994;37(2):181–6.
15. Arend WP, Michel BA, Bloch DA, et al. The American College of Rheumatology 1990 criteria for the classification of Takayasu arteritis. Arthritis Rheum 1990;33(8):1129–34.
16. Leavitt RY, Fauci AS, Bloch DA, et al. The American College of Rheumatology 1990 criteria for the classification of Wegener's granulomatosis. Arthritis Rheum 1990;33(8):1101–7.
17. Masi AT, Hunder GG, Lie JT, et al. The American College of Rheumatology 1990 criteria for the classification of Churg-Strauss syndrome (allergic granulomatosis and angiitis). Arthritis Rheum 1990;33(8):1094–100.
18. Lightfoot RW Jr, Michel BA, Bloch DA, et al. The American College of Rheumatology 1990 criteria for the classification of polyarteritis nodosa. Arthritis Rheum 1990;33(8):1088–93.
19. Mills JA, Michel BA, Bloch DA, et al. The American College of Rheumatology 1990 criteria for the classification of Henoch-Schonlein purpura. Arthritis Rheum 1990;33(8):1114–21.
20. Calabrese LH, Michel BA, Bloch DA, et al. The American College of Rheumatology 1990 criteria for the classification of hypersensitivity vasculitis. Arthritis Rheum 1990;33(8):1108–13.
21. Jennette JC, Falk RJ, Andrassy K, et al. Nomenclature of systemic vasculitides. Proposal of an international consensus conference. Arthritis Rheum 1994;37(2):187–92.
22. Waller R, Ahmed A, Patel I, et al. Update on the classification of vasculitis. Best Pract Res Clin Rheumatol 2013;27(1):3–17.
23. Grateau G, Hentgen V, Stojanovic KS, et al. How should we approach classification of autoinflammatory diseases? Nat Rev Rheumatol 2013;9(10):624–9.

24. Craven A, Robson J, Ponte C, et al. ACR/EULAR-endorsed study to develop Diagnostic and Classification Criteria for Vasculitis (DCVAS). Clin Exp Nephrol 2013;17(5):619–21.

25. Brugiere O, Mal H, Sleiman C, et al. Isolated pulmonary arteries involvement in a patient with Takayasu's arteritis. Eur Respir J 1998;11(3): 767–70.

26. Riancho-Zarrabeitia L, Zurbano F, Gomez-Roman J, et al. Isolated pulmonary vasculitis: case report and literature review. Semin Arthritis Rheum 2015;44(5):514–7.

27. Masuda S, Ishii T, Asuwa N, et al. Isolated pulmonary giant cell vasculitis. Pathol Res Pract 1994; 190(11):1095–100.

28. Dellaripa PF, Fischer A, Flaherty KR, editors. Pulmonary manifestations of rheumatic disease: a comprehensive guide. New York: Springer-Verlag; 2014.

29. Johnston SL, Lock RJ, Gompels MM. Takayasu arteritis: a review. J Clin Pathol 2002;55(7):481–6.

30. Sugiyama K, Ijiri S, Tagawa S, et al. Takayasu disease on the centenary of its discovery. Jpn J Ophthalmol 2009;53(2):81–91.

31. Lupi-Herrera E, Sanchez-Torres G, Marcushamer J, et al. Takayasu's arteritis. Clinical study of 107 cases. Am Heart J 1977;93(1):94–103.

32. Ishikawa K. Diagnostic approach and proposed criteria for the clinical diagnosis of Takayasu's arteriopathy. J Am Coll Cardiol 1988;12(4):964–72.

33. Numano F, Okawara M, Inomata H, et al. Takayasu's arteritis. Lancet 2000;356(9234):1023–5.

34. Sharma S, Kamalakar T, Rajani M, et al. The incidence and patterns of pulmonary artery involvement in Takayasu's arteritis. Clin Radiol 1990; 42(3):177–81.

35. Castañer E, Alguersuari A, Gallardo X, et al. When to suspect pulmonary vasculitis: radiologic and clinical clues. Radiographics 2010;30(1):33–53.

36. Yamada I, Numano F, Suzuki S. Takayasu arteritis: evaluation with MR imaging. Radiology 1993; 188(1):89–94.

37. Park JH, Chung JW, Im JG, et al. Takayasu arteritis: evaluation of mural changes in the aorta and pulmonary artery with CT angiography. Radiology 1995;196(1):89–93.

38. Matsunaga N, Hayashi K, Sakamoto I, et al. Takayasu arteritis: protean radiologic manifestations and diagnosis. Radiographics 1997;17(3):579–94.

39. Leavitt RY, Fauci AS. Pulmonary vasculitis. Am Rev Respir Dis 1986;134(1):149–66.

40. Meller J, Strutz F, Siefker U, et al. Early diagnosis and follow-up of aortitis with [(18)F]FDG PET and MRI. Eur J Nucl Med Mol Imaging 2003;30(5):730–6.

41. Ness T, Bley TA, Schmidt WA, et al. The diagnosis and treatment of giant cell arteritis. Dtsch Arztebl Int 2013;110(21):376–85.

42. Gonzalez-Gay MA, Miranda-Filloy JA, Lopez-Diaz MJ, et al. Giant cell arteritis in northwestern Spain: a 25-year epidemiologic study. Medicine (Baltimore) 2007;86(2):61–8.

43. Salvarani C, Gabriel SE, O'Fallon WM, et al. The incidence of giant cell arteritis in Olmsted County, Minnesota: apparent fluctuations in a cyclic pattern. Ann Intern Med 1995;123(3):192–4.

44. Gonzalez-Gay MA, Garcia-Porrua C, Piñeiro A, et al. Aortic aneurysm and dissection in patients with biopsy-proven giant cell arteritis from northwestern Spain: a population-based study. Medicine (Baltimore) 2004;83(6):335–41.

45. Gilden D, White T, Khmeleva N, et al. Prevalence and distribution of VZV in temporal arteries of patients with giant cell arteritis. Neurology 2015; 84(19):1948–55.

46. Papaioannou CC, Gupta RC, Hunder GG, et al. Circulating immune complexes in giant cell arteritis and polymyalgia rheumatica. Arthritis Rheum 1980; 23(9):1021–5.

47. Tatò F, Hoffmann U. Giant cell arteritis: a systemic vascular disease. Vasc Med 2008;13(2):127–40 [Erratum appears in Vasc Med 2008;13(3):299].

48. Hunder GG, Bloch DA, Michel BA, et al. The American College of Rheumatology 1990 criteria for the classification of giant cell arteritis. Arthritis Rheum 1990;33(8):1122–8.

49. Larson TS, Hall S, Hepper NG, et al. Respiratory tract symptoms as a clue to giant cell arteritis. Ann Intern Med 1984;101(5):594–7.

50. Marten K, Schnyder P, Schirg E, et al. Pattern-based differential diagnosis in pulmonary vasculitis using volumetric CT. AJR Am J Roentgenol 2005; 184(3):720–33.

51. Prieto-González S, Arguis P, García-Martínez A, et al. Large vessel involvement in biopsy-proven giant cell arteritis: prospective study in 40 newly diagnosed patients using CT angiography. Ann Rheum Dis 2012;71(7):1170–6.

52. Blockmans D, de Ceuninck L, Vanderschueren S, et al. Repetitive 18F-fluorodeoxyglucose positron emission tomography in giant cell arteritis: a prospective study of 35 patients. Arthritis Rheum 2006;55(1):131–7.

53. Guillevin L, Lhote F, Amouroux J, et al. Antineutrophil cytoplasmic antibodies, abnormal angiograms and pathological findings in polyarteritis nodosa and Churg-Strauss syndrome: indications for the classification of vasculitides of the polyarteritis Nodosa Group. Br J Rheumatol 1996; 35(10):958–64.

54. Frankel SK, Sullivan EJ, Brown KK. Vasculitis: Wegener granulomatosis, Churg-Strauss syndrome, microscopic polyangiitis, polyarteritis nodosa, and Takayasu arteritis. Crit Care Clin 2002;18(4): 855–79.

55. Jennette JC, Falk RJ. Nosology of primary vasculitis. Curr Opin Rheumatol 2007;19(1):10–6.

56. Hansell DM. Small-vessel diseases of the lung: CT-pathologic correlates. Radiology 2002;225(3):639–53.

57. Falk RJ, Gross WL, Guillevin L, et al, American College of Rheumatology, American Society of Nephrology, European League Against Rheumatism. Granulomatosis with polyangiitis (Wegener's): an alternative name for Wegener's granulomatosis. Arthritis Rheum 2011;63(4):863–4.

58. Seo P, Stone JH. The antineutrophil cytoplasmic antibody-associated vasculitides. Am J Med 2004;117(1):39–50.

59. Travis WD, Hoffman GS, Leavitt RY, et al. Surgical pathology of the lung in Wegener's granulomatosis. Review of 87 open lung biopsies from 67 patients. Am J Surg Pathol 1991;15(4):315–33.

60. Chung MP, Yi CA, Lee HY, et al. Imaging of pulmonary vasculitis. Radiology 2010;255(2):322–41.

61. Anderson G, Coles ET, Crane M, et al. Wegener's granuloma. A series of 265 British cases seen between 1975 and 1985. A report by a subcommittee of the British Thoracic Society Research Committee. Q J Med 1992;83(302):427–38.

62. Fauci AS, Haynes BF, Katz P, et al. Wegener's granulomatosis: prospective clinical and therapeutic experience with 85 patients for 21 years. Ann Intern Med 1983;98(1):76–85.

63. Hoffman GS, Kerr GS, Leavitt RY, et al. Wegener granulomatosis: an analysis of 158 patients. Ann Intern Med 1992;116(6):488–98.

64. Tervaert JW, van der Woude FJ, Fauci AS, et al. Association between active Wegener's granulomatosis and anticytoplasmic antibodies. Arch Intern Med 1989;149(11):2461–5.

65. Kerr GS, Fleisher TA, Hallahan CW, et al. Limited prognostic value of changes in antineutrophil cytoplasmic antibody titer in patients with Wegener's granulomatosis. Arthritis Rheum 1993;36(3):365–71.

66. Boomsma MM, Stegeman CA, van der Leij MJ, et al. Prediction of relapses in Wegener's granulomatosis by measurement of antineutrophil cytoplasmic antibody levels: a prospective study. Arthritis Rheum 2000;43(9):2025–33.

67. Nolle B, Specks U, Ludemann J, et al. Anticytoplasmic autoantibodies: their immunodiagnostic value in Wegener granulomatosis. Ann Intern Med 1989;111(1):28–40.

68. Bligny D, Mahr A, Toumelin PL, et al. Predicting mortality in systemic Wegener's granulomatosis: a survival analysis based on 93 patients. Arthritis Rheum 2004;51(1):83–91.

69. Neumann I, Kain R, Regele H, et al. Histological and clinical predictors of early and late renal outcome in ANCA-associated vasculitis. Nephrol Dial Transplant 2005;20(1):96–104.

70. Holle JU, Gross WL, Holl-Ulrich K, et al. Prospective long-term follow-up of patients with localised Wegener's granulomatosis: does it occur as persistent disease stage? Ann Rheum Dis 2010;69(11):1934–9.

71. Reuter M, Schnabel A, Wesner F, et al. Pulmonary Wegener's granulomatosis: correlation between high-resolution CT findings and clinical scoring of disease activity. Chest 1998;114(2):500–6.

72. Cordier JF, Valeyre D, Guillevin L, et al. Pulmonary Wegener's granulomatosis. A clinical and imaging study of 77 cases. Chest 1990;97(4):906–12.

73. Lee KS, Kim TS, Fujimoto K, et al. Thoracic manifestation of Wegener's granulomatosis: CT findings in 30 patients. Eur Radiol 2003;13(1):43–51.

74. Aberle DR, Gamsu G, Lynch D. Thoracic manifestations of Wegener granulomatosis: diagnosis and course. Radiology 1990;174(3 Pt 1):703–9.

75. Komócsi A, Reuter M, Heller M, et al. Active disease and residual damage in treated Wegener's granulomatosis: an observational study using pulmonary high-resolution computed tomography. Eur Radiol 2003;13(1):36–42.

76. Ananthakrishnan L, Sharma N, Kanne JP. Wegener's granulomatosis in the chest: high-resolution CT findings. AJR Am J Roentgenol 2009;192(3):676–82.

77. Lohrmann C, Uhl M, Kotter E, et al. Pulmonary manifestations of Wegener granulomatosis: CT findings in 57 patients and a review of the literature. Eur J Radiol 2005;53(3):471–7.

78. Comarmond C, Crestani B, Tazi A, et al. Pulmonary fibrosis in antineutrophil cytoplasmic antibodies (ANCA)-associated vasculitis: a series of 49 patients and review of the literature. Medicine (Baltimore) 2014;93(24):340–9 [Erratum appears in Medicine (Baltimore) 2014;93(24):414].

79. Attali P, Begum R, Ban Romdhane H, et al. Pulmonary Wegener's granulomatosis: changes at follow-up CT. Eur Radiol 1998;8(6):1009–113.

80. Pretorius ES, Stone JH, Hellman DB, et al. Wegener's granulomatosis: CT evolution of pulmonary parenchymal findings in treated disease. Crit Rev Comput Tomogr 2004;45(1):67–85.

81. Pretorius ES, Stone JH, Hellmann DB, et al. Wegener's granulomatosis: spectrum of CT findings in diagnosis, disease progression, and response to therapy. Crit Rev Diagn Imaging 2000;41(4):279–313.

82. Niles JL, Böttinger EP, Saurina GR, et al. The syndrome of lung hemorrhage and nephritis is usually an ANCA-associated condition. Arch Intern Med 1996;156(4):440–5.

83. Guillevin L, Durand-Gasselin B, Cevallos R, et al. Microscopic polyangiitis: clinical and laboratory findings in eighty-five patients. Arthritis Rheum 1999;42(3):421–30.

84. Lhote F, Cohen P, Guillevin L. Polyarteritis nodosa, microscopic polyangiitis and Churg-Strauss syndrome. Lupus 1998;7(4):238–58.

85. Akikusa B, Sato T, Ogawa M, et al. Necrotizing alveolar capillaritis in autopsy cases of microscopic polyangiitis. Incidence, histopathogenesis, and relationship with systemic vasculitis. Arch Pathol Lab Med 1997;121(2):144–9.

86. Primack SL, Miller RR, Müller NL. Diffuse pulmonary hemorrhage: clinical, pathologic, and imaging features. AJR Am J Roentgenol 1995;164(2):295–300.

87. Comarmond C, Pagnoux C, Khellaf M, et al, French Vasculitis Study Group. Eosinophilic granulomatosis with polyangiitis (Churg-Strauss): clinical characteristics and long-term followup of the 383 patients enrolled in the French Vasculitis Study Group cohort. Arthritis Rheum 2013;65(1):270–81.

88. Neumann T, Manger B, Schmid M, et al. Cardiac involvement in Churg-Strauss syndrome: impact of endomyocarditis. Medicine (Baltimore) 2009;88(4):236–43.

89. Guillevin L, Cohen P, Gayraud M, et al. Churg-Strauss syndrome. Clinical study and long-term follow-up of 96 patients. Medicine (Baltimore) 1999;78(1):26–37.

90. Guillevin L, Guittard T, Bletry O, et al. Systemic necrotizing angiitis with asthma: causes and precipitating factors in 43 cases. Lung 1987;165(3):165–72.

91. Lanham JG, Elkon KB, Pusey CD, et al. Systemic vasculitis with asthma and eosinophilia: a clinical approach to the Churg-Strauss syndrome. Medicine (Baltimore) 1984;63(2):65–81.

92. Guillevin L, Thi Huong Du Le, Godeau P, et al. Clinical findings and prognosis of polyarteritis nodosa and Churg-Strauss angiitis: a study in 165 patients. Br J Rheumatol 1988;27(4):258–64.

93. Katzenstein AL. Diagnostic features and differential diagnosis of Churg-Strauss syndrome in the lung. A review. Am J Clin Pathol 2000;114(5):767–72.

94. Keogh KA, Specks U. Churg-Strauss syndrome: clinical presentation, antineutrophil cytoplasmic antibodies, and leukotriene receptor antagonists. Am J Med 2003;115(4):284–90.

95. Chumbley LC, Harrison EG Jr, DeRemee RA. Allergic granulomatosis and angiitis (Churg-Strauss syndrome). Report and analysis of 30 cases. Mayo Clin Proc 1977;52(8):477–84.

96. Buschman DL, Waldron JA Jr, King TE Jr. Churg-Strauss pulmonary vasculitis. High-resolution computed tomography scanning and pathologic findings. Am Rev Respir Dis 1990;142(2):458–61.

97. Degesys GE, Mintzer RA, Vrla RF. Allergic granulomatosis: Churg-Strauss syndrome. AJR Am J Roentgenol 1980;135(6):1281–2.

98. Worthy SA, Müller NL, Hansell DM, et al. Churg-Strauss syndrome: the spectrum of pulmonary CT findings in 17 patients. AJR Am J Roentgenol 1998;170(2):297–300.

99. Silva CI, Müller NL, Fujimoto K, et al. Churg-Strauss syndrome: high resolution CT and pathologic findings. J Thorac Imaging 2005;20(2):74–80.

100. Kim YK, Lee KS, Chung MP, et al. Pulmonary involvement in Churg-Strauss syndrome: an analysis of CT, clinical, and pathologic findings. Eur Radiol 2007;17(12):3157–65.

101. Choi YH, Im JG, Han BK, et al. Thoracic manifestation of Churg-Strauss syndrome: radiologic and clinical findings. Chest 2000;117(1):117–24.

102. Pusey CD. Anti-glomerular basement membrane disease. Kidney Int 2003;64(4):1535–50.

103. Tarzi RM, Cook HT, Pusey CD. Crescentic glomerulonephritis: new aspects of pathogenesis. Semin Nephrol 2011;31(4):361–8.

104. Lombard CM, Colby TV, Elliott CG. Surgical pathology of the lung in anti-basement membrane antibody-associated Goodpasture's syndrome. Hum Pathol 1989;20(5):445–51.

105. Donaghy M, Rees AJ. Cigarette smoking and lung haemorrhage in glomerulonephritis caused by autoantibodies to glomerular basement membrane. Lancet 1983;2(8364):1390–3.

106. García-Rostan y Pérez GM, García Bragado F, Puras Gil AM. Pulmonary hemorrhage and antiglomerular basement membrane antibody-mediated glomerulonephritis after exposure to smoked cocaine (crack): a case report and review of the literature. Pathol Int 1997;47(10):692–7.

107. Rigante D, Castellazzi L, Bosco A, et al. Is there a crossroad between infections, genetics, and Henoch-Schönlein purpura? Autoimmun Rev 2013;12(10):1016–21.

108. Pillebout E, Thervet E, Hill G, et al. Henoch-Schönlein purpura in adults: outcome and prognostic factors. J Am Soc Nephrol 2002;13(5):1271–8.

109. Nadrous HF, Yu AC, Specks U, et al. Pulmonary involvement in Henoch-Schönlein purpura. Mayo Clin Proc 2004;79(9):1151–7.

110. Cream JJ, Gumpel JM, Peachey RD. Schönlein-Henoch purpura in the adult. A study of 77 adults with anaphylactoid or Schönlein-Henoch purpura. Q J Med 1970;39(156):461–84.

111. Wisnieski JJ, Baer AN, Christensen J, et al. Hypocomplementemic urticarial vasculitis syndrome. Clinical and serologic findings in 18 patients. Medicine (Baltimore) 1995;74(1):24–41.

112. Grotz W, Baba HA, Becker JU, et al. Hypocomplementemic urticarial vasculitis syndrome: an interdisciplinary challenge. Dtsch Arztebl Int 2009;106(46):756–63.

113. Schwartz HR, McDuffie FC, Black LF, et al. Hypocomplementemic urticarial vasculitis: association

with chronic obstructive pulmonary disease. Mayo Clin Proc 1982;57(4):231–8.

114. Paira SO. Bilateral pleural effusion in a patient with urticarial vasculitis. Clin Rheumatol 1994;13(3): 504–6.

115. Ramos-Casals M, Robles A, Brito-Zerón P, et al. Life-threatening cryoglobulinemia: clinical and immunological characterization of 29 cases. Semin Arthritis Rheum 2006;36(3):189–96.

116. Direskeneli H. Behçet's disease: infectious aetiology, new autoantigens, and HLA-B51. Ann Rheum Dis 2001;60(11):996–1002.

117. Sakane T, Takeno M, Suzuki N, et al. Behçet's disease. N Engl J Med 1999;341(17):1284–91.

118. Erkan F, Gül A, Tasali E. Pulmonary manifestations of Behçet's disease. Thorax 2001;56(7):572–8.

119. Uzun O, Akpolat T, Erkan L. Pulmonary vasculitis in Behcet disease: a cumulative analysis. Chest 2005;127(6):2243–53.

120. Erkan F, Cavdar T. Pulmonary vasculitis in Behçet's disease. Am Rev Respir Dis 1992;146(1):232–9.

121. Chae EJ, Do KH, Seo JB, et al. Radiologic and clinical findings of Behçet disease: comprehensive review of multisystemic involvement. Radiographics 2008;28(5):e31.

122. Efthimiou J, Johnston C, Spiro SG, et al. Pulmonary disease in Behçet's syndrome. Q J Med 1986; 58(227):259–80.

123. Ahn JM, Im JG, Ryoo JW, et al. Thoracic manifestations of Behçet syndrome: radiographic and CT findings in nine patients. Radiology 1995;194(1): 199–203.

124. Grenier P, Bletry O, Cornud F, et al. Pulmonary involvement in Behcet disease. AJR Am J Roentgenol 1981;137(3):565–9.

125. Numan F, Islak C, Berkmen T, et al. Behçet disease: pulmonary arterial involvement in 15 cases. Radiology 1994;192(2):465–8.

126. Cöplü L, Emrí S, Selçuk ZT, et al. Life threatening chylous pleural and pericardial effusion in a patient with Behçet's syndrome. Thorax 1992;47(1): 64–5.

127. Durieux P, Bletry O, Huchon G, et al. Multiple pulmonary arterial aneurysms in Behcet's disease and Hughes-Stovin syndrome. Am J Med 1981; 71(4):736–41.

128. Rockall AG, Rickards D, Shaw PJ. Imaging of the pulmonary manifestations of systemic disease. Postgrad Med J 2001;77(912):621–38.

129. Franks TJ, Koss MN. Pulmonary capillaritis. Curr Opin Pulm Med 2000;6(5):430–5.

130. Toyoshima H, Kusaba T, Yamaguchi M. Cause of death in autopsied RA patients. Ryumachi 1993; 33(3):209–14 [in Japanese].

131. Schwarz MI, Zamora MR, Hodges TN, et al. Isolated pulmonary capillaritis and diffuse alveolar hemorrhage in rheumatoid arthritis and mixed connective tissue disease. Chest 1998;113(6): 1609–15.

132. Hunninghake GW, Fauci AS. Pulmonary involvement in the collagen vascular diseases. Am Rev Respir Dis 1979;119(3):471–503.

133. Webb WR, Gamsu G. Cavitary pulmonary nodules with systemic lupus erythematosus: differential diagnosis. AJR Am J Roentgenol 1981;136(1): 27–31.

134. Miller LR, Greenberg SD, McLarty JW. Lupus lung. Chest 1985;88(2):265–9.

135. Zamora MR, Warner ML, Tuder R, et al. Diffuse alveolar hemorrhage and systemic lupus erythematosus. Clinical presentation, histology, survival, and outcome. Medicine (Baltimore) 1997;76(3): 192–202.

136. Haupt HM, Moore GW, Hutchins GM. The lung in systemic lupus erythematosus. Analysis of the pathologic changes in 120 patients. Am J Med 1981;71(5):791–8.

137. Albelda SM, Gefter WB, Epstein DM, et al. Diffuse pulmonary hemorrhage: a review and classification. Radiology 1985;154(2):289–97.

138. Asherson RA. Pulmonary hypertension in systemic lupus erythematosus. J Rheumatol 1990;17(3): 414–5.

139. Pope J. An update in pulmonary hypertension in systemic lupus erythematosus: do we need to know about it? Lupus 2008;17(4):274–7.

Imaging of Acute Lung Injury

 CrossMark

Brett M. Elicker, MD[a],*, Kirk T. Jones, MD[b], David M. Naeger, MD[c], James A. Frank, MD[d]

KEYWORDS

- Acute lung injury (ALI) • Acute respiratory distress syndrome (ARDS)
- Diffuse alveolar damage (DAD) • Acute interstitial pneumonia (AIP)
- Acute fibrinous organizing pneumonia (AFOP) • Acute eosinophilic pneumonia (AEP)

KEY POINTS

- Acute lung injury (ALI) is the clinical syndrome associated with patients who have diffuse alveolar damage on histopathology.
- A variety of diseases may mimic ALI, including hydrostatic edema, infection, aspiration, organizing pneumonia, interstitial lung disease, and acute eosinophilic pneumonia.
- Treatment of ALI is mainly supportive, and no pharmacologic treatment (eg, corticosteroids) has been shown to be convincingly beneficial.
- The key role of imaging is to identify diseases that mimic ALI so that appropriate specific treatment may be instituted.

INTRODUCTION

Acute lung injury (ALI) is a common cause of acute respiratory symptoms in the hospitalized patient, accounting for more than 10% of admissions to the intensive care unit[1] and affecting nearly 200,000 people in the United States yearly.[2] ALI is unique from other causes of dyspnea in its pathophysiologic mechanism of disease. Injury to the alveolar epithelium and capillary endothelium increases alveolar barrier permeability, resulting in airspace edema and inflammation. Because of this unique pattern of injury, the natural history, treatment, and prognosis of ALI differs significantly from other acute lung diseases. The diagnosis of ALI is typically based on clinical and radiographic criteria; however, because these criteria can be nonspecific, diagnostic uncertainty is common. A multidisciplinary approach that synthesizes clinical, imaging, and pathologic data, when available, can ensure an accurate diagnosis. Imaging represents a cornerstone modality in the detection, characterization, and follow-up of patients with suspected ALI, but radiologists must also have a comprehensive knowledge of the clinical and pathologic findings seen in patients with ALI. The goal of this article is to provide a review of ALI with an emphasis on this multidisciplinary approach.

CLINICAL
Definitions

ALI, acute respiratory distress syndrome (ARDS), and diffuse alveolar damage (DAD) all refer to a similar pathophysiologic process; however, they are not synonymous. The first challenge in understanding this topic is to be aware of the subtle, yet important, differences between these 3 terms (Table 1). DAD is a histopathologic pattern of injury

No disclosures for any of the authors.
[a] Cardiac and Pulmonary Imaging Section, Department of Radiology and Biomedical Imaging, University of California, 505 Parnassus Avenue, Box 0628, San Francisco, CA 94143, USA; [b] Department of Pathology, University of California, 505 Parnassus Avenue, Box 0102, San Francisco, CA 94143, USA; [c] Department of Radiology and Biomedical Imaging, University of California, 505 Parnassus Avenue, Box 0628, San Francisco, CA 94143, USA; [d] Division of Pulmonary, Critical Care, Allergy and Sleep, San Francisco VA Medical Center, 4150 Clement Street, Box 111D, San Francisco, CA 94121, USA
* Corresponding author.
E-mail address: brett.elicker@ucsf.edu

Radiol Clin N Am 54 (2016) 1119–1132
http://dx.doi.org/10.1016/j.rcl.2016.05.006
0033-8389/16/$ – see front matter © 2016 Elsevier Inc. All rights reserved.

Table 1	
Definitions of diffuse alveolar damage, acute lung injury, and acute respiratory distress syndrome	
Term	**Definition**
DAD	A histopathologic pattern of injury characterized by alveolar epithelial injury, proteinaceous edema, hyaline membranes, edema, and eventually fibroplasia
ALI	The clinical syndrome associated with any patient that has DAD pathologically

ARDS	A clinical syndrome defined by 4 criteria:
	1. Acute onset (occurring within 1 wk of an insult or after the onset of symptoms)
	2. Bilateral opacities on chest radiography (opacities not explained by effusions, collapse, or nodules)
	3. Exclusion of cardiac failure or fluid overload as a cause of symptoms (echocardiography often obtained, particularly when there are no risk factors for hydrostatic edema)
	4. Reduced oxygenation (3 levels of severity)
	   a. Mild: 200 mm Hg < Pao_2/Fio_2 ≤300 mm Hg
	   b. Moderate: 100 mm Hg < Pao_2/Fio_2 ≤200 mm Hg
	   c. Severe: Pao_2/Fio_2 ≤100 mm Hg

characterized by alveolar epithelial injury, proteinaceous edema, hyaline membranes, edema, and eventually, fibroplasia. The pathologic manifestations of DAD are discussed in greater detail later.

ALI and ARDS, on the other hand, are both clinical syndromes. ARDS was most recently defined in a 2012 consensus statement.[3] It is characterized by the acute onset of hypoxemia and diffuse parenchymal opacities on chest radiograph not explained by cardiogenic edema or fluid overload. ARDS is further categorized into mild, moderate, and severe forms based on the severity of hypoxemia as defined by the ratio of the partial pressure of oxygen in arterial blood to the fraction of inspired oxygen (Pao_2/Fio_2 ratio). ALI, on the other hand, refers to the clinical syndrome associated with any patient who has DAD pathologically, but its use is not limited by the strict clinical criteria that define ARDS. To add further confusion, an older consensus paper[4] defined ALI using similar criteria to ARDS, except with less severe hypoxemia. This definition of ALI was subsequently removed in the 2012 classification because practitioners had been using the term ALI to describe patients who clinically appeared to have ARDS, but did not meet the oxygenation criteria. Presently, the most accurate use of the term ALI is to describe any clinical symptoms or findings that are associated with histopathologic DAD, which include both cases that meet criteria for ARDS and those that do not meet criteria for ARDS.

In many cases, a definitive pathologic diagnosis is not available in patients with ALI or ARDS; thus, the diagnosis is often presumed and based on the exclusion of other causes of acute lung symptoms. As discussed earlier, DAD and ARDS are not synonymous. Not all patients who meet clinical and radiographic criteria for ARDS will have DAD on

pathology. DAD mimics that may meet clinical criteria for ARDS are shown in **Box 1**. In a study of ARDS patients undergoing autopsy,[5] only 45% of patients who met criteria for ARDS had DAD on pathology. In the group with mild ARDS, only 14% had DAD on pathology. The most common alternative (non-DAD) diagnoses in this study included pneumonia (49%), no significant lung abnormality (14%), emphysema (7%), pulmonary hemorrhage (6%), and malignancy (5.5%). In another study of open lung biopsy in patients with nonresolving ARDS (persistent hypoxemic respiratory failure >1 week after admission),[6] 58% had DAD on pathology. The most common alternative (non-DAD) diagnoses in this study were interstitial fibrosis (37%), organizing pneumonia (OP; 26%), and alveolar hemorrhage (14%). It is also important to note that not all patients with DAD on histopathology meet clinical

Box 1
Clinical and radiographic mimics of acute lung injury
Hydrostatic pulmonary edema
Rare causes of pulmonary edema (high altitude, high permeability such as interleukin-2 infusion, neurogenic, postobstructive)
Pneumonia without ALI
Aspiration
Diffuse alveolar hemorrhage
Acute hypersensitivity pneumonitis
Organizing pneumonia
Acute eosinophilic pneumonia
Acute fibrinous organizing pneumonia

criteria for ARDS, although they can still be considered to have ALI.

Demographics and Causes of Acute Lung Injury

ALI may affect patients of any age, including pediatric patients,[7] but its highest incidence is seen in patients over the age of 75.[2] There are a variety of causes that may be pulmonary or extrapulmonary in origin (Box 2). The most common causes vary depending on referral patterns and specialties at different institutions. In an analysis of 21 academic and community hospitals in the state of Washington, the most common causes of ARDS were pneumonia with sepsis (46%), sepsis from a non-pulmonary source (33%), aspiration (11%), transfusion (3%), drug overdose (3%), pancreatitis (3%), and other (14%).[2] In a study of ARDS patients at the Mayo Clinic in Rochester, Minnesota, the most common causes were idiopathic (21%), stem-cell or solid organ transplantation (17%), connective tissue disease (16%), acute exacerbation of idiopathic pulmonary fibrosis (IPF; 12%), drugs (10%), and radiation therapy (2%).[8]

As ALI and ARDS are diagnoses of exclusion, a search for alternative causes of dyspnea and diffuse lung opacities is important. This is particularly true in patients without common risk factors for ALI or ARDS, such as pneumonia or sepsis, because these patients have a higher mortality than those with common risk factors but may have steroid-responsive disease.[9] There are currently no pharmacologic

---

Box 2
Pulmonary and extrapulmonary causes of acute lung injury and acute respiratory distress syndrome associated with diffuse alveolar damage pathologically

Pulmonary

Pneumonia

Aspiration

Inhalational injury

Pulmonary contusion

Extrapulmonary

Sepsis (extrapulmonary)

Surgery

Drugs

Pancreatitis

Transfusion

Connective tissue disease

Trauma

---

therapies for ALI or ARDS. Therefore, an aggressive diagnostic workup early after presentation, and the identification of steroid-responsive diseases that clinically mimic ALI may have a significant impact on outcomes.[10] Diagnostic studies that may be obtained in the evaluation of patients with suspected ALI or ARDS are focused on clinical entities that may mimic DAD. Diagnostic evaluation may include echocardiography, pulmonary artery pressure measurements obtained from pulmonary artery catheterization, bronchoalveolar lavage, blood cultures, sputum analysis, connective tissue disease serologies, and other laboratory tests. Imaging is a vital component of this diagnostic evaluation. Although chest radiographs are routinely obtained in all hospitalized patients with acute dyspnea and comprise one of the principal criteria for ARDS, computed tomography (CT) may also be helpful in the detection of treatable causes of acute respiratory failure.

Bronchoscopy often represents the first invasive diagnostic test obtained when an initial clinical evaluation is unrevealing. In particular, bronchoscopy with alveolar lavage increases diagnostic accuracy for certain infections, diffuse alveolar hemorrhage, and acute eosinophilic pneumonia (AEP). Open lung biopsy is often helpful, although only occasionally obtained. In a study of 57 patients meeting clinical criteria for ARDS, but without a clear precipitant, open lung biopsy led to the initiation of new treatments in 60% of patients and the termination of unnecessary treatment in 37% of patients.[11] The most common changes in treatment included the administration of corticosteroids (46%), cyclophosphamide (14%), and antimicrobial therapies (9%). One caveat in interpreting this study: corticosteroids were given to patients with DAD on lung biopsy, but this is not currently considered the standard of care.

Mortality

Studies of mortality are heterogeneous with regards to the population studied. Some studies have evaluated patients with clinical ARDS, whereas others have evaluated those with pathologic evidence of DAD. The studies that included ARDS patients were undoubtedly a mix of those with and without DAD. Regardless, the average mortality of these entities is high compared with other common causes of hypoxemia, such as cardiogenic pulmonary edema. Recent advances in supportive techniques, such as the introduction of low tidal volume ventilation, would predict an improvement in outcomes compared with prior decades; however, despite the positive results from randomized trials, adherence to lung-protective ventilation strategies is less than complete.[12]

Although some observational trials[13] and a systematic review[14] have shown a reduction in ARDS mortality over time, another review of the literature[15] reported no significant change in mortality between 1994 and 2006. The overall pooled mortality in this review was 44.3%. More recent data comparing ARDS mortality by severity, based on the 2012 criteria, reported 28-day mortalities of 30%, 35%, and 43% for mild, moderate, and severe ARDS, respectively.[1] Among patients who meet the clinical criteria for ARDS in whom histopathology was obtained, mortality also varies depending on the presence or absence of DAD. In one recent study, the odds ratio for mortality in patients with ARDS and DAD was 1.8 compared with patients who had ARDS without DAD.[16] Although most patients who die with ARDS succumb to multiorgan failure or shock, the presence of DAD on histopathology was associated with a higher risk of death from respiratory failure.[17] Among patients with DAD, mortality may also vary depending on the clinical context. For example, the mortality of patients with DAD due to an acute exacerbation of IPF is as high as 86%.[8]

Treatment

Treatment of ALI is primarily supportive through supplemental oxygen and mechanical ventilation, if necessary. The main pharmacologic treatment is aimed at any underlying cause, if one can be identified, such as infection. The use of corticosteroids in patients with protracted hypoxemic respiratory failure is controversial. Although one study demonstrated a benefit of using corticosteroids for a subset of ARDS patients with persistent respiratory failure of at least 7 days' duration,[18] a multicenter, double-blind randomized controlled trial of steroids versus placebo in patients with ARDS of at least 7 days' duration[19] showed no significant difference in the 60-day mortality comparing the corticosteroid group (29.2% mortality) with the placebo group (28.6% mortality). Interestingly, the steroid group in this study showed a greater number of ventilator-free days, improved oxygenation, and improved blood pressure compared with the placebo group. It is possible that the benefits of steroid therapy in this population may have been counteracted by drug-related complications of this therapy. Alternatively, there may be a subset of patients for whom steroid therapy was beneficial. For example, because DAD and OP often coexist, it is possible that a subset of patients had steroid-responsive OP following ARDS, but this remains to be investigated.

PATHOLOGY

DAD is the main pathologic correlate to the clinical entity ALI. The term diffuse in this setting refers to the global involvement of the alveolus such that both the endothelial (alveolar capillary) and the epithelial (pneumocyte) components are affected. The histologic appearance of this process evolves over the course of the injury from an early exudative or injury phase, through a proliferative or organizing phase, and finally into a healed or resolved phase.[20]

The proliferative phase is characterized by alveolar septal thickening from interstitial edema and mild inflammation. Ultrastructural analysis by electron microscopy reveals that this phase is initially characterized by necrosis of type 1 pneumocytes, endothelial cell damage, and sloughing of the alveolar basement membranes. This loss of the alveolar integrity results in leaking of fibrin-rich proteinaceous fluid into airspaces. After 1 or 2 days from the initial injury, this fluid admixes with the cytoplasm and nucleoplasm of the dead cells and forms homogeneous eosinophilic hyaline membranes, which lie in close apposition to the alveolar septa (**Fig. 1**). Hyaline membranes become better developed over the course of the next 3 to 5 days. During this time, there is recruitment of inflammatory cells into the region.

The organizing phase begins near the end of the first week following injury and is characterized by re-epithelialization and fibroplasia. The alveoli show growth of type 2 pneumocytes along their surface. These cells are thought to differentiate into type 1 pneumocytes as the repair process continues. The alveolar septa are thickened by

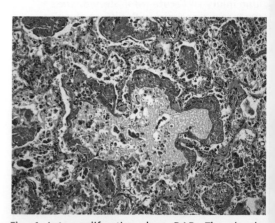

Fig. 1. Late proliferative phase DAD. The alveolar septa are thickened by edema and mild chronic inflammation. There are well-developed hyaline membranes along the alveolar septal surface. The airspaces show filling with edema (hematoxylin eosin, original magnification ×200).

interstitial accumulation of granulation tissuelike fibrosis composed of fibroblasts, myofibroblasts, and small vessels. These fibroblasts and myofibroblasts can also extend into the airspaces, resulting in consolidated regions of OP. It is important in pathology to recognize this overlap of OP and DAD because the nonspecific presence of OP may be a sign of either a steroid-responsive process (as in cryptogenic OP) or organizing DAD that may not be as easily treatable.

The healed or resolved phase is characterized by either a return to normal pulmonary alveolar architecture or a progression to fibrosis. As the type 2 pneumoctyes proliferate, the regions of OP may be incorporated into the interstitium where the fibroblasts undergo apoptosis. Apoptosis results in a relatively normal-appearing lung following resolution of the injury. Alternately, the involved regions may show extensive architectural remodeling by fibrosis, which may be manifest as either large areas of alveolar lobular collapse with fibrosis, airspace enlargement with fibrosis, or microscopic honeycomb fibrosis.

A second pattern of lung injury that may occur in isolation or may be associated with DAD is OP. This nonspecific injury pattern is characterized by consolidation of alveolar ducts and alveolar spaces by branching rounded polypoid plugs of granulation tissue (**Fig. 2**).[21,22] The underlying lung architecture is preserved, and the regions of alveolar consolidation are often patchy and frequently bronchiolocentric. The fibrous plugs are rich in mucopolysaccharides and have a slight basophilic appearance on hematoxylin and eosin staining (rather than the eosinophilic appearance seen with established dense fibrosis in scar tissue). There are often numerous associated intra-alveolar macrophages with foamy cytoplasm. Alveolar septal inflammation is variable, but may be nearly absent.

Acute fibrinous organizing pneumonia (AFOP) is a term used to describe a pattern of ALI that histologically lies within the spectrum between DAD and OP. Similar to DAD, the airspaces show accumulation of fibrin, and similar to OP, this fibrin-rich material is arranged into polypoid plugs.[23] Like the other 2 patterns of ALI, AFOP is histologically nonspecific and may be observed in several types of toxic insults. Identification of hyaline membranes should prompt the diagnosis of DAD rather than AFOP, and identification of numerous eosinophils should prompt a diagnosis of eosinophilic pneumonia (which frequently shows abundant intra-alveolar fibrin).

IMAGING
Radiographic Findings of Acute Lung Injury

Chest radiographs typically are the first imaging modality obtained in patients with suspected ALI. Although the chest radiograph is a fast and inexpensive test, its findings are nonspecific and interobserver agreement for ALI is only moderate.[24] Figueroa-Casas and colleagues[25] assessed the diagnostic performance of chest radiographs for ARDS compared with CT and found that chest radiographs had a sensitivity of 73%, specificity of 70%, positive predictive value of 47%, and negative predictive value of 88%.

Bilateral lung opacities are one of the primary criteria for ARDS (**Fig. 3**) and will be seen,

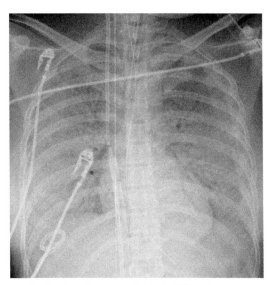

Fig. 3. Chest radiograph of ARDS. Diffuse lung consolidation with air bronchograms is present on a frontal chest radiograph of a patient with ARDS. Diffuse lung opacity on chest radiograph comprises one of the principal criteria for the diagnosis of ARDS.

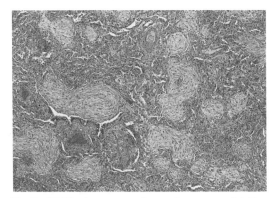

Fig. 2. OP. The lung parenchyma shows consolidation by numerous rounded polypoid plugs of granulation tissuelike fibrosis. There is mild alveolar septal interstitial inflammation (hematoxylin-eosin, original magnification ×40).

therefore, in all patients with ARDS whether or not it is associated with DAD pathologically. The differential of bilateral lung opacities on chest radiographs is thus broad and includes ALI, infection without ALI, aspiration, hydrostatic pulmonary edema, diffuse alveolar hemorrhage, acute hypersensitivity pneumonitis, OP, and AEP.

The distinction between diffuse lung consolidation and layering pleural effusions or bilateral atelectasis may be challenging. Good radiographic technique is important in avoiding this pitfall. Ideally, patients should be imaged in an upright or semiupright position at maximal inspiration. In the supine position, pleural effusions may layer posteriorly and extend from base to apex, mimicking diffuse lung consolidation (Fig. 4). When the patient is imaged in an upright position, the pleural effusions layer toward the lung bases and cause more typical blunting of the costophrenic angles. Atelectasis may be distinguished from consolidation by signs of volume loss, such as fissural displacement, diaphragmatic elevation and mediastinal/hilar deviation. In many cases of atelectasis, however, these signs are lacking.

Computed Tomography Findings of Acute Lung Injury

Compared with chest radiographs, CT is more sensitive in the detection of early disease and is more accurate in the characterization of abnormalities and formulation of a differential diagnosis. The typical CT findings of ALI are symmetric or diffuse ground-glass opacities and/or consolidation (Fig. 5). Smooth interlobular septal thickening may be seen in association with ground-glass opacity (ie, crazy paving) (Fig. 6); however, interlobular septal thickening as an isolated finding is not typical. These findings overlap significantly with hydrostatic pulmonary edema, certain infections (particularly viruses, atypical bacteria, and *Pneumocystis jirovecii*), diffuse alveolar hemorrhage, acute hypersensitivity pneumonitis, and AEP.

The distribution of abnormalities on CT varies depending on the cause of ALI: pulmonary versus extrapulmonary. ALI from an extrapulmonary cause (eg, pancreatitis) classically shows an even gradient of lung opacity from anterior to posterior (Fig. 7). The anterior lung is normal or shows ground-glass opacity, whereas the posterior lung shows confluent consolidation. The specificity of this pattern for ALI is unclear, however. ALI from a pulmonary cause does not tend to show this gradient, but instead demonstrates more heterogeneous opacities and nondependent areas of consolidation (Fig. 8).

Role of Computed Tomography in Patients with Acute Lung Injury and Acute Respiratory Distress Syndrome

The results of CT scans in patients meeting clinical criteria for ARDS have been shown to change management in greater than 25% of cases. Management changes in the study by Simon and colleagues[26] included changes in antibiotic therapy against bacteria or fungi (12.7%), drainage of pleural effusions (7.8%), correction of misplaced lines or tubes (4.9%), diuresis (2.9%), and anticoagulation (2.5%). The role of CT scan in patients with ALI or ARDS is 2-fold. First, CT is able to confirm the presence of abnormalities that are compatible with ALI. As discussed previously, chest radiographs are limited in their ability to

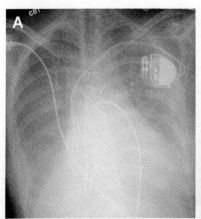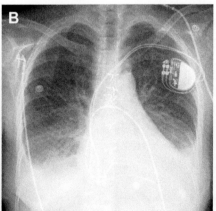

Fig. 4. Pleural effusions mimicking ARDS. Supine frontal chest radiograph (*A*) shows diffuse opacities. The distinction between lung consolidation and layering effusions is difficult when imaging patients in the supine position. An upright chest radiograph (*B*) in the same patient shows that these opacities represent layering effusions and there is no significant lung consolidation.

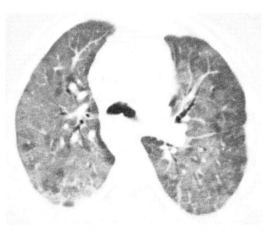

Fig. 5. DAD without ARDS. Extensive bilateral ground-glass opacity is seen on this axial CT image in a patient with DAD due to drug toxicity. Although DAD was present on open lung biopsy, the patient did not meet clinical criteria for ARDS because of a Pao_2/Fio_2 ratio greater than 300 mm Hg.

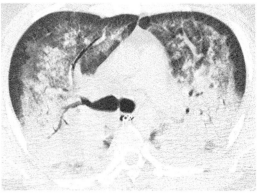

Fig. 7. ALI from an extrapulmonary cause. Axial CT shows a gradient of density from anterior to posterior. The anterior lung is nearly normal, and the posterior lung shows dense consolidation. This distribution suggests an extrapulmonary cause of ALI. The cause of ALI in this patient was sepsis from an abdominal source.

distinguish diffuse lung opacities from pleural effusions and atelectasis. CT is more specific in this distinction and thus may target patients who will benefit from drainage of pleural effusions or recruitment techniques to reduce atelectasis.

Second, CT may identify patients with lung disease that is incompatible with ALI and suggestive of an alternative cause. A careful search for CT findings suggestive of these alternative causes has the potential to change management by detecting a disease that may be responsive to specific pharmacologic intervention. Infection should be considered in cases in which nondependent areas of consolidation are present. Greater than 90% of patients with pneumonia will show these nondependent opacities.[27] Tree-in-bud opacities are strongly suggestive of infection or aspiration[28]

(Fig. 9). Pulmonary edema should be considered in patients with smooth interlobular septal thickening, pleural effusions, or cardiomegaly. In the study by Komiya and colleagues,[29] findings suggesting hydrostatic pulmonary edema over ALI included an upper lung or central distribution of ground-glass opacity and the presence of peribronchovascular interstitial thickening (Fig. 10). Findings of fibrosis (irregular reticulation, traction bronchiectasis, and honeycombing) suggest interstitial lung disease (ILD). Of note, CT findings of fibrosis may develop in patients with ALI over time; however, they are not usually present within the first week after clinical presentation.

OP is another entity that may clinically mimic ALI. Both OP and ALI may have an acute or subacute clinical presentation with hypoxemia and

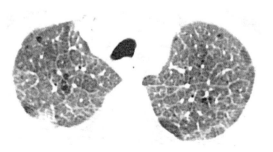

Fig. 6. Crazy paving in ALI. Axial CT image demonstrates a combination of ground-glass opacity and interlobular septal thickening, also known as the crazy-paving pattern. In the acute setting, this pattern is most commonly seen with pulmonary edema, ALI, infection, and hemorrhage. This patient had DAD from sepsis.

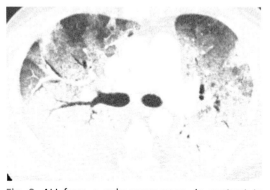

Fig. 8. ALI from a pulmonary cause. In contrast to Fig. 7, this axial CT image shows more heterogeneous opacities with focal nondependent areas of consolidation. This distribution suggests a pulmonary cause of ALI. The cause of ALI in this patient was pneumonia.

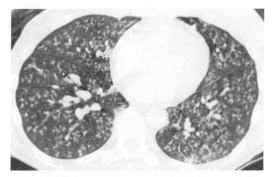

Fig. 9. ARDS due to infection without ALI. An axial CT image shows extensive bilateral centrilobular nodules and tree-in-bud opacities in a patient with viral infection. Although this patient met clinical criteria for ARDS, they did not have DAD on pathology.

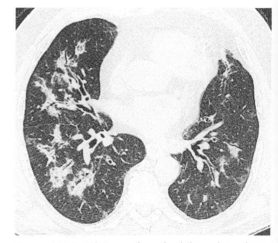

Fig. 11. OP. Focal areas of patchy, bilateral, peribronchovascular consolidation are seen on this axial CT of a patient with OP.

bilateral opacities on chest radiographs. On CT, OP shows characteristic findings of patchy, bilateral, often rounded areas of peribronchovascular and subpleural consolidation (Fig. 11). As OP tends to be a highly steroid-responsive disease, distinction from ALI has a significant impact on treatment. It is important to note that DAD and OP show significant pathologic overlap and often coexist (Fig. 12). This overlap is termed organizing DAD. In most cases, DAD is the predominant finding and OP is a secondary finding; however, in rare cases, the opposite is true. CT may be helpful in determining the relative contributions of DAD versus OP to the overall disease burden and may be able to predict steroid responsiveness in cases of organizing DAD.

The Subacute to Chronic Appearance of Acute Lung Injury

ALI shows a typical evolution over time on CT that mirrors the pathologic stages of DAD.[30,31] Initially, ground-glass opacity and/or consolidation are seen in isolation. Over time (1–4 weeks), findings

of fibrosis may develop, including irregular reticulation and traction bronchiectasis (Fig. 13). In diseases such as IPF, reticulation and traction bronchiectasis represent irreversible fibrosis; however, in the setting of ALI, these findings may eventually resolve over time. Despite this fact, the development of bronchiectasis, in particular, is a poor prognostic sign. In the study by Chung and colleagues,[32] the development of varcoid bronchiectasis was associated with higher mortality, seen in 43% of patients who died but only 7% of survivors.

ALI may eventually lead to permanent fibrosis with or without honeycombing; however, in most cases, the extent of fibrosis is limited. As many as 90% of patients who survive the acute stage of clinical ARDS will show some signs of fibrosis 6 to 10 months after the onset of symptoms.[33] The presence and extent of these findings correlate with the severity of ARDS and duration of mechanical ventilation using high peak inspiratory

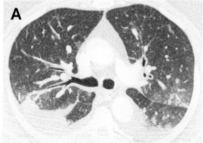
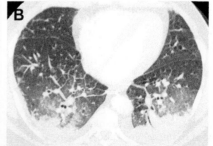

Fig. 10. ARDS due to edema without ALI. Two axial CT images through the upper (A) and lower (B) lungs show bilateral ground-glass opacity and consolidation. The presence of peribronchovascular interstitial thickening and interlobular septal thickening suggests hydrostatic pulmonary edema over ALI.

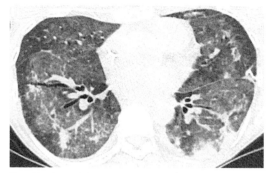

Fig. 12. Organizing DAD. An axial CT image shows bilateral ground-glass opacity and focal areas of consolidation. Open lung biopsy showed features of both DAD and OP. The focal areas of peribronchovascular and subpleural consolidation on CT corresponded to OP, whereas the more symmetric ground-glass opacities corresponded to DAD.

pressures or high oxygen levels. This fibrosis typically has an anterior, subpleural distribution (Fig. 14). This distribution may be a result of barotrauma and oxygen toxicity in an area of lung that is relatively resistant to atelectasis.

SPECIFIC CAUSES OF ACUTE LUNG INJURY

ALI is most often caused by common etiologies, such as pneumonia. There are several uncommon causes of ALI that deserve specific mention because of their unique clinical, pathologic, or radiographic features.

Acute Interstitial Pneumonia

Acute interstitial pneumonia (AIP), previously known as Hamman-Rich syndrome, is the idiopathic clinical disorder associated with histopathologic DAD. Patients are given a diagnosis of AIP when they meet clinical criteria for ARDS, but no cause is identified. Lung biopsy is required to confidently confirm the diagnosis and exclude mimics of AIP. Given that many patients with AIP have a prodromal illness, viral infection may be one of the potential inciting factors. The demographics and clinical course are similar to ARDS from an identifiable cause. Information on mortality is limited by small sample sizes and varies significantly from 20% to 100%.[10,34]

Radiographic findings are similar or identical to nonidiopathic ARDS (Fig. 15). Chest radiographs demonstrate extensive bilateral lung opacities, and CT demonstrates diffuse ground-glass opacity and consolidation evolving over time to reticulation, traction bronchiectasis, and honeycombing.[35] In one study comparing AIP to nonidiopathic cases of ARDS,[36] AIP more frequently showed a lower lung and symmetric distribution. Honeycombing was also more common in the evolution of AIP,

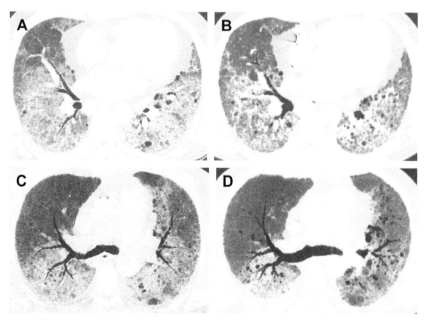

Fig. 13. Evolution of CT findings of ALI over time. A baseline CT (*A*) at the onset of acute symptoms demonstrates extensive bilateral ground-glass opacity and consolidation. Three weeks later, a CT at the same level (*B*) shows the interval development of irregular reticulation. Axial minimum intensity projection images show the development of traction bronchiectasis over time when comparing images at the onset of symptoms (*C*) and 3 weeks later (*D*). This is the typical evolution of the CT findings of ALI over time.

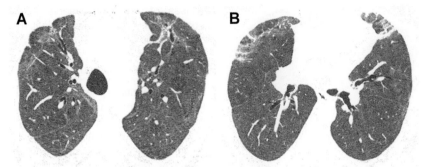

Fig. 14. Post-ARDS fibrosis. Two axial CT images though the mid (*A*) and lower (*B*) lungs demonstrate an anterior distribution of irregular reticulation and traction bronchiectasis. This is a typical distribution of fibrosis from prior ARDS.

although this may have been due to the inclusion of patients with an acute exacerbation of ILD. Corticosteroids are often administered given the lack of any other effective treatment; however, they are unlikely to provide a significant benefit.

Acute Exacerbation of Interstitial Lung Disease

Over the past 2 decades, there has been an increased awareness of patients with ILD presenting with acute symptoms not attributable to infection, edema, or other identifiable causes. The cause of these acute symptoms is presumably related to the underlying ILD, although the trigger for the acute acceleration of disease is unknown. Although an acute exacerbation may be seen with any ILD, it is most common in patients with IPF. Silva and colleagues[37] reviewed 24 patients

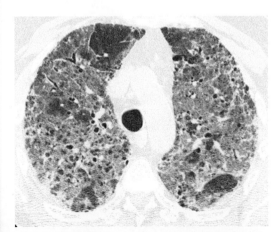

Fig. 15. AIP. Diffuse ground-glass opacity is present on this axial CT image. This appearance is indistinguishable from nonidiopathic ALI, edema, infection, hemorrhage, acute hypersensitivity pneumonitis, and AEP. The lucencies that underlie the ground-glass represent pre-existing emphysema in a smoker.

with a diagnosis of acute exacerbation of interstitial pneumonia. This cohort was composed of patients with IPF (50%), connective tissue disease (33.3%), and idiopathic nonspecific interstitial pneumonia (16.7%). In a retrospective review of 147 patients with IPF, 9.6% developed an acute exacerbation during the 2-year observational period.[38] Thoracic surgery is one risk factor for the development of an acute exacerbation. Sakamoto and colleagues[39] showed a 7.7% incidence of acute exacerbation in IPF patients immediately after thoracic surgery.

Pathology in patients with acute exacerbation of ILD showed 1 of 3 patterns: (1) DAD, (2) OP, or (3) progressive fibrosis.[40] DAD comprises most cases. Criteria for the diagnosis of acute exacerbation of IPF include the following[41]:

1. Acute worsening of symptoms over 30 days or less
2. New bilateral radiographic abnormalities
3. Absence of infection or other identifiable abnormality

The radiographic findings of acute exacerbation of ILD are similar to those of ALI except the findings are often superimposed on the pre-existing fibrosis.[37] Signs of fibrosis may be present on imaging obtained before the onset of acute symptoms. If no prior films are available, the signs of fibrosis may be present at the onset of acute symptoms (**Fig. 16**), as opposed to other causes of DAD in which these signs may develop 1 to 4 weeks later. Three variants of acute exacerbation have been described based on the distribution of ground-glass opacity and consolidation on CT[42]: (1) diffuse, (2) multifocal, and (3) peripheral (**Fig. 17**). In the study of Akira and colleagues,[42] there were significant differences in survival based on this distribution, as follows: diffuse (0% at 100 days), multifocal (50% at 500 days), and peripheral (75% at 500 days).

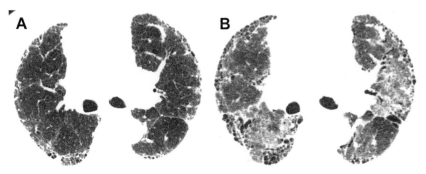

Fig. 16. Acute exacerbation of IPF. Baseline axial CT (*A*) shows peripheral fibrosis with honeycombing in a patient with IPF. Two years later, the patient presents with acute dyspnea. A follow-up CT (*B*) shows both worsening of fibrosis and the development of diffuse ground-glass opacity, compatible with an acute exacerbation.

Acute Fibrinous Organizing Pneumonia

AFOP is a unique form of ALI.[23] Although its histopathologic features share features with DAD and OP, they do not meet strict criteria for either one; however, AFOP likely represents a variant of these patterns of injury. There are a variety of associations including rejection in lung transplantation,[43] connective tissue disease, drug toxicity, and infection. The clinical presentation may be acute or subacute. The CT findings include symmetric, bilateral ground-glass opacity, and nodular areas of consolidation.[44] These findings may be seen in isolation or in combination. These radiographic findings mirror those of both DAD and OP (Fig. 18). The clinical course ranges from rapid progression and death to complete recovery, similar to the wide clinical spectrum seen in patients with DAD or OP.

Acute Eosinophilic Pneumonia

AEP is a disorder that shares many characteristics with ALI. Most patients with AEP present with acute respiratory symptoms requiring admission to the intensive care unit. Characteristic findings on histopathology include DAD associated with an increased number of tissue eosinophils.[45] Interestingly, a more recent review of the pathology of AEP showed findings resembling AFOP,[46] further emphasizing the close relationship between DAD and AFOP.

There are some important differences between AEP and ALI. Rhee and colleagues[47] performed a retrospective analysis of the clinical characteristics of 137 patients with AEP. Ninety-nine percent of patients were current smokers. Of these, 90% of patients described a change in smoking habits in the 1 month before developing AEP. This change in smoking habits included starting smoking, restarting smoking, or increasing the number of cigarettes smoked per day. The association between smoking and AEP was confirmed in the study by Uchiyama and colleagues,[48] in which 97% of patients were smokers. Another important difference between AEP and ALI is the significant clinical and radiographic response to corticosteroid treatment. In the study by Rhee and colleagues,[47] the average time to complete symptom resolution after

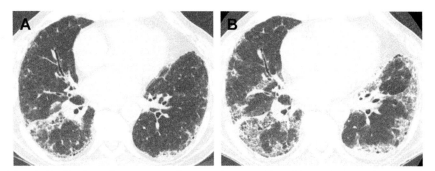

Fig. 17. Peripheral distribution of acute exacerbation of IPF. Peripheral irregular reticulation and early honeycombing are present on a baseline axial CT image (*A*) in a patient with IPF. Six months later, the patient presents with worsening cough and acute dyspnea. A follow-up CT (*B*) shows a peripheral distribution of new ground-glass opacity, compatible with acute exacerbation. This distribution has a significantly better prognosis than the diffuse or patchy distributions.

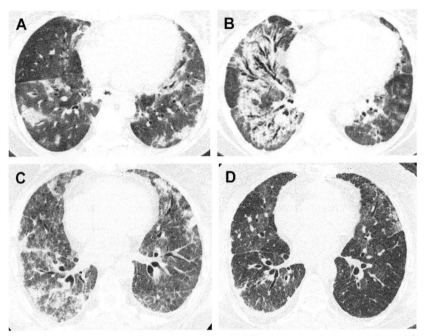

Fig. 18. AFOP. Axial CT (*A*) shows typical findings of AFOP with bilateral ground-glass opacity and focal, rounded areas of consolidation. Six months later (*B*), this progresses to severe fibrosis. In another patient with AFOP, the initial CT (*C*) shows similar findings to (*A*). In this patient, the follow-up CT (*D*) shows significant improvement in the findings. These 2 patients demonstrate the spectrum of changes over time in AFOP.

corticosteroid treatment was 7 days. In addition, 85% of chest radiographs showed complete clearing by 7 days.

The diagnosis of AEP presents several challenges. With the exception of the smoking history, the clinical presentation of AEP is nearly identical

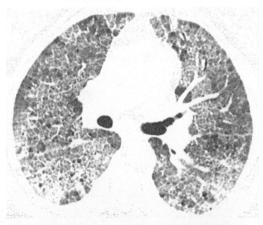

Fig. 19. AEP. Single axial CT through the mid lung in a patient who began smoking 1 month ago shows diffuse ground-glass opacity associated with interlobular septal thickening. Although the CT findings in isolation are nonspecific, when interpreted in the context of the clinical history, AEP is a leading diagnosis.

to ALI. Peripheral eosinophilia is only seen in approximately 30% of patients. In addition, there is significant overlap between AEP and ALI on imaging. Chest radiographs in both show extensive bilateral lung opacities. The main findings of AEP on CT are ground-glass opacity (97% of patients) and interlobular septal thickening (68% of patients)[47] (**Fig. 19**). This combination of findings is more commonly seen in patients with pulmonary edema; however, AEP should be suspected in patients in whom edema is unlikely (eg, younger age, normal echocardiogram). The diagnosis of AEP is most often confirmed by the presence of an increased number of eosinophils on bronchoscopy or characteristic pathologic findings on lung biopsy. As opposed to ALI/ARDS, corticosteroids are routinely administered given the rapid response seen in most patients.

SUMMARY

ALI is a clinical entity that requires input from clinicians, radiologists, and pathologists. Multidisciplinary input is vital in ensuring appropriate diagnosis and treatment. The main role of imaging is to evaluate for diseases that may mimic ALI clinically, including infection, edema, hemorrhage, OP, ILDs, and AEP. Radiologists need to be aware of the typical findings of ALI, and how these findings evolve over time, in addition to the features that distinguish ALI from these alternative causes.

REFERENCES

1. Bellani G, Laffey JG, Pham T, et al. Epidemiology, patterns of care, and mortality for patients with acute respiratory distress syndrome in intensive care units in 50 countries. JAMA 2016;315:788–800.
2. Rubenfeld GD, Caldwell E, Peabody E, et al. Incidence and outcomes of acute lung injury. N Engl J Med 2005;353:1685–93.
3. ARDS Definition Task Force, Ranieri VM, Rubenfeld GD, et al. Acute respiratory distress syndrome: the Berlin definition. JAMA 2012;307:2526–33.
4. Bernard GR, Artigas A, Brigham KL, et al. The American-European Consensus Conference on ARDS. Definitions, mechanisms, relevant outcomes, and clinical trial coordination. Am J Respir Crit Care Med 1994;149:818–24.
5. Thille AW, Esteban A, Fernández-Segoviano P, et al. Comparison of the Berlin definition for acute respiratory distress syndrome with autopsy. Am J Respir Crit Care Med 2013;187:761–7.
6. Guerin C, Bayle F, Leray V, et al. Open lung biopsy in nonresolving ARDS frequently identifies diffuse alveolar damage regardless of the severity stage and may have implications for patient management. Intensive Care Med 2015;41:222–30.
7. Flori HR, Glidden DV, Rutherford GW, et al. Pediatric acute lung injury: prospective evaluation of risk factors associated with mortality. Am J Respir Crit Care Med 2005;171:995–1001.
8. Parambil JG, Myers JL, Aubry M-C, et al. Causes and prognosis of diffuse alveolar damage diagnosed on surgical lung biopsy. Chest 2007; 132:50–7.
9. Gibelin A, Parrot A, Maitre B, et al. Acute respiratory distress syndrome mimickers lacking common risk factors of the Berlin definition. Intensive Care Med 2016;42:164–72.
10. Suh GY, Kang EH, Chung MP, et al. Early intervention can improve clinical outcome of acute interstitial pneumonia. Chest 2006;129:753–61.
11. Patel SR, Karmpaliotis D, Ayas NT, et al. The role of open-lung biopsy in ARDS. Chest 2004;125:197–202.
12. Weinert CR, Gross CR, Marinelli WA. Impact of randomized trial results on acute lung injury ventilator therapy in teaching hospitals. Am J Respir Crit Care Med 2003;167:1304–9.
13. Erickson SE, Martin GS, Davis JL, et al, NIH NHLBI ARDS Network. Recent trends in acute lung injury mortality: 1996-2005. Crit Care Med 2009;37:1574–9.
14. Zambon M, Vincent J-L. Mortality rates for patients with acute lung injury/ARDS have decreased over time. Chest 2008;133:1120–7.
15. Phua J, Badia JR, Adhikari NKJ, et al. Has mortality from acute respiratory distress syndrome decreased over time?: a systematic review. Am J Respir Crit Care Med 2009;179:220–7.
16. Cardinal-Fernández P, Bajwa EK, Dominguez-Calvo A, et al. The presence of diffuse alveolar damage on open lung biopsy is associated with mortality in patients with acute respiratory distress syndrome: a systematic review and meta-analysis. Chest 2016; 149(5):1155–64.
17. Lorente JA, Cardinal-Fernández P, Muñoz D, et al. Acute respiratory distress syndrome in patients with and without diffuse alveolar damage: an autopsy study. Intensive Care Med 2015;41:1921–30.
18. Meduri GU, Golden E, Freire AX, et al. Methylprednisolone infusion in early severe ARDS: results of a randomized controlled trial. Chest 2007;131: 954–63.
19. Steinberg KP, Hudson LD, Goodman RB, et al. Efficacy and safety of corticosteroids for persistent acute respiratory distress syndrome. N Engl J Med 2006;354:1671–84.
20. Castro CY. ARDS and diffuse alveolar damage: a pathologist's perspective. Semin Thorac Cardiovasc Surg 2006;18:13–9.
21. Lohr RH, Boland BJ, Douglas WW, et al. Organizing pneumonia. Features and prognosis of cryptogenic, secondary, and focal variants. Arch Intern Med 1997;157:1323–9.
22. Colby TV. Pathologic aspects of bronchiolitis obliterans organizing pneumonia. Chest 1992;102: 38S–43S.
23. Beasley MB, Franks TJ, Galvin JR, et al. Acute fibrinous and organizing pneumonia: a histological pattern of lung injury and possible variant of diffuse alveolar damage. Arch Pathol Lab Med 2002;126: 1064–70.
24. Rubenfeld GD, Caldwell E, Granton J, et al. Interobserver variability in applying a radiographic definition for ARDS. Chest 1999;116:1347–53.
25. Figueroa-Casas JB, Brunner N, Dwivedi AK, et al. Accuracy of the chest radiograph to identify bilateral pulmonary infiltrates consistent with the diagnosis of acute respiratory distress syndrome using computed tomography as reference standard. J Crit Care 2013; 28:352–7.
26. Simon M, Braune S, Laqmani A, et al. Value of computed tomography of the chest in subjects with ARDS: a retrospective observational study. Respir Care 2015;61(3):316–23.
27. Winer-Muram HT, Steiner RM, Gurney JW, et al. Ventilator-associated pneumonia in patients with adult respiratory distress syndrome: CT evaluation. Radiology 1998;208:193–9.
28. Miller WT, Panosian JS. Causes and imaging patterns of tree-in-bud opacities. Chest 2013;144: 1883–92.

29. Komiya K, Ishii H, Murakami J, et al. Comparison of chest computed tomography features in the acute phase of cardiogenic pulmonary edema and acute respiratory distress syndrome on arrival at the emergency department. J Thorac Imaging 2013; 28:322–8.

30. Ichikado K, Johkoh T, Ikezoe J, et al. Acute interstitial pneumonia: high-resolution CT findings correlated with pathology. AJR Am J Roentgenol 1997; 168:333–8.

31. Ichikado K, Suga M, Gushima Y, et al. Hyperoxia-induced diffuse alveolar damage in pigs: correlation between thin-section CT and histopathologic findings. Radiology 2000;216:531–8.

32. Chung JH, Kradin RL, Greene RE, et al. CT predictors of mortality in pathology confirmed ARDS. Eur Radiol 2011;21:730–7.

33. Nöbauer-Huhmann IM, Eibenberger K, Schaefer-Prokop C, et al. Changes in lung parenchyma after acute respiratory distress syndrome (ARDS): assessment with high-resolution computed tomography. Eur Radiol 2001;11:2436–43.

34. Avnon LS, Pikovsky O, Sion-Vardy N, et al. Acute interstitial pneumonia-Hamman-Rich syndrome: clinical characteristics and diagnostic and therapeutic considerations. Anesth Analg 2009;108:232–7.

35. Johkoh T, Müller NL, Taniguchi H, et al. Acute interstitial pneumonia: thin-section CT findings in 36 patients. Radiology 1999;211:859–63.

36. Tomiyama N, Müller NL, Johkoh T, et al. Acute respiratory distress syndrome and acute interstitial pneumonia: comparison of thin-section CT findings. J Comput Assist Tomogr 2001;25:28–33.

37. Silva CIS, Müller NL, Fujimoto K, et al. Acute exacerbation of chronic interstitial pneumonia: high-resolution computed tomography and pathologic findings. J Thorac Imaging 2007;22:221–9.

38. Kim DS, Park JH, Park BK, et al. Acute exacerbation of idiopathic pulmonary fibrosis: frequency and clinical features. Eur Respir J 2006;27:143–50.

39. Sakamoto S, Homma S, Mun M, et al. Acute exacerbation of idiopathic interstitial pneumonia following lung surgery in 3 of 68 consecutive patients: a retrospective study. Intern Med 2011;50:77–85.

40. Churg A, Müller NL, Silva CIS, et al. Acute exacerbation (acute lung injury of unknown cause) in UIP and other forms of fibrotic interstitial pneumonias. Am J Surg Pathol 2007;31:277–84.

41. Collard HR, Moore BB, Flaherty KR, et al. Acute exacerbations of idiopathic pulmonary fibrosis. Am J Respir Crit Care Med 2007;176:636–43.

42. Akira M, Kozuka T, Yamamoto S, et al. Computed tomography findings in acute exacerbation of idiopathic pulmonary fibrosis. Am J Respir Crit Care Med 2008;178:372–8.

43. Paraskeva M, McLean C, Ellis S, et al. Acute fibrinoid organizing pneumonia after lung transplantation. Am J Respir Crit Care Med 2013;187:1360–8.

44. Feinstein MB, DeSouza SA, Moreira AL, et al. A comparison of the pathological, clinical and radiographical, features of cryptogenic organising pneumonia, acute fibrinous and organising pneumonia and granulomatous organising pneumonia. J Clin Pathol 2015;68:441–7.

45. Tazelaar HD, Linz LJ, Colby TV, et al. Acute eosinophilic pneumonia: histopathologic findings in nine patients. Am J Respir Crit Care Med 1997;155: 296–302.

46. Mochimaru H, Fukuda Y, Azuma A, et al. Reconsideration of discrepancies between clinical and histopathological features in acute eosinophilic pneumonia. Sarcoidosis Vasc Diffuse Lung Dis 2014;31:325–35.

47. Rhee CK, Min KH, Yim NY, et al. Clinical characteristics and corticosteroid treatment of acute eosinophilic pneumonia. Eur Respir J 2013;41:402–9.

48. Uchiyama H, Suda T, Nakamura Y, et al. Alterations in smoking habits are associated with acute eosinophilic pneumonia. Chest 2008;133:1174–80.

Imaging of Pulmonary Hypertension

Christopher J. François, MD*, Mark L. Schiebler, MD

KEYWORDS

- Pulmonary hypertension • Pulmonary arterial hypertension
- Chronic thromboembolic pulmonary hypertension • Systemic sclerosis • Cor pulmonale
- Magnetic resonance imaging • Computed tomography

KEY POINTS

- Pulmonary hypertension from worsening of left ventricular function is a common disease and is becoming more of a public health issue as the world's population ages.
- The critical issue with all noninvasive imaging modalities is that there is no ability to measure pulmonary artery pressure.
- Noninvasive imaging has a critical role in the initial diagnosis and follow-up of patients with pulmonary hypertension.
- Computed tomography and magnetic resonance (MR) imaging can help identify the specific cause of pulmonary hypertension.
- Cardiac MR imaging is increasingly used to assess the impact of pulmonary hypertension treatment on right ventricular function.

INTRODUCTION

Pulmonary hypertension (PH) is a diverse group of entities that affect the pulmonary vasculature. These diseases can secondarily affect the right heart by causing a chronic increase in right heart pressure, or primary heart disease of the left ventricle (LV) can be a secondary cause of PH.[1,2] PH is defined as a mean pulmonary artery pressure (mPAP) of 25 mm Hg or greater, determined from right heart catheterization. Further classification of PH is based on additional hemodynamic parameters, including cardiac output and pulmonary capillary wedge pressure. The most recent update to the classification of the different categories of PH is based on conditions that have similar hemodynamic and pathologic findings and management.[3] Five groups are included in the updated classification from 2013 (Table 1):

group 1 (pulmonary arterial hypertension [PAH]), group 2 (PH secondary to left heart disease), group 3 (PH secondary to diffuse lung disease or chronic hypoxia), group 4 (chronic thromboembolic PH [CTEPH]), and group 5 (PH caused by unclear or multifactorial mechanisms).

A complete analysis of the clinical presentation, treatment, and all the subtypes of PH and their respective imaging findings is beyond the scope of this article. Imaging often provides the initial evidence that PH may be present and can help to identify the specific cause of PH in many cases. It is important to recognize that PH secondary to left heart disease (group 2) is the most common cause of PH[4] and to be aware of specific radiological findings that can have a critical impact on management, such as CTEPH, pulmonary veno-occlusive disease (PVOD), and pulmonary capillary hemangiomatosis (PCH). Furthermore, cross-sectional imaging is

Disclosure: The authors have nothing to disclose.
Department of Radiology, University of Wisconsin – Madison, 600 Highland Avenue, E1/Clinical Science Center, Madison, WI 53792, USA
* Corresponding author.
E-mail address: cfrancois@uwhealth.org

Radiol Clin N Am 54 (2016) 1133–1149
http://dx.doi.org/10.1016/j.rcl.2016.05.011
0033-8389/16/$ – see front matter © 2016 Elsevier Inc. All rights reserved.

Table 1
2013 Classification of PH

Group	Type	Examples
1	PAH	Idiopathic PAH; heritable PAH; drug-induced PAH; PAH associated with CTD, HIV, portal hypertension, CHD, schistosomiasis
1′	PVOD PCH	—
1″	PPHN	—
2	PH 2° to left heart disease	LV systolic dysfunction; LV diastolic dysfunction; valvular disease; cardiomyopathies
3	PH 2° to lung disease and/or hypoxia	COPD, ILD, sleep apnea, altitude, and so forth
4	CTEPH	—
5	Unclear cause or multifactorial	Hematological diseases, systemic diseases, and so forth

Abbreviations: CHD, congenital heart disease; COPD, chronic obstructive pulmonary disease; CTD, connective tissue disease; CTEPH, chronic thromboembolic PH; HIV, human immunodeficiency virus; ILD, interstitial lung disease; PAH, pulmonary arterial hypertension; PCH, pulmonary capillary hemangiomatosis; PPHN, persistent PH of newborn; PVOD, pulmonary veno-occlusive disease.

Adapted from Simonneau G, Gatzoulis MA, Adatia I, et al. Updated clinical classification of pulmonary hypertension. J Am Coll Cardiol 2013;62:D34–41.

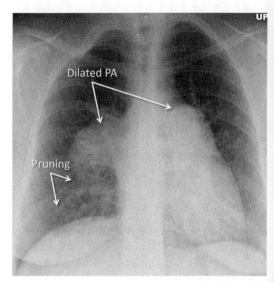

Fig. 1. Frontal chest radiograph of a patient with PAH (group 1) secondary to uncorrected atrial septal defect. The central PAs are severely dilated and there is abrupt tapering of the branch pulmonary arteries resulting in a pruning appearance.

used to assess the right ventricle (RV) and measure the effects of PH on RV function. The underlying pathophysiology and the roles of right heart catheterization, pulmonary angiography, and PET in PH are not discussed here. This article highlights the use of computed tomography (CT) and magnetic resonance (MR) imaging in the diagnosis and management of PH.

CHEST RADIOGRAPHY

Chest radiographs can detect the characteristic changes in the pulmonary arteries (PAs) and RV in patients with advanced PH.[5,6] The central PAs are typically dilated (**Figs. 1** and **2**) and the right heart (atrium and ventricle) may be enlarged (see **Fig. 2**). Abnormalities in the lungs may be detected with chest radiography in patients with PAH

secondary to systemic sclerosis (SSc) or PH secondary to diffuse lung disease, such as emphysema or diffuse lung disease. Chest radiography is appropriate for the initial evaluation of patients with unexplained dyspnea or symptoms that could be attributable to PH. However, chest radiography is insensitive for the identification of patients with mild to moderate PH.[7]

ECHOCARDIOGRAPHY

Transthoracic two-dimensional (2D) Doppler echocardiography (TTE) is the most commonly used noninvasive imaging modality for estimating PA pressures and assessing cardiac function in PH. TTE can be used to screen for PH and may be appropriate in patients with a family history of PAH, congenital heart disease (CHD) and systemic to pulmonary shunts, portal hypertension, or systemic diseases associated with PH.[8,9] Furthermore, serial TTE is routinely performed to monitor the effects of therapy on estimated PA pressures and cardiac function. However, TTE is limited in its ability to comprehensively and accurately evaluate the entire pulmonary vasculature and RV. TTE is particularly useful in determining whether left heart disease or CHD is the cause of PH, but is more restricted in its ability to completely characterize the extent of disease in other causes of PH.

The systolic PA pressure can be estimated with 2D Doppler (**Fig. 3**) using the simplified Bernoulli equation, $\Delta P = 4v^2$,[10] in which v is the peak velocity of the tricuspid regurgitation (TR) jet. The systolic

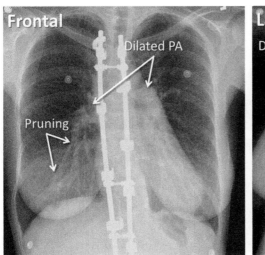
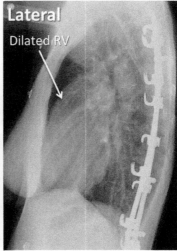

Fig. 2. Frontal and lateral chest radiographs of a patient with idiopathic PAH (group 1). The frontal radiograph confirms dilatation of the central PA and abrupt tapering of the branch PA resulting in a pruning appearance. The lateral radiograph shows an enlarged RV.

PA pressure is then calculated by adding the result of the simplified Bernoulli equation to the estimate of right atrial pressure, determined from the size and collapsibility of the inferior vena cava during respiration.[2,10] Systolic PA pressure calculated in this way correlates well with pressures measured invasively. However, substantial differences between noninvasive and invasive pressure measurements are frequent. Causes of inaccurate PA pressure measurement with TTE include poor acoustic windows, Doppler alignment with the TR jet, observer variability in measuring the peak TR velocity, and breakdown in the assumptions inherent in the simplified Bernoulli equation.

In spite of these limitations of TTE in the estimation of PA pressure, TTE remains critical in the initial assessment and follow-up of patients with suspected or known PH. In addition to the estimate of systolic PA pressure, an initial assessment of patients with PH with TTE includes an evaluation of RV size and function, evaluation of the left heart for signs of left heart disease, and an evaluation for intracardiac shunts.[9] In patients with established PH, TTE is frequently relied on to detect the onset of RV dysfunction because of the relationship between progressive RV dysfunction and morbidity and mortality.[11]

VENTILATION/PERFUSION SCANNING

Ventilation/perfusion (V/Q) scanning is recommended in the evaluation of patients with unexplained PH, primarily to identify patients who may have CTEPH (Fig. 4). CTEPH occurs in up to 3.8% of

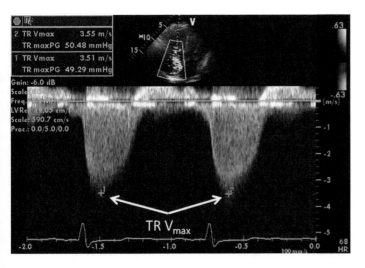

Fig. 3. In this patient with PAH (group 1) secondary to SSc, Doppler echocardiography was used to estimate the systolic PA pressure from the peak velocity (V_{max}) of the tricuspid regurgitation (TR) jet. Using the modified Bernoulli equation in this example, the systolic PA pressure would be approximately 53 to 54 mm Hg assuming that right atrial pressure is 4 mm Hg.

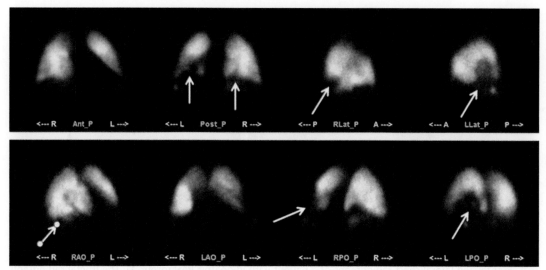

Fig. 4. In this patient with PH, V/Q scanning confirms the presence of segmental perfusion defects (*arrows*) consistent with chronic thromboembolic PH.

patients following an initial acute pulmonary embolism and is more common in patients with multiple thromboembolic events.[12] Because of the serious morbidity and mortality associated with CTEPH and the potential for significant improvement after pulmonary endarterectomy,[13] if identified appropriately, the accurate diagnosis of CTEPH is imperative. V/Q scanning has sensitivity greater than 96% and specificity greater than 90%[14,15] when interpreted using the modified PIOPED (Prospective Investigation of Pulmonary Embolism Diagnosis) criteria. CTEPH can be excluded with a sensitivity of 90% to 100% and specificity of 94% to 100% if the V/Q scan is normal or of low probability.[16]

COMPUTED TOMOGRAPHY
Computed Tomography Techniques

Noncontrast CT (NCCT) and CT angiography (CTA) are routinely used in the clinical evaluation and management of patients with PH. CT is indicated for the evaluation of the lungs in patients with chronic unexplained dyspnea.[7] NCCT is used to assess the extent and severity of diffuse lung diseases (**Fig. 5**)[17,18] and chronic obstructive pulmonary disease.[19–22] NCCT is also helpful in identifying pulmonary arteriovenous malformations (AVMs), PVOD, and PCH. CTA, which requires the intravenous administration of iodinated contrast material, has become the reference standard for the diagnosis of acute pulmonary embolism given its ability to routinely assess main, lobar, segmental, and subsegmental PAs.

However, the role of CTA in CTEPH is less well established.

New-generation CT scanners have the ability to perform dual-energy CT (DECT), either with 2 x-ray sources and 2 detectors (dual-source CT [DSCT]) or with a single x-ray source and single detector. Single-source DECT is performed with advanced, rapidly switching kilovoltage at the x-ray tube anode and with advanced detectors that can simultaneously separate photons with different energies. DECT allows the scanner to quantitatively characterize the soft tissue material properties. In patients with PH, DECT has been used to acquire quantitative lung perfusion and pulmonary blood volume maps, using a standard pulmonary CTA acquisition.[23–26]

Characterization of Pulmonary Hypertension Causes

Both NCCT and CTA can accurately characterize specific causes of PH. In emphysema, CT characterizes the type of emphysema, the presence of airway disease, and secondary features associated with smoking-related pulmonary disease.[19–22,27–29] Recently developed quantitative CT methods of assessing emphysema severity correlate with clinical[30–33] and histologic[34–36] parameters. Pulmonary AVMs can be accurately detected with CT. Pulmonary AVMs appear as a nodular opacity with a feeding artery and a draining vein (**Fig. 6**).[37,38] In most patients with hereditary hemorrhagic telangiectasia, NCCT is sufficient and CTA is not necessary in the identification of pulmonary AVMs. CTA is typically necessary

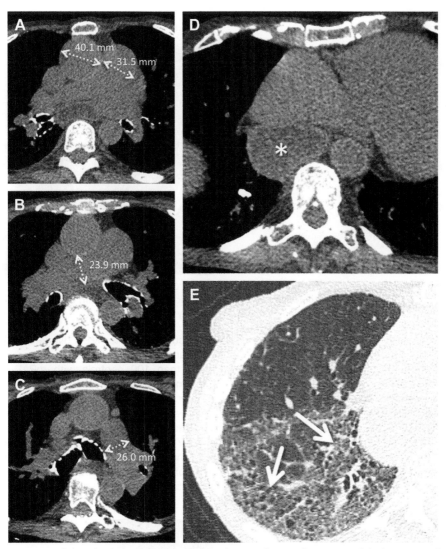

Fig. 5. Noncontrast-enhanced CT of a patient with PAH (group 1) secondary to SSc. (*A*) The main pulmonary artery (MPA)/ascending aorta (AAo) ratio is less than 1 because the AAo is dilated (4.0 cm). However, the (*B*) right pulmonary artery and (*C*) left pulmonary artery are all dilated. Other findings of SSc include (*D*) patulous esophagus (*asterisk*) and (*E*) pulmonary fibrosis (*arrows*).

only in characterizing larger pulmonary AVMs or to help determine the success of embolization therapy for this disorder.[39] The CT findings in PVOD and PCH (group 1′) reflect the underlying hemodynamic alterations. The distinction of PVOD and PCH (presence of smooth septal lines, geographic and nodular ground-glass opacities, and pleural effusions; **Fig. 7**)[40,41] from other causes of PH is critical to ensuring appropriate treatment and evaluation for lung transplant. The diagnosis of PVOD is critical, because the pharmacologic therapy for PH uses agents that dilate the pulmonary arterial vascular bed. These agents can in turn cause a catastrophic collapse in perfusion pressure to the

left heart in cases of PVOD, potentially resulting in death. CTA abnormalities suggestive of CTEPH are present in approximately 90% of patients[42] and include right ventricular hypertrophy, interventricular septal straightening, complete PA luminal obstruction, intimal irregularities, bands, webs (**Fig. 8**), mural thrombus (**Fig. 9**), and mosaic lung attenuation (**Fig. 10**).

Characterization of Pulmonary Hypertension Severity

Dilatation of the main, right, and left PAs is the most conspicuous finding on CT (see **Fig. 5**). Other

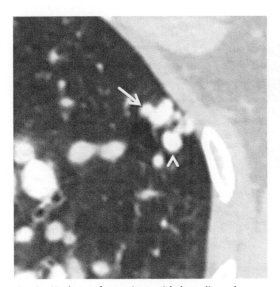

Fig. 6. CT chest of a patient with hereditary hemor-rhagic telangiectasia and multiple pulmonary AVMs. Lung windows show an arteriovenous malformation with feeding artery (*arrow*) and draining vein (*arrow-head*) in the anterior left upper lobe.

findings of PH include calcification, tortuosity, and rapid tapering of the PAs. RV dilatation and hyper-trophy, flattening or bowing of the interventricular septum (**Figs. 11** and **12**), reflux of intravenous contrast into the hepatic veins, and bronchial artery dilatation of the bronchial arteries are addi-tional CT findings of PH. Data from the Framing-ham Heart Study indicate that the normal main PA (MPA) diameter is 25.1 ± 2.8 mm and the

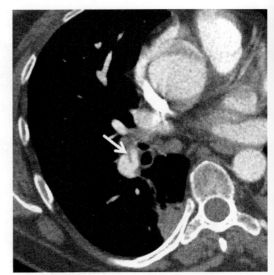

Fig. 8. CTA chest of a patient with chronic thrombo-embolic PH reveals a web in the right lower lobe pul-monary artery (*arrow*).

90% cutoff value for MPA diameter is 29 mm in men and 27 mm in women.[43] From a study in more than 100 controls with mPAP less than 25 mm Hg and nearly 300 subjects with mPAP greater than 25 mm Hg, Mahammedi and col-leagues[44] concluded that mean MPA diameter in patients without PH is 25.7 ± 0.4 mm in women and 27.5 ± 0.5 mm in men, with a threshold of 29.0 mm having a sensitivity of 52% and speci-ficity of 90% for the prediction of mPAP greater than 25 mm Hg.

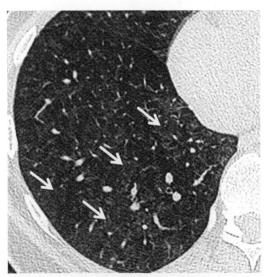

Fig. 7. Noncontrast chest CT of a patient with PCH re-veals diffuse centrilobular ground-glass opacities (several representative areas are indicated with *arrows*).

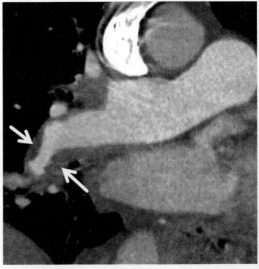

Fig. 9. Multiplanar reformatted CTA images of a pa-tient with chronic thromboembolic PH shows chronic mural thrombus in the right lower lobe pulmonary ar-tery (*arrows*).

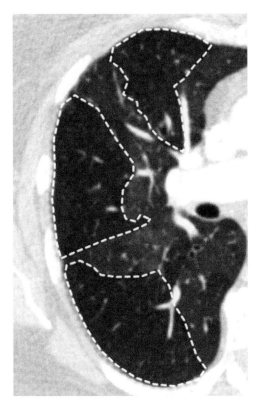

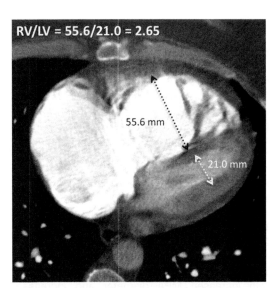

Fig. 10. CT chest of a patient with chronic thromboembolic PH shows mosaic lung attenuation caused by heterogeneous lung perfusion with darker areas enclosed by the dashed lines indicating hypoperfusion.

Fig. 12. CTA chest of a patient with idiopathic PAH (group 1). The RV is dilated and the RV to LV diameter ratio (2.65) is greater than 1.

Another method of assessing MPA size is to compare the MPA diameter with the diameter of the ascending aorta (AAo) (Fig. 13). In the Framingham Heart Study, MPA/AAo diameter ratio was 0.77 ± 0.09, with a 90% cutoff value for MPA/AAo ratio of 0.9 in both men and women.[43] Mahammedi and colleagues[44] reported that an MPA/AAo ratio greater than 1.0 was 70.8% sensitive and 76.5% specific in predicting mPAP greater than 25 mm Hg. The problem with using

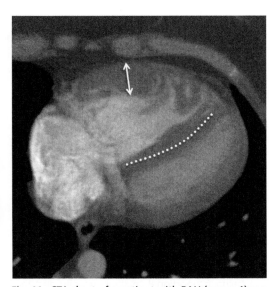

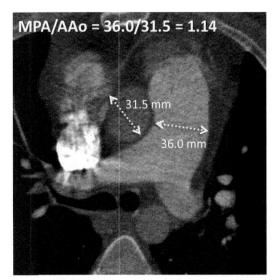

Fig. 11. CTA chest of a patient with PAH (group 1) secondary to CHD. CTA of the chest shows severe right ventricular free wall hypertrophy (double arrow) and bowing of the interventricular septum to the left (dashed line).

Fig. 13. CT chest of a patient with PAH (group 1) with multiple findings of chronic increased pulmonary arterial pressures. The MPA diameter is greater than 33 mm, the MPA/AAo diameter ratio is greater than 1, and the RV/LV diameter ratio is greater than 1.

aortic measurements in the diagnosis of PH by CT is that diseases unrelated to PH can cause dilatation of the ascending aorta (see Fig. 5).

Increased MPA and RV diameters and increased MPA/AAo and RV/LV ratios are correlated with increased pulmonary vascular resistance in patients with PAH secondary to SSc (group 1 PAH).[45] However, these CT-based metrics are less predictive of PAH severity than MR imaging and TTE-based metrics.[46]

Kam and colleagues[47] reported that patients with group 2 PH (PH secondary to left heart disease) have larger MPA diameters (mild to moderate PH, 34.9 ± 1.0 mm; severe PH, 38.3 ± 0.9 mm) than those without PH (27.4 ± 0.9 mm).

Iyer and colleagues[48] reported that patients with group 3 PH (PH secondary to lung disease) have both increased MPA diameter and increased MPA/AAo ratio, with MPA/AAo greater than 1 being most strongly correlated with increased systolic PA pressure in multivariate analysis. Additional parameters that are highly associated with PH include enlarged descending right and left PAs, thickened RV free wall, increased RV/LV wall thickness ratio, and increased RV/LV diameter ratios.[49] Caution is needed when using MPA dilatation as a criterion for PH in patients with pulmonary fibrosis, because MPA dilatation can occur in the absence of PH in patients with chronic pulmonary disease.[50]

Although the Qanadli and Mastora indices[51] have been developed to quantify the overall obstructive burden of chronic pulmonary emboli in patients with group 4 PH (CTEPH), these CTA measures of PA obstruction do not correlate with RV function or pulmonary vascular resistance in these patients.[51,52] MPA diameter, RV/LV diameter ratio, and RV wall thickness have been found to be correlated with mPAP in CTEPH.[51]

MAGNETIC RESONANCE IMAGING
Magnetic Resonance Imaging Techniques

The wide variety of techniques available to assess anatomy and function is an advantage of MR imaging, relative to other imaging modalities. This variety includes MR angiography (MRA) sequences for PA anatomy, MR imaging perfusion and flow sequences for pulmonary blood flow quantification, and cardiac MR imaging sequences for cardiac morphology and function. Pulmonary MRA is primarily performed using contrast-enhanced MRA techniques (Fig. 14) because of the much faster acquisition times relative to non–contrast-enhanced MRA techniques. With current, commercially available, accelerated acquisition

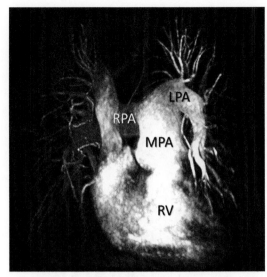

Fig. 14. Contrast-enhanced MRA of a patient with PAH (group 1) showing dilated central pulmonary arteries and abrupt tapering (pruning) of the segmental pulmonary arteries.

techniques it is now routinely feasible to obtain whole-chest, high-spatial-resolution images in a short (15–18 seconds) breath hold.[53]

Dynamic contrast-enhanced (DCE) MR imaging using advanced image acceleration methods have been used to qualitatively and quantitatively measure global and regional pulmonary perfusion.[54–64] DCE MR imaging for quantitative lung perfusion is usually performed during the first pass of contrast through the pulmonary vasculature and with a breath hold, although free-breathing DCE MR imaging methods are also available.[65,66] Although DCE MR imaging methods are primarily used for lung perfusion, non–contrast-enhanced lung perfusion methods have also been investigated.[67–69] There are methods currently under investigation for the evaluation of lung structure and function using MR imaging. These methods include ultrashort echo time perfusion acquisitions,[70] Fourier decomposition MR imaging,[71] and combining DCE MR imaging lung perfusion scans with hyperpolarized gas for ventilation imaging using MR imaging.[72]

PA blood flow can also be measured using 2D phase contrast (PC) flow MR imaging sequences.[73] 2D PC MR imaging quantifies flow based on the phase shifts induced by magnetic field gradients, with the phase shifts in moving protons being proportional to their velocity and the strength of the velocity encoding gradient that is used. The 2D PC MR imaging sequence can be prescribed such that it is sensitive to flow through the plane or within the plan of acquisition. For quantitative 2D PC MR imaging, flow sensitivity is set up to be through the imaging plane, with the most accurate quantification achieved when the imaging plane is perpendicular to the vessel of interest. With newer hardware and faster MR imaging acquisition techniques, 2D PC MR imaging has been extended to time-resolved, three-dimensional (3D), three-directional flow-sensitive acquisitions, typically referred to as four-dimensional (4D) flow MR imaging.[74]

Cardiac MR (CMR) imaging has become the standard of reference for quantifying RV size and function[75,76] using electrocardiographically gated, cine balanced, steady state free precession (bSSFP) sequences. RV size and function can be quantified from short-axis or transaxial bSSFP images. The transaxial orientation has been shown to have improved reproducibility and precision for the measurements of RV volumes and RV ejection fraction.[77] Additional CMR techniques that have been used to characterize the changes in the myocardium in patients with PH include T1 mapping, late gadolinium enhancement (LGE), and myocardial strain imaging. Myocardial T1 mapping is an approach to measuring the T1 recovery characteristics of the heart, which are determined by the exponential time constant for MR imaging longitudinal relaxation.[78] LGE CMR is performed using inversion recovery prepared spoiled gradient echo or bSSFP sequences and can be acquired as multiple 2D acquisitions or using 3D techniques.

Characterization of Pulmonary Hypertension Causes

Indications for using MR imaging to establish the cause of PH is primarily limited to evaluating for the possibility of CHD with left-to-right shunts, such as atrial and ventricular septal defects and patent ductus arteriosus. In addition to cine bSSFP imaging for cardiac morphology and function, the evaluation of known or potential CHD includes pulmonary MRA and 2D flow MR imaging through the MPA and AAo to calculate the pulmonary to systemic flow (Qp/Qs) ratio.

Although the use of contrast-enhanced pulmonary MRA in the detection of acute pulmonary thromboembolism is well established,[53,79] its use in confirming the diagnosis of CTEPH or other causes of PH is not established. Compared with CTA and V/Q scanning, DCE MRA is highly sensitive and specific for the diagnosis of CTEPH.[80]

Characterization of Pulmonary Hypertension Severity

Increasing evidence is now available supporting the use of MR imaging in measuring the effects of PH on PA hemodynamics and RV function (**Figs. 15** and **16**). Because of the importance of RV function in determining prognosis in PH,[81] CMR in particular is having an increasing role in the management of PH. Increased RV end-diastolic and end-systolic volumes and decreased RV ejection fraction indicate the changes that are associated with a poorer prognosis in patients with PH, despite optimized medical therapy. As systolic PA pressures increase, RV systolic pressure can be greater than LV systolic pressure, which can impede LV function because of shifting of the interventricular septum into the LV outflow tract[82] and asynchrony of the RV and LV.[83,84] With more severe and prolonged PH, RV diastolic function can also be impaired, leading to flattening or bowing of the interventricular septum during diastole and impaired LV filling (**Fig. 17**). The dynamic changes that occur in the function of the interventricular septum are hypothesized to be a cause for the fibrosis and abnormal LGE that is present at the RV insertion points.[85,86]

Numerous studies have documented the clinical utility of 2D PC MR imaging in patients with PH. Peak systolic MPA flow is more spatially heterogeneous, with a greater degree of retrograde flow.[87] Subsequently, other investigators confirmed that patients with PH have reduced pulmonary blood flow velocities, volumes, and distensibility,[88,89] and increased retrograde flow.[89–91]

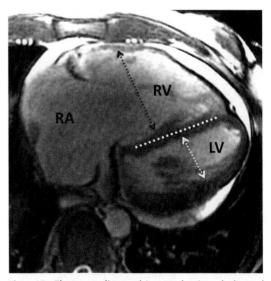

Fig. 15. Electrocardiographic-gated cine balanced steady state free precession imaging is used to assess right ventricular size, thickness, and function in patients with PH. In this patient with PAH (group 1), the RV is dilated and the RV/LV diameter ratio is greater than 1.

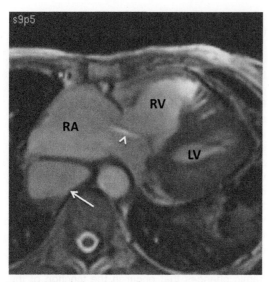

Fig. 16. Cine balanced steady state free precession image from end systole shows TR (*arrowhead*), dilated RV and right atrium (RA), RV/LV diameter ratio greater than 1, and patulous esophagus (*arrow*).

The distensibility of the MPA is defined as the relative change in the cross-sectional area of the MPA throughout the cardiac cycle multiplied by the pulse pressure required to induce that change. Because the MPA pulse pressure is typically not known, the pulsatility, or relative area change (RAC; RAC = $\frac{\text{CSA}_{max} - \text{CSA}_{min}}{\text{CSA}_{min}}$, in which CSA_{max} and

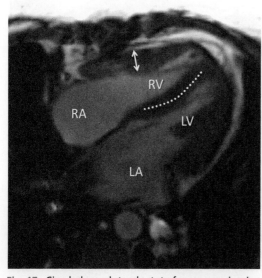

Fig. 17. Cine balanced steady state free precession image from end diastole shows a thickened (*double arrow*) RV and bowing of the interventricular septum to the left (*dashed line*). LA, left atrium.

CSA_{min} are the maximum and minimum MPA cross-sectional areas, respectively), is used as a surrogate marker of MPA stiffness (**Fig. 18**).[92] Decreased MPA RAC indicates increased MPA stiffening and is associated with increased mortality.[93] Recently, Forouzan and colleagues[94] reported on the use of exercise stress CMR to measure the changes in MPA RAC, and a surrogate of MPA stiffness. The methodology described by these investigators offers the opportunity to better understand the mechanisms that lead to exercise-induced PH[95] and exercise tolerance in patients with PH. Furthermore, these techniques could help bridge the gap in the understanding of the mechanisms for developing PH in patients with left heart disease.[4]

MPA RAC can be combined with right heart catheterization hemodynamic data to calculate additional indices of proximal PA stiffness, including compliance, distensibility, elastic modulus, and stiffness index (β).[92,96] Essentially all categories of PH result in proximal PA stiffening and contribute to progressive RV dysfunction.

Another noninvasive correlate of MPA stiffness is the pulse wave velocity, which is the rate at which the systolic wave propagates through the vasculature, in the central PAs.[97,98] Because of the short length of the MPA and the low temporal resolution of MR imaging, the pulse wave velocity in the MPA is typically estimated using the flow-area method.[94,98]

The severity of TR can also be quantified with 2D PC MR imaging. From the peak TR velocity, the peak systolic pulmonary artery pressure can be estimated using the simplified Bernoulli equation, analogous to the method used in Doppler TTE (**Fig. 19**).

4D flow MR imaging has been used to assess the hemodynamic changes in the pulmonary circulation, including in studies of PH.[99–103] One of the most striking findings on 4D flow MR imaging in PH is the development of an abnormal vortex in the MPA (**Fig. 20**),[99,100] with the persistence of the vortices being related to the mPAP at right heart catheterization[100] and the degree of vorticity being associated with multiple TTE measures of RV dysfunction.[102] In a canine model of acute thromboembolic PH, 4D flow MR imaging was used to comprehensively quantify RV and LV function, MPA and AAo flow, and tricuspid valve regurgitation velocity.[101] Another parameter that can be estimated with 4D flow MR imaging is MPA wall shear stress (WSS),[103] which has been reported to affect smooth muscle tone through mechanical transduction and influence on vascular remodeling.[104–106] A recently published 2 center study using 4D flow MR imaging in subjects with PH found

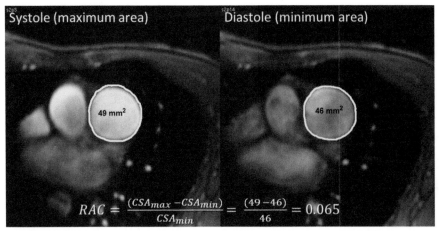

Fig. 18. Stiffening of the proximal PA is reflected in decreased RAC in CSA, which can be quantified from electrocardiographic-gated cine images through the central pulmonary arteries.

that MPA WSS was significantly lower ($P<.05$) in patients with PH compared with healthy volunteers.[103] Prolonged pulmonary mean transit time and decreased pulmonary blood flow measured with DCE MR imaging are more common in patients with PH[61,107] and are associated with poorer outcomes.[108]

Abnormal midmyocardial LGE, especially at the insertion points of the RV on the interventricular septum (Fig. 21), is a frequent finding in PH. Swift and colleagues[109] reported that more than 80% of patients with PH have some degree of LGE and almost 30% have LGE involving the RV insertion points and interventricular septum. The presence of LGE in PH is strongly associated with increased MPA pressures, RV dilatation, and RV hypertrophy,[110] with LGE involving the interventricular septum being more strongly associated with other indices of RV failure.[109] More importantly, an increased incidence of adverse outcomes is associated with the presence of abnormal LGE.[111] Similarly, T1-mapping studies have reported a strong correlation between RV dysfunction and T1 values at the interventricular septum RV insertion points.[112] The role of T1 mapping in the detection of changes in T1 values within the hypertrophied RV free wall may be of greater significance.[113,114]

Addetia and colleagues[115] reported that, owing to its superior reproducibility in measuring RV volumes and function, CMR can be used effectively with lower costs compared with TTE. Other smaller[116] and larger[76] trials have begun to use MR imaging to study the effects of PH therapy on the RV.

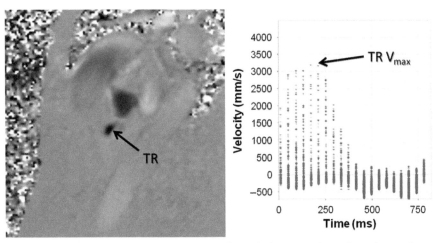

Fig. 19. Two-dimensional flow-sensitive, PC MR imaging through the TR jet (*arrow*) can be used to estimate the systolic pulmonary artery pressure from the TR V_{max}.

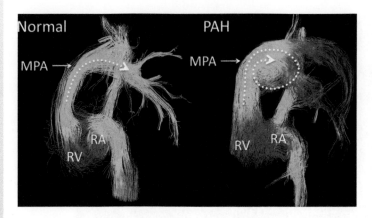

Fig. 20. 4D flow MR imaging in normal vessels and PAH showing smooth, laminar flow in the MPA of the healthy volunteer (*dashed arrow*) and abnormal vortex formation in the MPA in the patient with PAH (*dashed arrow*).

SUMMARY

At present, the 6-minute walk distance (6MWD) is used to monitor the effects of treatment on PH,[117] but in a recent meta-analysis of more than 20 clinical trials the 6MWD was not found to be predictive of outcomes.[118] Therefore, additional quantitative, imaging-based markers of PH severity that can be used to document response to therapy are increasingly being used in clinical trials and clinically.

Multimodality diagnostic imaging continues to have an integral role in the evaluation and management of PH. Both MR imaging and CT are valuable in determining the cause and are helping to noninvasively study the pathophysiology of PH. These methods are also increasingly being used to guide

the management and follow-up of these patients after medical and/or surgical therapy. Advances in CT perfusion, MR imaging perfusion, MR imaging tissue characterization, and 4D flow MR imaging open new opportunities for these modalities to improve the understanding of the vascular biology in PH, enhance clinical trials using new therapies, and improve patient outcomes for this deadly disease.

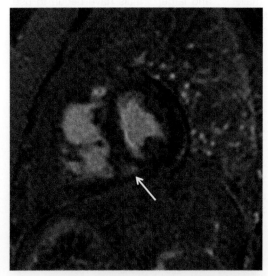

Fig. 21. LGE MR imaging of a patient with PAH (group 1) secondary to SSc. LGE is present in the inferior interventricular septum at the insertion of the right ventricular free wall (*arrow*).

REFERENCES

1. McLaughlin VV, Shah SJ, Souza R, et al. Management of pulmonary arterial hypertension. J Am Coll Cardiol 2015;65:1976–97.
2. Shah SJ. Pulmonary hypertension. JAMA 2012; 308:1366–74.
3. Simonneau G, Gatzoulis MA, Adatia I, et al. Updated clinical classification of pulmonary hypertension. J Am Coll Cardiol 2013;62:D34–41.
4. Vachiery JL, Adir Y, Barbera JA, et al. Pulmonary hypertension due to left heart diseases. J Am Coll Cardiol 2013;62:D100–8.
5. Matthay RA, Schwarz MI, Ellis JH Jr, et al. Pulmonary artery hypertension in chronic obstructive pulmonary disease: determination by chest radiography. Invest Radiol 1981;16:95–100.
6. Schmidt HC, Kauczor HU, Schild HH, et al. Pulmonary hypertension in patients with chronic pulmonary thromboembolism: chest radiograph and CT evaluation before and after surgery. Eur Radiol 1996;6:817–25.
7. Brown K, Gutierrez AJ, Mohammed TL, et al. ACR Appropriateness Criteria® pulmonary hypertension. J Thorac Imaging 2013;28:W57–60.
8. Barst RJ, McGoon M, Torbicki A, et al. Diagnosis and differential assessment of pulmonary arterial hypertension. J Am Coll Cardiol 2004; 43:40S–7S.
9. McGoon M, Gutterman D, Steen V, et al. Screening, early detection, and diagnosis of pulmonary

arterial hypertension: ACCP evidence-based clinical practice guidelines. Chest 2004;126:14S–34S.

10. Rudski LG, Lai WW, Afilalo J, et al. Guidelines for the echocardiographic assessment of the right heart in adults: a report from the American Society of Echocardiography endorsed by the European Association of Echocardiography, a registered branch of the European Society of Cardiology, and the Canadian Society of Echocardiography. J Am Soc Echocardiogr 2010;23:685–713 [quiz: 786–8].

11. Sanchez O, Trinquart L, Colombet I, et al. Prognostic value of right ventricular dysfunction in patients with haemodynamically stable pulmonary embolism: a systematic review. Eur Heart J 2008; 29:1569–77.

12. Pengo V, Lensing AW, Prins MH, et al. Incidence of chronic thromboembolic pulmonary hypertension after pulmonary embolism. N Engl J Med 2004; 350:2257–64.

13. Madani MM, Auger WR, Pretorius V, et al. Pulmonary endarterectomy: recent changes in a single institution's experience of more than 2,700 patients. Ann Thorac Surg 2012;94:97–103 [discussion: 103].

14. Tunariu N, Gibbs SJ, Win Z, et al. Ventilation-perfusion scintigraphy is more sensitive than multidetector CTPA in detecting chronic thromboembolic pulmonary disease as a treatable cause of pulmonary hypertension. J Nucl Med 2007;48:680–4.

15. He J, Fang W, Lv B, et al. Diagnosis of chronic thromboembolic pulmonary hypertension: comparison of ventilation/perfusion scanning and multidetector computed tomography pulmonary angiography with pulmonary angiography. Nucl Med Commun 2012;33:459–63.

16. Galie N, Hoeper MM, Humbert M, et al. Guidelines for the diagnosis and treatment of pulmonary hypertension: the Task Force for the Diagnosis and Treatment of Pulmonary Hypertension of the European Society of Cardiology (ESC) and the European Respiratory Society (ERS), endorsed by the International Society of Heart and Lung Transplantation (ISHLT). Eur Heart J 2009;30:2493–537.

17. Mueller-Mang C, Grosse C, Schmid K, et al. What every radiologist should know about idiopathic interstitial pneumonias. Radiographics 2007;27: 595–615.

18. Ferguson EC, Berkowitz EA. Lung CT: part 2, the interstitial pneumonias–clinical, histologic, and CT manifestations. AJR Am J Roentgenol 2012;199: W464–76.

19. Lynch DA, Austin JH, Hogg JC, et al. CT-definable subtypes of chronic obstructive pulmonary disease: a statement of the Fleischner Society. Radiology 2015;277:192–205.

20. Smith BM, Austin JH, Newell JD Jr, et al. Pulmonary emphysema subtypes on computed tomography: the MESA COPD study. Am J Med 2014;127(94): e7–23.

21. Klein JS, Gamsu G, Webb WR, et al. High-resolution CT diagnosis of emphysema in symptomatic patients with normal chest radiographs and isolated low diffusing capacity. Radiology 1992;182: 817–21.

22. McDonough JE, Yuan R, Suzuki M, et al. Small-airway obstruction and emphysema in chronic obstructive pulmonary disease. N Engl J Med 2011;365:1567–75.

23. Nakazawa T, Watanabe Y, Hori Y, et al. Lung perfused blood volume images with dual-energy computed tomography for chronic thromboembolic pulmonary hypertension: correlation to scintigraphy with single-photon emission computed tomography. J Comput Assist Tomogr 2011;35: 590–5.

24. Ameli-Renani S, Rahman F, Nair A, et al. Dual-energy CT for imaging of pulmonary hypertension: challenges and opportunities. Radiographics 2014;34:1769–90.

25. Ameli-Renani S, Ramsay L, Bacon JL, et al. Dual-energy computed tomography in the assessment of vascular and parenchymal enhancement in suspected pulmonary hypertension. J Thorac Imaging 2014;29:98–106.

26. Dournes G, Verdier D, Montaudon M, et al. Dual-energy CT perfusion and angiography in chronic thromboembolic pulmonary hypertension: diagnostic accuracy and concordance with radionuclide scintigraphy. Eur Radiol 2014;24:42–51.

27. Mets OM, Schmidt M, Buckens CF, et al. Diagnosis of chronic obstructive pulmonary disease in lung cancer screening computed tomography scans: independent contribution of emphysema, air trapping and bronchial wall thickening. Respir Res 2013;14:59.

28. Schroeder JD, McKenzie AS, Zach JA, et al. Relationships between airflow obstruction and quantitative CT measurements of emphysema, air trapping, and airways in subjects with and without chronic obstructive pulmonary disease. AJR Am J Roentgenol 2013;201:W460–70.

29. Mohamed Hoesein FA, Schmidt M, Mets OM, et al. Discriminating dominant computed tomography phenotypes in smokers without or with mild COPD. Respir Med 2014;108:136–43.

30. Galban CJ, Han MK, Boes JL, et al. Computed tomography-based biomarker provides unique signature for diagnosis of COPD phenotypes and disease progression. Nat Med 2012;18:1711–5.

31. Group COCW, Barr RG, Berkowitz EA, et al. A combined pulmonary-radiology workshop for visual evaluation of COPD: study design, chest CT findings and concordance with quantitative evaluation. COPD 2012;9:151–9.

32. Martinez CH, Chen YH, Westgate PM, et al. Relationship between quantitative CT metrics and health status and BODE in chronic obstructive pulmonary disease. Thorax 2012;67:399–406.

33. Mohamed Hoesein FA, de Jong PA, Lammers JW, et al. Contribution of CT quantified emphysema, air trapping and airway wall thickness on pulmonary function in male smokers with and without COPD. COPD 2014;11:503–9.

34. Muller NL, Staples CA, Miller RR, et al. "Density mask". An objective method to quantitate emphysema using computed tomography. Chest 1988; 94:782–7.

35. Coxson HO, Rogers RM, Whittall KP, et al. A quantification of the lung surface area in emphysema using computed tomography. Am J Respir Crit Care Med 1999;159:851–6.

36. Madani A, Zanen J, de Maertelaer V, et al. Pulmonary emphysema: objective quantification at multi-detector row CT–comparison with macroscopic and microscopic morphometry. Radiology 2006;238:1036–43.

37. Cottin V, Chinet T, Lavole A, et al. Pulmonary arteriovenous malformations in hereditary hemorrhagic telangiectasia: a series of 126 patients. Medicine (Baltimore) 2007;86:1–17.

38. Cottin V, Plauchu H, Bayle JY, et al. Pulmonary arteriovenous malformations in patients with hereditary hemorrhagic telangiectasia. Am J Respir Crit Care Med 2004;169:994–1000.

39. Remy J, Remy-Jardin M, Wattinne L, et al. Pulmonary arteriovenous malformations: evaluation with CT of the chest before and after treatment. Radiology 1992;182:809–16.

40. Resten A, Maitre S, Humbert M, et al. Pulmonary hypertension: CT of the chest in pulmonary venoocclusive disease. AJR Am J Roentgenol 2004;183: 65–70.

41. Frazier AA, Franks TJ, Mohammed TL, et al. From the archives of the AFIP: pulmonary veno-occlusive disease and pulmonary capillary hemangiomatosis. Radiographics 2007;27:867–82.

42. Reichelt A, Hoeper MM, Galanski M, et al. Chronic thromboembolic pulmonary hypertension: evaluation with 64-detector row CT versus digital subtraction angiography. Eur J Radiol 2009;71:49–54.

43. Truong QA, Massaro JM, Rogers IS, et al. Reference values for normal pulmonary artery dimensions by noncontrast cardiac computed tomography: the Framingham Heart Study. Circ Cardiovasc Imaging 2012;5:147–54.

44. Mahammedi A, Oshmyansky A, Hassoun PM, et al. Pulmonary artery measurements in pulmonary hypertension: the role of computed tomography. J Thorac Imaging 2013;28:96–103.

45. Condliffe R, Radon M, Hurdman J, et al. CT pulmonary angiography combined with echocardiography in suspected systemic sclerosis-associated pulmonary arterial hypertension. Rheumatology (Oxford) 2011;50:1480–6.

46. Rajaram S, Swift AJ, Capener D, et al. Comparison of the diagnostic utility of cardiac magnetic resonance imaging, computed tomography, and echocardiography in assessment of suspected pulmonary arterial hypertension in patients with connective tissue disease. J Rheumatol 2012;39:1265–74.

47. Kam JC, Pi J, Doraiswamy V, et al. CT scanning in the evaluation of pulmonary hypertension. Lung 2013;191:321–6.

48. Iyer AS, Wells JM, Vishin S, et al. CT scan-measured pulmonary artery to aorta ratio and echocardiography for detecting pulmonary hypertension in severe COPD. Chest 2014;145:824–32.

49. Chan AL, Juarez MM, Shelton DK, et al. Novel computed tomographic chest metrics to detect pulmonary hypertension. BMC Med Imaging 2011;11:7.

50. Devaraj A, Wells AU, Meister MG, et al. The effect of diffuse pulmonary fibrosis on the reliability of CT signs of pulmonary hypertension. Radiology 2008;249:1042–9.

51. Liu M, Ma Z, Guo X, et al. Computed tomographic pulmonary angiography in the assessment of severity of chronic thromboembolic pulmonary hypertension and right ventricular dysfunction. Eur J Radiol 2011;80:e462–9.

52. Liu M, Ma Z, Guo X, et al. Cardiovascular parameters of computed tomographic pulmonary angiography to assess pulmonary vascular resistance in patients with chronic thromboembolic pulmonary hypertension. Int J Cardiol 2013;164:295–300.

53. Schiebler ML, Nagle SK, Francois CJ, et al. Effectiveness of MR angiography for the primary diagnosis of acute pulmonary embolism: clinical outcomes at 3 months and 1 year. J Magn Reson Imaging 2013;38:914–25.

54. Wang K, Schiebler ML, Francois CJ, et al. Pulmonary perfusion MRI using interleaved variable density sampling and HighlY constrained cartesian reconstruction (HYCR). J Magn Reson Imaging 2013;38:751–6.

55. Bell LC, Wang K, Munoz Del Rio A, et al. Comparison of models and contrast agents for improved signal and signal linearity in dynamic contrast-enhanced pulmonary magnetic resonance imaging. Invest Radiol 2015;50:174–8.

56. Silverman JM, Julien PJ, Herfkens RJ, et al. Quantitative differential pulmonary perfusion: MR imaging versus radionuclide lung scanning. Radiology 1993;189:699–701.

57. Hatabu H, Tadamura E, Levin DL, et al. Quantitative assessment of pulmonary perfusion with dynamic contrast-enhanced MRI. Magn Reson Med 1999; 42:1033–8.

58. Fink C, Puderbach M, Ley S, et al. Contrast-enhanced three-dimensional pulmonary perfusion magnetic resonance imaging: intraindividual comparison of 1.0 M gadobutrol and 0.5 M Gd-DTPA at three dose levels. Invest Radiol 2004;39:143–8.

59. Ohno Y, Hatabu H, Murase K, et al. Quantitative assessment of regional pulmonary perfusion in the entire lung using three-dimensional ultrafast dynamic contrast-enhanced magnetic resonance imaging: preliminary experience in 40 subjects. J Magn Reson Imaging 2004;20:353–65.

60. Ley S, Mereles D, Risse F, et al. Quantitative 3D pulmonary MR-perfusion in patients with pulmonary arterial hypertension: correlation with invasive pressure measurements. Eur J Radiol 2007;61:251–5.

61. Ohno Y, Hatabu H, Murase K, et al. Primary pulmonary hypertension: 3D dynamic perfusion MRI for quantitative analysis of regional pulmonary perfusion. AJR Am J Roentgenol 2007;188:48–56.

62. Jang YM, Oh YM, Seo JB, et al. Quantitatively assessed dynamic contrast-enhanced magnetic resonance imaging in patients with chronic obstructive pulmonary disease: correlation of perfusion parameters with pulmonary function test and quantitative computed tomography. Invest Radiol 2008;43:403–10.

63. Oechsner M, Muhlhausler M, Ritter CO, et al. Quantitative contrast-enhanced perfusion measurements of the human lung using the prebolus approach. J Magn Reson Imaging 2009;30:104–11.

64. Hansch A, Kohlmann P, Hinneburg U, et al. Quantitative evaluation of MR perfusion imaging using blood pool contrast agent in subjects without pulmonary diseases and in patients with pulmonary embolism. Eur Radiol 2012;22:1748–56.

65. Maxien D, Ingrisch M, Meinel FG, et al. Quantification of pulmonary perfusion with free-breathing dynamic contrast-enhanced MRI–a pilot study in healthy volunteers. Rofo 2013;185:1175–81.

66. Ingrisch M, Maxien D, Schwab F, et al. Assessment of pulmonary perfusion with breath-hold and free-breathing dynamic contrast-enhanced magnetic resonance imaging: quantification and reproducibility. Invest Radiol 2014;49:382–9.

67. Hatabu H, Tadamura E, Prasad PV, et al. Noninvasive pulmonary perfusion imaging by STAR-HASTE sequence. Magn Reson Med 2000;44:808–12.

68. Bolar DS, Levin DL, Hopkins SR, et al. Quantification of regional pulmonary blood flow using ASL-FAIRER. Magn Reson Med 2006;55:1308–17.

69. Martirosian P, Boss A, Fenchel M, et al. Quantitative lung perfusion mapping at 0.2 T using FAIR True-FISP MRI. Magn Reson Med 2006;55:1065–74.

70. Bell LC, Johnson KM, Fain SB, et al. Simultaneous MRI of lung structure and perfusion in a single breathhold. J Magn Reson Imaging 2015;41:52–9.

71. Kjorstad A, Corteville DM, Fischer A, et al. Quantitative lung perfusion evaluation using Fourier decomposition perfusion MRI. Magn Reson Med 2014;72:558–62.

72. Rizi RR, Saha PK, Wang B, et al. Co-registration of acquired MR ventilation and perfusion images–validation in a porcine model. Magn Reson Med 2003;49:13–8.

73. Gefter WB, Hatabu H. Evaluation of pulmonary vascular anatomy and blood flow by magnetic resonance. J Thorac Imaging 1993;8:122–36.

74. Frydrychowicz A, Francois CJ, Turski PA. Four-dimensional phase contrast magnetic resonance angiography: potential clinical applications. Eur J Radiol 2011;80:24–35.

75. Grothues F, Moon JC, Bellenger NG, et al. Interstudy reproducibility of right ventricular volumes, function, and mass with cardiovascular magnetic resonance. Am Heart J 2004;147:218–23.

76. Peacock AJ, Crawley S, McLure L, et al. Changes in right ventricular function measured by cardiac magnetic resonance imaging in patients receiving pulmonary arterial hypertension-targeted therapy: the EURO-MR study. Circ Cardiovasc Imaging 2014;7:107–14.

77. Jauhiainen T, Jarvinen VM, Hekali PE. Evaluation of methods for MR imaging of human right ventricular heart volumes and mass. Acta Radiol 1987;2002(43):587–92.

78. Moon JC, Messroghli DR, Kellman P, et al. Myocardial T1 mapping and extracellular volume quantification: a Society for Cardiovascular Magnetic Resonance (SCMR) and CMR Working Group of the European Society of Cardiology consensus statement. J Cardiovasc Magn Reson 2013;15:92.

79. Nagle SK, Schiebler ML, Repplinger MD, et al. Contrast enhanced pulmonary magnetic resonance angiography for pulmonary embolism: building a successful program. Eur J Radiol 2016;85:553–63.

80. Rajaram S, Swift AJ, Telfer A, et al. 3D contrast-enhanced lung perfusion MRI is an effective screening tool for chronic thromboembolic pulmonary hypertension: results from the ASPIRE Registry. Thorax 2013;68:677–8.

81. van Wolferen SA, van de Veerdonk MC, Mauritz GJ, et al. Clinically significant change in stroke volume in pulmonary hypertension. Chest 2011;139:1003–9.

82. Gan C, Lankhaar JW, Marcus JT, et al. Impaired left ventricular filling due to right-to-left ventricular interaction in patients with pulmonary arterial hypertension. Am J Physiol Heart Circ Physiol 2006;290:H1528–33.

83. Marcus JT, Gan CT, Zwanenburg JJ, et al. Interventricular mechanical asynchrony in pulmonary arterial hypertension: left-to-right delay in peak shortening is related to right ventricular overload

and left ventricular underfilling. J Am Coll Cardiol 2008;51:750–7.

84. Haddad F, Guihaire J, Skhiri M, et al. Septal curvature is marker of hemodynamic, anatomical, and electromechanical ventricular interdependence in patients with pulmonary arterial hypertension. Echocardiography 2014;31:699–707.

85. Sato T, Tsujino I, Ohira H, et al. Paradoxical interventricular septal motion as a major determinant of late gadolinium enhancement in ventricular insertion points in pulmonary hypertension. PLoS One 2013;8:e66724.

86. Shehata ML, Lossnitzer D, Skrok J, et al. Myocardial delayed enhancement in pulmonary hypertension: pulmonary hemodynamics, right ventricular function, and remodeling. AJR Am J Roentgenol 2011;196:87–94.

87. Pelc NJ, Sommer FG, Li KCP, et al. Quantitative magnetic-resonance flow imaging. Magn Reson Q 1994;10:125–47.

88. Ley S, Mereles D, Puderbach M, et al. Value of MR phase-contrast flow measurements for functional assessment of pulmonary arterial hypertension. Eur Radiol 2007;17:1892–7.

89. Bogren HG, Klipstein RH, Mohiaddin RH, et al. Pulmonary artery distensibility and blood flow patterns: a magnetic resonance study of normal subjects and of patients with pulmonary arterial hypertension. Am Heart J 1989;118:990–9.

90. Kondo C, Caputo GR, Masui T, et al. Pulmonary hypertension: pulmonary flow quantification and flow profile analysis with velocity-encoded cine MR imaging. Radiology 1992;183:751–8.

91. Mousseaux E, Tasu JP, Jolivet O, et al. Pulmonary arterial resistance: noninvasive measurement with indexes of pulmonary flow estimated at velocity-encoded MR imaging - preliminary experience. Radiology 1999;212:896–902.

92. Sanz J, Kariisa M, Dellegrottaglie S, et al. Evaluation of pulmonary artery stiffness in pulmonary hypertension with cardiac magnetic resonance. JACC Cardiovasc Imaging 2009;2:286–95.

93. Gan CT, Lankhaar JW, Westerhof N, et al. Noninvasively assessed pulmonary artery stiffness predicts mortality in pulmonary arterial hypertension. Chest 2007;132:1906–12.

94. Forouzan O, Warczytowa J, Wieben O, et al. Noninvasive measurement using cardiovascular magnetic resonance of changes in pulmonary artery stiffness with exercise. J Cardiovasc Magn Reson 2015;17:109.

95. Naeije R, Vanderpool R, Dhakal BP, et al. Exercise-induced pulmonary hypertension: physiological basis and methodological concerns. Am J Respir Crit Care Med 2013;187:576–83.

96. Bellofiore A, Chesler NC. Methods for measuring right ventricular function and hemodynamic

coupling with the pulmonary vasculature. Ann Biomed Eng 2013;41:1384–98.

97. Poon CY, Edwards JM, Evans CJ, et al. Assessment of pulmonary artery pulse wave velocity in children: an MRI pilot study. Magn Reson Imaging 2013;31:1690–4.

98. Ibrahim el SH, Shaffer JM, White RD. Assessment of pulmonary artery stiffness using velocity-encoding magnetic resonance imaging: evaluation of techniques. Magn Reson Imaging 2011;29:966–74.

99. Reiter G, Reiter U, Kovacs G, et al. Magnetic resonance-derived 3-dimensional blood flow patterns in the main pulmonary artery as a marker of pulmonary hypertension and a measure of elevated mean pulmonary arterial pressure. Circ Cardiovasc Imaging 2008;1:23–30.

100. Reiter U, Reiter G, Kovacs G, et al. Evaluation of elevated mean pulmonary arterial pressure based on magnetic resonance 4D velocity mapping: comparison of visualization techniques. PLoS One 2013;8:e82212.

101. Roldan-Alzate A, Frydrychowicz A, Johnson KM, et al. Non-invasive assessment of cardiac function and pulmonary vascular resistance in an canine model of acute thromboembolic pulmonary hypertension using 4D flow cardiovascular magnetic resonance. J Cardiovasc Magn Reson 2014;16:23.

102. Fenster BE, Browning J, Schroeder JD, et al. Vorticity is a marker of right ventricular diastolic dysfunction. Am J Physiol Heart Circ Physiol 2015;309(6):H1087–93.

103. Barker AJ, Roldan-Alzate A, Entezari P, et al. Four-dimensional flow assessment of pulmonary artery flow and wall shear stress in adult pulmonary arterial hypertension: results from two institutions. Magn Reson Med 2015;73:1904–13.

104. Truong U, Fonseca B, Dunning J, et al. Wall shear stress measured by phase contrast cardiovascular magnetic resonance in children and adolescents with pulmonary arterial hypertension. J Cardiovasc Magn Reson 2013;15:81.

105. Tang BT, Pickard SS, Chan FP, et al. Wall shear stress is decreased in the pulmonary arteries of patients with pulmonary arterial hypertension: An image-based, computational fluid dynamics study. Pulm Circ 2012;2:470–6.

106. Wang Z, Lakes RS, Golob M, et al. Changes in large pulmonary arterial viscoelasticity in chronic pulmonary hypertension. PLoS One 2013;8:e78569.

107. Ohno Y, Murase K, Higashino T, et al. Assessment of bolus injection protocol with appropriate concentration for quantitative assessment of pulmonary perfusion by dynamic contrast-enhanced MR imaging. J Magn Reson Imaging 2007;25:55–65.

108. Swift AJ, Wild JM, Nagle SK, et al. Quantitative magnetic resonance imaging of pulmonary hypertension: a practical approach to the current state of the art. J Thorac Imaging 2014;29:68–79.

109. Swift AJ, Rajaram S, Capener D, et al. LGE patterns in pulmonary hypertension do not impact overall mortality. JACC Cardiovasc Imaging 2014; 7:1209–17.

110. Sanz J, Garcia-Alvarez A, Fernandez-Friera L, et al. Right ventriculo-arterial coupling in pulmonary hypertension: a magnetic resonance study. Heart 2012;98:238–43.

111. Freed BH, Gomberg-Maitland M, Chandra S, et al. Late gadolinium enhancement cardiovascular magnetic resonance predicts clinical worsening in patients with pulmonary hypertension. J Cardiovasc Magn Reson 2012;14:11.

112. Garcia-Alvarez A, Garcia-Lunar I, Pereda D, et al. Association of myocardial T1-mapping CMR with hemodynamics and RV performance in pulmonary hypertension. JACC Cardiovasc Imaging 2015;8: 76–82.

113. Mehta BB, Chen X, Bilchick KC, et al. Accelerated and navigator-gated look-locker imaging for cardiac t1 estimation (ANGIE): development and application to T1 mapping of the right ventricle. Magn Reson Med 2015;73(1):150–60.

114. Kawel-Boehm N, Dellas Buser T, Greiser A, et al. In-vivo assessment of normal T1 values of the right-ventricular myocardium by cardiac MRI. Int J Cardiovasc Imaging 2014;30:323–8.

115. Addetia K, Bhave NM, Tabit CE, et al. Sample size and cost analysis for pulmonary arterial hypertension drug trials using various imaging modalities to assess right ventricular size and function end points. Circ Cardiovasc Imaging 2014;7:115–24.

116. Wilkins MR, Paul GA, Strange JW, et al. Sildenafil versus Endothelin Receptor Antagonist for Pulmonary Hypertension (SERAPH) study. Am J Respir Crit Care Med 2005;171:1292–7.

117. Schulze-Neick I, Lange PE, Haas NA. Intravenous epoprostenol for primary pulmonary hypertension. N Engl J Med 1996;334:1477 [author reply: 1477–8].

118. Savarese G, Paolillo S, Costanzo P, et al. Do changes of 6-minute walk distance predict clinical events in patients with pulmonary arterial hypertension? A meta-analysis of 22 randomized trials. J Am Coll Cardiol 2012;60:1192–201.

Imaging of Eosinophilic Lung Diseases

Melissa Price, MD[a], Matthew D. Gilman, MD[a], Brett W. Carter, MD[b], Bradley S. Sabloff, MD[b], Mylene T. Truong, MD[b], Carol C. Wu, MD[b],*

KEYWORDS

- Eosinophilic pneumonia • Eosinophilic granulomatosis with polyangiitis
- Allergic bronchopulmonary aspergillosis • Hypereosinophilic syndromes

KEY POINTS

- The classic "photographic negative of pulmonary edema" pattern is only seen in a minority of patients with chronic eosinophilic pneumonia.
- Simple pulmonary eosinophilia is characterized by peripheral eosinophilia, minimal respiratory symptom, and transient pulmonary opacities.
- Eosinophilic granulomatosis and polyangiitis, formerly known as Churg-Strauss syndrome, typically occur in patients with history of asthma, allergic rhinitis, and/or sinusitis.
- Hyperdense mucus is pathognomonic for allergic bronchopulmonary aspergillosis.
- Drug-induced eosinophilic pneumonia can have clinical presentations and imaging features similar to acute eosinophilic pneumonia, chronic eosinophilic pneumonia, or rarely, eosinophilic granulomatosis and polyangiitis.

INTRODUCTION

Eosinophilic lung diseases encompass a varied group of pulmonary diseases that characteristically feature peripheral or tissue eosinophilia. The clinical presentation of these disorders varies markedly, and patients may be asymptomatic or experience life-threatening respiratory illness at the time of diagnosis.[1]

Eosinophilic lung disease traditionally can be diagnosed when one of the following criteria are met: (1) peripheral eosinophilia in the presence of opacities on a chest radiograph, (2) surgical or transbronchial lung biopsy demonstrating tissue eosinophilia, or (3) increase in the percentage of eosinophils in bronchoalveolar lavage (BAL) fluid.[2]

Imaging findings, particularly with thin-section computed tomography (CT), can sometimes suggest the diagnosis of an eosinophilic lung disease. In many cases, given the relatively rare nature and nonspecific clinical presentation of these diseases, the findings on CT may be the first clue to the diagnosis and may prompt further diagnostic workup. Alternatively, in patients with known peripheral eosinophilia, imaging can provide information regarding presence, severity, and distribution of pulmonary involvement, potentially narrow the differential possibilities, and serve as a guide for BAL or biopsy.

IMAGING PROTOCOLS

Standard chest CT protocol is preferably with thin slice thickness (<1.5 mm) and high spatial resolution image reconstruction algorithm.

The authors have nothing to disclose.
[a] Department of Radiology, Massachusetts General Hospital, 55 Fruit Street, Founders 202, Boston, MA 02114, USA; [b] Department of Diagnostic Radiology, University of Texas MD Anderson Cancer Center, 1515 Holcombe Boulevard, Unit 1478, Houston, TX 77030, USA
* Corresponding author.
E-mail address: carolcwu@gmail.com

radiologic.theclinics.com

DIAGNOSTIC CRITERIA

- Blood, tissue, or BAL fluid eosinophilia
- Pulmonary opacities

Acute Eosinophilic Pneumonia

The clinical diagnosis of acute eosinophilic pneumonia (AEP) is made in patients with an acute febrile illness lasting fewer than 5 days, hypoxemic respiratory failure, diffuse opacities on chest radiograph, and greater than 25% eosinophils in BAL fluid. Blood eosinophils may be normal or mildly elevated at initial presentation[2] but subsequently increase in the days after treatment.[3,4] The absence of a concurrent infection is necessary for the diagnosis.[2,5] Although the clinical presentation and imaging of findings of AEP may mimic acute respiratory distress syndrome (ARDS), the BAL fluid should demonstrate high neutrophils in ARDS.[2]

The cause of AEP has not been identified, but there is a reported association with cigarette smoking, particularly new-onset cigarette smoking.[4,6–9] The illness has also been reported to occur after inhalation of toxins[10] and use of certain medications.[11,12]

The chest radiograph findings in patients with AEP vary and include bilateral septal thickening and patchy or diffuse opacities.[4,13]

CT commonly shows ground-glass opacities, consolidation, interlobular septal thickening, bronchial wall thickening, and pleural effusions.[14] A CT pattern of crazy-paving with thickening of the interlobular septa and intralobular lines in the setting of ground-glass opacities[15] can be seen in patients with AEP[14] (Fig. 1). When present, pleural effusions are most commonly bilateral. In most cases, there is no overall lung zone predominance in the cephalocaudal plane.[14,16]

A peripheral distribution of the ground-glass and consolidative opacities has been described to occur in up to half of patients with AEP.[14] Cardiomegaly is not a feature of the illness.[17] In a minority of patients with AEP, lymphadenopathy may be observed at CT.[16]

AEP is extremely steroid responsive; however, there are patients who recover fully in the absence of corticosteroid treatment.[18]

Chronic Eosinophilic Pneumonia

Idiopathic chronic eosinophilic pneumonia (ICEP) is an uncommon entity with respiratory symptoms such as dyspnea and cough lasting more than 2 weeks. It is associated with alveolar eosinophilia 40% or greater at (BAL) differential cell count and/or blood eosinophilia 1000/mm^3 or more. Other known causes of eosinophilic lung disease must be excluded. The disease affects women twice as often as men. Up to 50% patients with ICEP have a history of asthma.[19] In distinction from eosinophilic granulomatosis with polyangiitis (EGPA) or hypereosinophilic syndrome (HES), patients with ICEP usually do not have extrathoracic manifestations.[19]

The classic radiographic finding has been described as the photographic negative of pulmonary edema with diffuse peripheral opacities and ill-defined margins.[20,21] However, this classic radiographic pattern is seen in fewer than one-third of patients.[22] The opacities usually do not have lobar or segmental distribution, can be unilateral or bilateral, and are often in an apical or axillary location without basilar involvement. These opacities can disappear and reappear in the exact same locations.[20] Pleural effusion is not commonly seen.

CT often shows bilateral subpleural consolidation and ground-glass opacities and can be associated

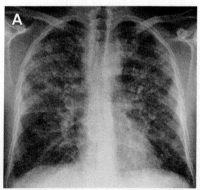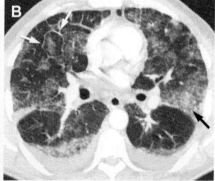

Fig. 1. AEP in a 41-year-old male firefighter who presented with severe dyspnea 6 days following a significant episode of occupational smoke inhalation. BAL specimen showed a heavy eosinophilic infiltrate with 36% eosinophils. (A) Chest radiograph shows patchy linear and nodular opacities. (B) CT demonstrates patchy ground-glass opacities (black arrow), interlobular septal thickening (white arrows), and small bilateral pleural effusions.

with enlarged mediastinal lymph nodes[23] (**Figs. 2** and **3**). In some cases, the peripheral nature of the opacities will not be apparent radiographically but are clearly demonstrated on CT.[24]

Chronic eosinophilic pneumonia (CEP) is very steroid responsive, and the opacities have been shown to resolve within 7 to 10 days of initiation of corticosteroid therapy.[21]

Simple Pulmonary Eosinophilia

Simple pulmonary eosinophilia (SPE), which was originally described by Löffler in 1932, occurs in the presence of blood eosinophilia, transient opacities on chest radiograph, and minimal associated respiratory symptoms. The cause of SPE is frequently parasitic infection or a drug reaction, but approximately one-third of cases are idiopathic. SPE has also been reported to occur as incidental findings on follow-up CT of 0.95% of oncologic patients[25] and in 0.9% of asymptomatic individuals undergoing low-dose CT for lung cancer screening.[26]

The plain radiographic findings of SPE are opacities with a nonsegmental peripheral distribution,[2] which can be unilateral or bilateral.[27] These opacities can be fleeting or migratory[27] (**Fig. 4**).

CT usually demonstrates peripheral patchy consolidations with scattered ground-glass opacities that have an upper and mid lung zone predominance (**Fig. 5**). As with the radiographic findings, the CT imaging features of the illness are often fleeting and migratory. Some patients may also have discrete pulmonary nodules, and bronchial wall thickening is commonly seen.[16] SPE and CEP have a similar pattern of distribution of opacities; however, the opacities in SPE often fluctuate over a period of days, whereas in CEP they persist for weeks to months.[24] In cases of SPE incidentally found during oncologic follow-up or screening, single or multiple pulmonary nodules with ground-glass halos are the most common findings. These lesions are reported to have lower lung zone predominance with peripheral distribution.[25,26] These lesions can have mild to moderate uptake on fludeoxyglucose-PET[28] and mimic primary or metastatic neoplasm. In patients with these findings, correlation with blood eosinophil count and short-term follow-up CT may help obviate more invasive procedures.[25,26,28]

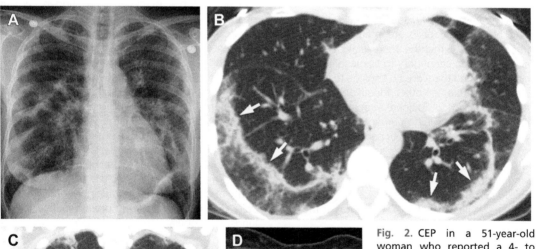

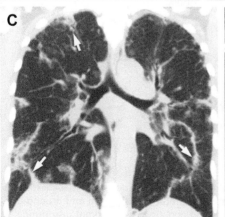

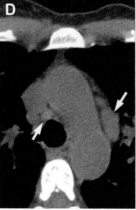

Fig. 2. CEP in a 51-year-old woman who reported a 4- to 6-week history of dyspnea and was found to have peripheral and bronchoalveolar fluid eosinophilia. (*A*) Chest radiograph shows peripheral predominant foci of nodular consolidation. Axial (*B*) and coronal (*C*) CT images demonstrate the characteristic subpleural consolidative and ground-glass opacities (*arrows*). (*D*) Axial CT image on soft tissue windows shows enlarged mediastinal lymph nodes (*arrows*).

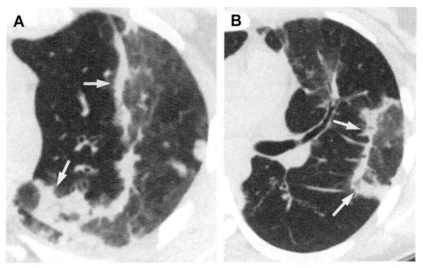

Fig. 3. A 31-year-old woman with CEP who initially presented with a chronic cough and had 71% eosinophils in BAL fluid. (*A*, *B*) CT images at 2 levels show peripheral ground-glass opacities and consolidation (*arrows*).

Individuals with idiopathic SPE often require no steroid therapy, and the pulmonary opacities and blood eosinophilia can often resolve within a month.[2]

Hypereosinophilic Syndrome

HES is a rare group of diseases that is diagnosed when blood eosinophils are greater than 1500/mm[3] for at least 6 months, there is evidence of organ dysfunction secondary to tissue infiltration by eosinophils, and there are no findings to suggest a parasitic, allergic, or other identifiable cause of the eosinophilia.[29] Additional subcategories have been identified, including primary HES, which occurs in the setting of clonal or neoplastic proliferation of eosinophils as well as secondary (reactive) HES, which is thought to be cytokine driven in response to a neoplastic or inflammatory condition.[30] HES is more common among men with a male-to-female ratio of 1.47:1 and has a median age at diagnosis of 52.5 years.[31]

In addition to hematologic abnormalities, cutaneous, neurologic, and cardiac involvement are common with HES.[32] Cardiac involvement is the primary cause of mortality in patients with HES and may result in complete heart block, eosinophilic myocarditis, restrictive cardiomyopathy, ventricular thrombus formation, and sudden cardiac death.[33,34] Pulmonary disease has been reported to occur in 40% of individuals with HES and can manifest as cough, dyspnea, and bronchospasm.[32]

Radiographs may show no abnormalities in patients with HES. In some patients, nodular opacities[35] or reticular opacities will be visible on plain radiograph.[29]

In individuals with HES and pulmonary involvement, CT often shows small nodules, frequently with a surrounding a ground-glass halo.[35] Patchy consolidation or ground-glass opacities may also be present, and pleural effusions are seen in a minority of cases.[16,36] The nodules or opacities typically do not have a zonal predominance in the lungs. Interlobular septal thickening and bronchial

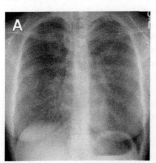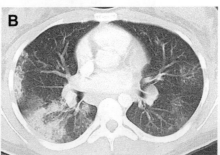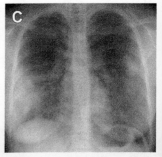

Fig. 4 Simple pulmonary eosinophilia in a 32-year-old woman with migratory opacities. (*A*) Initial chest radiograph shows bilateral multifocal consolidation. (*B*) CT demonstrates multifocal consolidation and ground-glass opacities. (*C*) Repeat chest radiograph 2 weeks later shows bilateral consolidation in a different distribution.

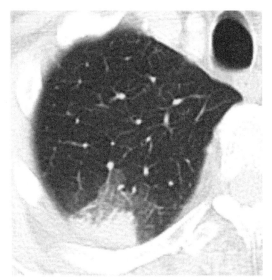

Fig. 5. Simple pulmonary eosinophilia in a 65-year-old man with peripheral eosinophilia. CT image shows right upper lobe subpleural nodular opacity with ground-glass halo, which improved spontaneously on follow-up imaging performed 4 weeks later.

wall thickening are commonly seen at CT.[16] Intrathoracic lymphadenopathy has been reported to occur in 12% to 33% of patients with HES.[16,36]

Treatment for lung involvement in HES includes corticosteroids often with an additional agent such as hydroxyurea, imatinib, interferon-α, or mepolizumab.[36]

Eosinophilic Granulomatosis with Polyangiitis (Churg-Strauss)

EGPA is a small-vessel antineutrophil cytoplasmic antibody (ANCA)-associated vasculitis with blood and tissue eosinophilia, which typically occurs in patients with asthma.[37,38] This disorder was previously known as Churg-Strauss syndrome, but the nomenclature was changed at the 2012 Revised International Chapel Hill Consensus Conference to highlight the histopathologic features of the disease.[38] In patients with EGPA, there is necrotizing granulomatous inflammation affecting the respiratory tract, necrotizing vasculitis, and eosinophilic organ infiltration.[39] ANCA is more frequently present in patients with glomerulonephritis.[38] Most affected patients are between 40 and 60 years of age.[35] Over the years, various diagnostic criteria have existed without widespread consensus.[40] The latest American College of Rheumatology criteria for the diagnosis of EGPA are listed in Box 1.[41]

EGPA usually occurs in 3 sequential phases. The first or allergic phase involves development of

Box 1
American College of Rheumatology classification criteria

- Asthma
- Eosinophilia (>10% on differential white blood cell count)
- Mononeuropathy or polyneuropathy
- Nonfixed pulmonary infiltrates
- Paranasal sinus abnormalities
- Extravascular eosinophils

4 out of 6 criteria = sensitivity of 85% and specificity of 99.7%

Data from Masi AT, Hunder GG, Lie JT, et al. The American College of Rheumatology 1990 criteria for the classification of Churg-Strauss syndrome (allergic granulomatosis and angiitis). Arthritis Rheum 1990;33(8):1094–100.

asthma, allergic rhinitis, and sinusitis. The second or eosinophilic phase is marked by an increase in peripheral eosinophilic count and eosinophilic infiltration of lungs, heart, or gastrointestinal system. Finally, the vasculitis phase is associated with necrotizing vasculitis resulting in purpura or neuropathy and constitutional symptoms such as fever, malaise, and weight loss.[39]

The most common radiographic finding in EGPA is bilateral nonsegmental multifocal consolidation. Diffuse reticulonodular opacities and bronchial wall thickening can also be seen. Less commonly, discrete pulmonary nodules may be visible.[42]

Common CT findings observed with EGPA include small (<10 mm) centrilobular nodules, ground-glass opacities, consolidation, and bronchial wall thickening[43] (Fig. 6). There is no overall zonal predominance. Pleural effusions occur in a minority of patients. Lymphadenopathy has been reported to present in approximately 25% of patients with EGPA.[16] EGPA is associated with increased risk of thromboembolic events including pulmonary embolism.[44,45] Therefore, if a contrast-enhanced CT is performed, an effort should be made to look for incidental pulmonary emboli.

Depending on the severity of disease, treatment usually involves corticosteroids with or without cyclophosphamide. Azathioprine or methotrexate can be used for maintenance therapy after remission has been achieved. Relapse occurs in approximately 25% to 30% of patients.[39,45]

Allergic Bronchopulmonary Aspergillosis

Allergic bronchopulmonary aspergillosis (ABPA) occurs mostly in patients with asthma or cystic fibrosis. *Aspergillus* is ubiquitous fungus in the

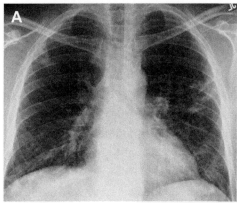
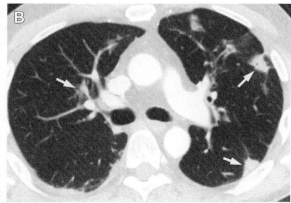
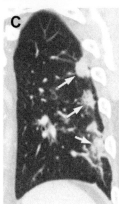
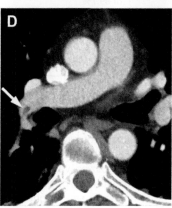

Fig. 6. EGPA in a 54-year-old man with severe asthma and eosinophilic rhinosinusitis. (*A*) Chest radiograph shows bilateral multifocal nonsegmental consolidation. Axial (*B*) and coronal (*C*) CT images demonstrate large nodules (*arrows*). (*D*) Axial CT image on soft tissue windows reveals a thrombus in the right interlobar pulmonary artery (*arrow*).

environment, and *Aspergillus fumigatus* is the most common pathogenic species in humans. It is thought that poor airway clearance in patients with asthma or cystic fibrosis allows noninvasive growth of *Aspergillus*, followed by hypersensitivity response in certain susceptible individuals, leading to airway injury in ABPA. Patients present with wheezing, dyspnea, cough, and hemoptysis. Occasionally patients will expectorate airway casts consisting of thick mucus and hyphae. Systemic symptoms such as fever, malaise, and weight loss are often reported. The combination of elevated serum *Aspergillus* immunoglubulin E (IgE) and positive skin testing is the most sensitive for making the diagnosis.[46] Allergic bronchopulmonary mycosis (ABPM) is a term used to describe patients who present with clinical features similar to ABPA caused by other fungi or yeasts.[47]

Radiographic findings of ABPA include consolidation, bronchial wall thickening, bronchiectasis, and mucoid impaction (tubular or gloved finger shadows).[48]

Classically, ABPA is associated with central or peripheral bronchiectasis and high attenuation mucoid impaction on CT.[49] High-attenuation mucus, which has been described as mucus plug that is visually denser than paraspinal skeletal muscle[50] or quantitatively with CT density greater than 70 HU,[51] is presumed to be due to calcium or metallic ions within the mucus. Although hyperdense mucus is a distinguishing CT feature of ABPA not seen in other entities associated with bronchiectasis and mucus plugging, it is present in only 28% to 36% of patients with ABPA.[50–52] The presence of high-attenuation mucoid impaction has been reported to correlate with higher peripheral eosinophil counts, serum total and *Aspergillus*-specific IgE levels,[49,51] and higher relapse rate.[49] Bronchiectasis in ABPA is often central, with predilection for the upper and middle lobes[50] (Fig. 7). The absence of bronchiectasis, however, should not prevent the diagnosis of ABPA in patients with other suggestive clinical findings. Bronchiectasis may not be present during the early stage of ABPA.[46,50,53] Other CT findings include consolidation, centrilobular nodules, and tree-in-bud opacities.[50]

Treatment is necessary to prevent further airway damage and decline in pulmonary function. Corticosteroids are used as first-line treatment for ABPA. The addition of antifungal agents has

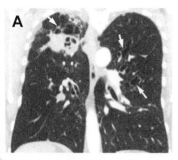 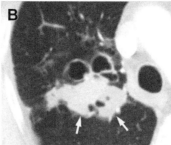 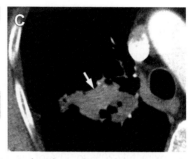

Fig. 7. ABPA in a 51-year-old woman with markedly elevated IgE levels treated with omalizumab, voriconazole, and chronic oral and inhaled corticosteroids. (*A*) Coronal CT image shows upper lobe predominant cystic and varicose bronchiectasis (*arrows*) with mucoid impaction and bronchial wall thickening. (*B*) CT image demonstrates mucus filling bronchiectatic airways in the right upper lobe (*arrows*). (*C*) A CT image at the same level on soft tissue windows shows the impacted area to have areas of internal high attenuation (*arrow*).

been shown to be useful. Omalizumab, an antibody to IgE, has also been introduced.[47] Patients are followed with serial assessment of total serum IgE level.[46,47]

Parasitic Infection

Eosinophilic pneumonia (EP) related to parasitic infection has been postulated to be a result of a combination of direct invasion and allergic reaction.[54] The prevalence and type of parasitic infection-related EP vary according to geographic locations. However, because of growing international travel and migration, these diseases are increasingly reported in nonendemic areas. Knowledge of world distribution of common parasites and the patient travel history is helpful in establishing the diagnosis. Some of the more common causes of parasitic eosinophilic diseases are detailed in later discussion.

Transient eosinophilic pulmonary pneumonia (Löffler syndrome)
Worldwide, the most common causes of transient eosinophilic pulmonary pneumonia (Löffler syndrome) are *Ascaris lumbricoides*, *Ancylostoma duodenale*, and *Necator americanus*. *Strongyloides stercoralis* is less common but is seen in the southeastern United States[55] and Puerto Rico.[56] Its ability to reproduce within the human hosts (autoinfection) can lead to prolonged disease and severe hyperinfection in immunocompromised individuals such as those on steroids or with human immunodeficiency virus infection.[56–58] Pulmonary symptoms in these parasitic infections are caused by hypersensitive response to larval migration through the lungs. Patients can be asymptomatic or present with fever, cough, dyspnea, and hemoptysis, with severity correlated to parasitic burden. Blood and sputum

eosinophilia is common.[55] The course tends to be self-limited.

Most common imaging findings are transient, migratory areas of consolidation.[59] Other findings include reticular or reticulonodular opacities, miliary nodules, and pleural effusions.[55,58,60] Pulmonary cavitation and abscess formation have also been reported with *Strongyloides*.[61,62]

Treatment is specific to the underlying parasitic infection.

Tropical pulmonary eosinophilia
Tropical pulmonary eosinophilia, a syndrome that results from immunologic response to filarial infection by *Wuchereria bancrofti and Brugia malayi*, is predominantly seen in the tropical and subtropical regions. It is the most serious parasitic eosinophilic lung disease.[55] Patients typically present with cough, dyspnea, and nocturnal wheezing, mimicking acute or refractory asthma. Marked peripheral eosinophilia is the norm with absolute blood eosinophil counts usually exceeding 3000 cells per cubic millimeter.[55,63] In the acute phase, interstitial eosinophilic infiltration occurs, and more chronically, interstitial fibrosis can develop.[63]

Radiographic findings of diffuse bilateral reticular or reticulonodular opacities have been described.[64–66] Bronchiectasis, air-trapping, and mediastinal lymphadenopathy can be seen on CT.[66]

Treatments include diethylcarbamazine, ivermectin, albendazole, and/or steroids. Because of the potential for relapses and persistent chronic inflammation and lung injuries, some patients require prolonged treatment.[55,63]

Echinococcosis
Echinococcus granulosus is mainly found in South and Central America, sub-Saharan Africa, Russia, and China and around the Mediterranean Sea. *Echinococcus multilocularis* is endemic in parts of

the United States, Canada, China, Northern Japan, and Europe. Humans are infected by eggs excreted in canine feces, and the larvae subsequently travel to the lungs and/or liver.[62] Peripheral eosinophilia is not always present. Patients with pulmonary involvement can be asymptomatic or present with cough, pain, fever, or hemoptysis.[55,67,68]

Echinococcosis usually presents as a solitary cyst in the lung, which usually appears as a sharply defined round or oval opacity on radiograph. Approximately 20% to 30% of patients have multiple pulmonary cysts.[62] A fluid-filled cyst with internal daughter cysts can be seen on CT. The water lily sign is seen when detached endocyst membrane floats within the pericyst. The cyst can also be completely air-filled (Fig. 8), referred to as the dry cyst sign, when it ruptures into an airway and expels its fluid content.[69] The cyst wall can calcify over time. Complications such as pneumothorax or empyema can also be observed on radiography or CT.[67,68]

Treatment options include surgical resection and/or albendazole.[67,68]

Paragonimiasis
Paragonimus westermani, endemic in Southeast Asia, can be contracted by ingestion of incompletely cooked freshwater crabs or crayfish. There are reported cases in the United States from ingestion of live crabs in sushi.[70] There are a few other species that are known to cause human infection.[55]

In the early stage of pleuropulmonary paragonimiasis, pneumothorax, hydropneumothorax, focal consolidation, and linear opacities are caused by migration of juvenile worms. Findings of thin-walled cysts, subpleural nodules (Fig. 9), masslike consolidation, bronchiectasis, and pleural thickening occur later in the disease process.[71,72] Compared with other parasitic infections, internal hypoattenuation or cavity within pulmonary lesions

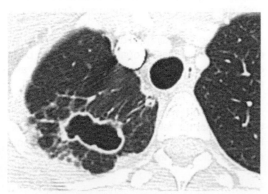

Fig. 8. Echinococcal cyst in a 31-year-old woman from South Africa. CT shows a lobulated air-containing cyst. The patient was treated with albendazole, and the cyst remained stable on subsequent CT.

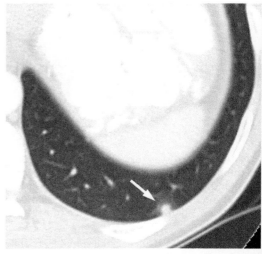

Fig. 9. Paragonimiasis in a 51-year-old Brazilian man with a history of gastric adenocarcinoma with peritoneal metastases. CT shows a 5-mm nodule in the left lower lobe with minimal surrounding ground-glass opacity (*arrow*), which was initially interpreted as suspicious for metastasis. The patient underwent a wedge resection of the nodule, which revealed necrotizing granulomatous inflammation due to degenerative trematodes with morphologic features of the *Paragonimus* species.

and perilesional centrilobular nodules occur more frequently in paragonimiasis.[73] Associated ascites, intraperitoneal or abdominal wall nodules, and low-attenuation hepatic lesions have also been reported.[74] Because nodules and masslike consolidation are frequent findings, pleuropulmonary paragonimiasis can mimic lung cancer as well as tuberculous or fungal infection.

Patients usually respond well to praziquantel or triclabendazole.[55]

Toxocariasis
Toxocariasis occurs worldwide, particularly in the tropics, and is caused by *Toxocara canis* or *Toxocara catis*.[55] Human infection occurs as the result of ingestion of embryonated eggs from soil or uncooked liver of cows, pigs, lambs, and chickens. The parasite larvae migrate to and invade various organs, including the liver, lung, and brain.[75] Patients can be asymptomatic or present with cough, dyspnea, or hemoptysis.

CT findings include ground-glass opacities, solid nodules, consolidation, and linear opacities with subpleural and lower lung predominance.[75] In one study, it was noted that a nodule with a ground-glass halo was more common in toxocariasis patients with eosinophilia than in those with normal eosinophil levels. Focal ground-glass opacity was more common in the normal eosinophil group.[76]

Patients can be treated with mebendazole, thiabendazole, or diethylcarbamazine with or without a short course of steroids.[55]

Drug- and Toxin-induced Eosinophilic Pneumonia

Multiple medications and toxins have been reported to cause EP. Drug- or toxin-induced EP is indistinguishable from idiopathic acute or CEP by symptoms, imaging, or histopathologic criteria. The diagnosis is based on temporal relationships of clinical signs and symptoms with recent use of or exposure to an associated causative agent. Resolution of symptoms with cessation of exposure is key to the diagnosis. Recurrence of the condition with re-exposure, although helpful in confirming the diagnosis, is usually not necessary and can be potentially dangerous.[77]

Nonsteroidal anti-inflammatory drugs (NSAIDs) and antibiotics such as nitrofurantoin[78–80] and dapsone[81,82] are some of the medications that most commonly cause EP. Antidepressants[12,83] and cardiovascular medications such as angiotensin conversion enzyme inhibitors[84,85] and β-blockers[86] have also been implicated. Oxaliplatin, an alkylating agent usually used in treatment of colorectal cancer, has been reported to cause EP.[87] Although most medications cause acute or chronic EP, zafirlukast, a leukotriene inhibitor used to treat asthma, is associated with EGPA.[88] It is unclear whether the medication induces vasculitis or its use allows steroid withdrawal and unmasking of the underlying vasculitis.[89,90] An extensive list of medications associated with EP can be found online at http://www.pneumotox.com, maintained by Department of Pulmonary and Intensive Care University Hospital Dijon France.[91] An abbreviated list of more commonly encountered medications associated with EP is provided in **Box 2**.

Imaging findings of drug-induced EP are similar to idiopathic forms of EP. Consolidation and ground-glass opacities (**Fig. 10**) with predominantly upper lung and peripheral distribution are the most common findings. The reversed halo sign (ground-glass opacity surrounded consolidation), small nodules, septal thickening, and reticulation are less common.[92]

Various toxin-induced EPs have been described. Cigarette smoking has been reported to cause AEP, usually in individuals who recently started smoking, restarted smoking, or have increased the quantity of cigarettes smoked.[8,93,94] High-level dust exposure, such as in the case of a firefighter exposed to World Trade Center dust

---

Box 2
Medications associated with eosinophilic pneumonia

Antibiotics
- Nitrofurantoin
- Daptomycin
- Dapsone
- Minocycline

NSAIDs (Cardiovascular medications)
- Amiodarone
- ACE inhibitor
- β-Blocker

Antidepressants
- Amitriptyline
- Velafaxine
- Fluoxetine

Anticonvulsants
- Phenytoin
- Carbamazepine

Others
- Mesalazine

Abbreviations: ACE, angiotensin converting enzyme; NSAIDs, nonsteroidal anti-inflammatory drugs.
Data from Bonniaud Ph, Baudouin N, Fanton A, et al. The drug-induced respiratory disease website. Dijon (France): Department of Pulmonary Medicine and Intensive Care University Hospital; 2016. Available at: http://www.pneumotox.com/.

---

consisting of silicates,[10] has also been reported to cause AEP. Crack cocaine inhalation has been reported to result in AEP,[95,96] eosinophilic pleural effusion,[97] and EGPA.[98]

Similar to idiopathic forms of AEP, CEP, and EGPA, corticosteroids are helpful in severe cases of drug- or toxin-induced eosinophilic lung diseases.[77]

RADIATION-INDUCED EOSINOPHILIC PNEUMONIA

There are reports of EP in women who received radiation therapy for breast cancer. These patients usually had a history of asthma and/or allergies and presented within 1 year of radiation treatment.[99,100] In one case, the patient developed CEP 6 years after completion of radiation treatment.[99] Pulmonary opacities can be seen in the irradiated lung or bilaterally (**Fig. 11**). It is postulated that the radiation causes an initial

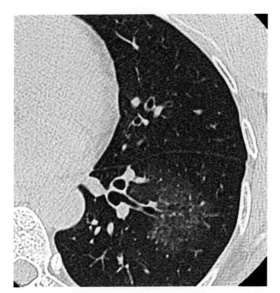

Fig. 10. Drug-induced EP in a 34-year-old woman who developed peripheral eosinophilia shortly after initiation of fluoxetine for treatment of depression. CT shows left lower lobe focal ground-glass opacity, which resolved after steroid treatment.

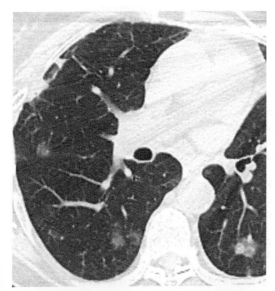

Fig. 11. Radiation-induced EP in a 72-year-old woman with a history of asthma and bilateral breast cancer who presented with cough, dyspnea, wheezing, and peripheral eosinophilia 3 months after completion of radiation treatment. CT image demonstrates bilateral nodular ground-glass opacities outside of the radiation field. The diagnosis of EP was confirmed after BAL showed elevated eosinophils in the lavage fluid and absence of pulmonary infection.

lymphocytic priming, which, when followed by antigenic stimulation, leads to development of CEP. The patients in reported cases had good response to systemic steroids.

DIFFERENTIAL DIAGNOSIS

- Infection
  - Bacterial
  - Mycobacterial
  - Fungal
- Organizing pneumonia
- Pulmonary alveolar hemorrhage
- Sarcoidosis
- ARDS
- Lung cancer
- Lymphoma

PEARLS, PITFALLS, VARIANTS

CT shows peripheral (subpleural) distribution of pulmonary opacities in CEP to better advantage than chest radiograph.

EGPA is associated with increased risk of pulmonary embolism, and efforts should be made to look for incidental pulmonary emboli if the chest CT was performed with intravenous contrast.

Hyperdense mucus is pathognomonic for ABPA.

WHAT THE REFERRING PHYSICIAN NEEDS TO KNOW

1. The distribution of pulmonary opacities to guide potential BAL or biopsy
2. Incidental nodules with ground-glass halos in patients with peripheral eosinophilia may represent SPE, and short-interval follow-up CT may help obviate more invasive procedures
3. The presence of hyperdense mucus in patients with ABPA because it can be associated with higher relapse rate

SUMMARY

Eosinophilic lung diseases can have a wide range of clinical presentations, which are often nonspecific. However, when certain clinical information (such as underlying asthma, travel history, or recent exposure to medications) is combined with the imaging characteristics (such as peripheral, upper lobe pulmonary opacities, or hyperdense mucus), differential diagnoses can be narrowed. Awareness of these uncommon entities allows radiologists to suggest these diagnoses in the appropriate situations. The main clinical and imaging features of various eosinophilic lung diseases are summarized in **Table 1**.

Table 1
Summary of clinical and imaging features of eosinophilic lung diseases

Eosinophilic Lung Disease	Clinical Feature	Imaging Feature
Acute EP	Acute onset fever, dyspnea	GGO, consolidation
Chronic EP	Subacute respiratory symptoms	Peripheral upper lobe predominant opacities
	Absence of extrapulmonary involvement	Photonegative of pulmonary edema
Simple pulmonary eosinophilia	Peripheral eosinophilia Minimum symptoms	Single or multiple pulmonary nodules with GG halos Transient GGO, consolidation
Hypereosinophilia syndrome	Marked peripheral eosinophilia Cutaneous, neurologic, or cardiac involvement	Pulmonary nodules with GG halos, consolidation, GGO
EGPA	Asthma, allergic rhinitis, sinusitis ANCA	GGO, consolidation, centrilobular nodules
ABPA	Asthma or cystic fibrosis *Aspergillus*-specific serum IgE	Bronchiectasis Hyperdense mucus
Parasitic infection	Travel to endemic region	Nodules, consolidation, subpleural linear opacities
Drug- or toxin-induced EP	Recent exposure to drug or toxin Improvement with cessation of exposure	Can be similar to AEP, CEP, or EGPA
Radiation-induced EP	Radiation treatment	Opacities outside of radiation field

Abbreviations: GG, ground-glass; GGO, ground-glass opacities.

REFERENCES

1. Fernandez Perez ER, Olson AL, Frankel SK. Eosinophilic lung diseases. Med Clin North Am 2011; 95(6):1163–87.
2. Allen JN, Davis WB. Eosinophilic lung diseases. Am J Respir Crit Care Med 1994;150(5 Pt 1): 1423–38.
3. Buelow BJ, Kelly BT, Zafra HT, et al. Absence of peripheral eosinophilia on initial clinical presentation does not rule out the diagnosis of acute eosinophilic pneumonia. J Allergy Clin Immunol Pract 2015;3(4):597–8.
4. Philit F, Etienne-Mastroianni B, Parrot A, et al. Idiopathic acute eosinophilic pneumonia: a study of 22 patients. Am J Respir Crit Care Med 2002;166(9): 1235–9.
5. Allen JN, Pacht ER, Gadek JE, et al. Acute eosinophilic pneumonia as a reversible cause of noninfectious respiratory failure. N Engl J Med 1989; 321(9):569–74.
6. Nakajima M, Manabe T, Niki Y, et al. Cigarette smoke-induced acute eosinophilic pneumonia. Radiology 1998;207(3):829–31.
7. Bok GH, Kim YK, Lee YM, et al. Cigarette smoking-induced acute eosinophilic pneumonia: a case report including a provocation test. J Korean Med Sci 2008;23(1):134–7.
8. Shorr AF, Scoville SL, Cersovsky SB, et al. Acute eosinophilic pneumonia among US Military personnel deployed in or near Iraq. JAMA 2004; 292(24):2997–3005.
9. Brackel CL, Ropers FG, Vermaas-Fricot SF, et al. Acute eosinophilic pneumonia after recent start of smoking. Lancet 2015;385(9973):1150.
10. Rom WN, Weiden M, Garcia R, et al. Acute eosinophilic pneumonia in a New York City firefighter exposed to World Trade Center dust. Am J Respir Crit Care Med 2002;166(6):797–800.
11. Rizos E, Tsigkaropoulou E, Lambrou P, et al. Risperidone-induced acute eosinophilic pneumonia. In Vivo 2013;27(5):651–3.
12. Tsigkaropoulou E, Hatzilia D, Rizos E, et al. Venlafaxine-induced acute eosinophilic pneumonia. Gen Hosp Psychiatry 2011;33(4):411.e7-9.
13. King MA, Pope-Harman AL, Allen JN, et al. Acute eosinophilic pneumonia: radiologic and clinical features. Radiology 1997;203(3):715–9.
14. Daimon T, Johkoh T, Sumikawa H, et al. Acute eosinophilic pneumonia: thin-section CT findings in 29 patients. Eur J Radiol 2008;65(3):462–7.
15. Hansell DM, Bankier AA, MacMahon H, et al. Fleischner Society: glossary of terms for thoracic imaging. Radiology 2008;246(3):697–722.
16. Johkoh T, Muller NL, Akira M, et al. Eosinophilic lung diseases: diagnostic accuracy of thin-

section CT in 111 patients. Radiology 2000;216(3): 773–80.

17. Cheon JE, Lee KS, Jung GS, et al. Acute eosinophilic pneumonia: radiographic and CT findings in six patients. AJR Am J Roentgenol 1996;167(5):1195–9.

18. Jhun BW, Kim SJ, Son RC, et al. Clinical outcomes in patients with acute eosinophilic pneumonia not treated with corticosteroids. Lung 2015;193(3): 361–7.

19. Marchand E, Cordier JF. Idiopathic chronic eosinophilic pneumonia. Semin Respir Crit Care Med 2006;27(2):134–41.

20. Gaensler EA, Carrington CB. Peripheral opacities in chronic eosinophilic pneumonia: the photographic negative of pulmonary edema. AJR Am J Roentgenol 1977;128(1):1–13.

21. Carrington CB, Addington WW, Goff AM, et al. Chronic eosinophilic pneumonia. N Engl J Med 1969;280(15):787–98.

22. Jederlinic PJ, Sicilian L, Gaensler EA. Chronic eosinophilic pneumonia. A report of 19 cases and a review of the literature. Medicine (Baltimore) 1988;67(3):154–62.

23. Marchand E, Reynaud-Gaubert M, Lauque D, et al. Idiopathic chronic eosinophilic pneumonia. A clinical and follow-up study of 62 cases. The Groupe d'Etudes et de Recherche sur les Maladies "Orphelines" Pulmonaires (GERM"O"P). Medicine (Baltimore) 1998;77(5):299–312.

24. Mayo JR, Muller NL, Road J, et al. Chronic eosinophilic pneumonia: CT findings in six cases. AJR Am J Roentgenol 1989;153(4):727–30.

25. Kim SJ, Bista AB, Park KJ, et al. Simple pulmonary eosinophilia found on follow-up computed tomography of oncologic patients. Eur J Radiol 2014; 83(10):1977–82.

26. Kim HY, Naidich DP, Lim KY, et al. Transient pulmonary eosinophilia incidentally found on low-dose computed tomography: findings in 40 individuals. J Comput Assist Tomogr 2008;32(1):101–7.

27. Citro LA, Gordon ME, Miller WT. Eosinophilic lung disease (or how to slice P.I.E.). Am J Roentgenol Radium Ther Nucl Med 1973;117(4):787–97.

28. Kim TJ, Lee KW, Kim HY, et al. Simple pulmonary eosinophilia evaluated by means of FDG PET: the findings of 14 cases. Korean J Radiol 2005;6(4): 208–13.

29. Chusid MJ, Dale DC. Eosinophilic leukemia. Remission with vincristine and hydroxyurea. Am J Med 1975;59(2):297–300.

30. Valent P, Klion AD, Horny HP, et al. Contemporary consensus proposal on criteria and classification of eosinophilic disorders and related syndromes. J Allergy Clin Immunol 2012;130(3):607–12.e9.

31. Crane MM, Chang CM, Kobayashi MG, et al. Incidence of myeloproliferative hypereosinophilic syndrome in the United States and an estimate

of all hypereosinophilic syndrome incidence. J Allergy Clin Immunol 2010;126(1):179–81.

32. Fauci AS, Harley JB, Roberts WC, et al. NIH conference. The idiopathic hypereosinophilic syndrome. Clinical, pathophysiologic, and therapeutic considerations. Ann Intern Med 1982;97(1):78–92.

33. Podjasek JC, Butterfield JH. Mortality in hypereosinophilic syndrome: 19 years of experience at Mayo Clinic with a review of the literature. Leuk Res 2013; 37(4):392–5.

34. Mankad R, Bonnichsen C, Mankad S. Hypereosinophilic syndrome: cardiac diagnosis and management. Heart 2016;102(2):100–6.

35. Kang EY, Shim JJ, Kim JS, et al. Pulmonary involvement of idiopathic hypereosinophilic syndrome: CT findings in five patients. J Comput Assist Tomogr 1997;21(4):612–5.

36. Dulohery MM, Patel RR, Schneider F, et al. Lung involvement in hypereosinophilic syndromes. Respir Med 2011;105(1):114–21.

37. Mouthon L, Dunogue B, Guillevin L. Diagnosis and classification of eosinophilic granulomatosis with polyangiitis (formerly named Churg-Strauss syndrome). J Autoimmun 2014;48–49:99–103.

38. Jennette JC, Falk RJ, Bacon PA, et al. 2012 revised International Chapel Hill Consensus Conference Nomenclature of Vasculitides. Arthritis Rheum 2013;65(1):1–11.

39. Gioffredi A, Maritati F, Oliva E, et al. Eosinophilic granulomatosis with polyangiitis: an overview. Front Immunol 2014;5:549.

40. Greco A, Rizzo MI, De Virgilio A, et al. Churg-Strauss syndrome. Autoimmun Rev 2015;14(4): 341–8.

41. Masi AT, Hunder GG, Lie JT, et al. The American College of Rheumatology 1990 criteria for the classification of Churg-Strauss syndrome (allergic granulomatosis and angiitis). Arthritis Rheum 1990;33(8): 1094–100.

42. Choi YH, Im JG, Han BK, et al. Thoracic manifestation of Churg-Strauss syndrome: radiologic and clinical findings. Chest 2000;117(1):117–24.

43. Kim YK, Lee KS, Chung MP, et al. Pulmonary involvement in Churg-Strauss syndrome: an analysis of CT, clinical, and pathologic findings. Eur Radiol 2007;17(12):3157–65.

44. Comarmond C, Pagnoux C, Khellaf M, et al. Eosinophilic granulomatosis with polyangiitis (Churg-Strauss): clinical characteristics and long-term followup of the 383 patients enrolled in the French Vasculitis Study Group cohort. Arthritis Rheum 2013;65(1):270–81.

45. Groh M, Pagnoux C, Baldini C, et al. Eosinophilic granulomatosis with polyangiitis (Churg-Strauss) (EGPA) Consensus Task Force recommendations for evaluation and management. Eur J Intern Med 2015;26(7):545–53.

46. Patterson KC, Strek ME. Diagnosis and treatment of pulmonary aspergillosis syndromes. Chest 2014;146(5):1358–68.
47. Greenberger PA, Bush RK, Demain JG, et al. Allergic bronchopulmonary aspergillosis. J Allergy Clin Immunol Pract 2014;2(6):703–8.
48. Mintzer RA, Rogers LF, Kruglik GD, et al. The spectrum of radiologic findings in allergic bronchopulmonary aspergillosis. Radiology 1978;127(2):301–7.
49. Agarwal R, Gupta D, Aggarwal AN, et al. Clinical significance of hyperattenuating mucoid impaction in allergic bronchopulmonary aspergillosis: an analysis of 155 patients. Chest 2007;132(4): 1183–90.
50. Kaur M, Sudan DS. Allergic bronchopulmonary aspergillosis (ABPA)—the high resolution computed tomography (HRCT) chest imaging scenario. J Clin Diagn Res 2014;8(6):RC05–7.
51. Phuyal S, Garg MK, Agarwal R, et al. High-attenuation mucus impaction in patients with allergic bronchopulmonary aspergillosis: objective criteria on high-resolution computed tomography and correlation with serologic parameters. Curr Probl Diagn Radiol 2015;45(3):168–73.
52. Logan PM, Muller NL. High-attenuation mucous plugging in allergic bronchopulmonary aspergillosis. Can Assoc Radiol J 1996;47(5):374–7.
53. Agarwal R, Chakrabarti A, Shah A, et al. Allergic bronchopulmonary aspergillosis: review of literature and proposal of new diagnostic and classification criteria. Clin Exp Allergy 2013;43(8):850–73.
54. Jeong YJ, Kim KI, Seo IJ, et al. Eosinophilic lung diseases: a clinical, radiologic, and pathologic overview. Radiographics 2007;27(3):617–37 [discussion: 37–9].
55. Chitkara RK, Krishna G. Parasitic pulmonary eosinophilia. Semin Respir Crit Care Med 2006;27(2): 171–84.
56. Woodring JH, Halfhill H 2nd, Reed JC. Pulmonary strongyloidiasis: clinical and imaging features. AJR Am J Roentgenol 1994;162(3):537–42.
57. Lessnau KD, Can S, Talavera W. Disseminated Strongyloides stercoralis in human immunodeficiency virus-infected patients. Treatment failure and a review of the literature. Chest 1993;104(1): 119–22.
58. Namisato S, Motomura K, Haranaga S, et al. Pulmonary strongyloidiasis in a patient receiving prednisolone therapy. Intern Med 2004;43(8):731–6.
59. Reeder MM, Palmer PE. Acute tropical pneumonias. Semin Roentgenol 1980;15(1):35–49.
60. Woodring JH, Halfhill H 2nd, Berger R, et al. Clinical and imaging features of pulmonary strongyloidiasis. South Med J 1996;89(1):10–9.
61. Ford J, Reiss-Levy E, Clark E, et al. Pulmonary strongyloidiasis and lung abscess. Chest 1981; 79(2):239–40.
62. Seabury JH, Abadie S, Savoy F Jr. Pulmonary strongyloidiasis with lung abscess. Ineffectiveness of thiabendazole therapy. Am J Trop Med Hyg 1971;20(2):209–11.
63. Vijayan VK. Tropical pulmonary eosinophilia: pathogenesis, diagnosis and management. Curr Opin Pulm Med 2007;13(5):428–33.
64. Herlinger H. Pulmonary changes in tropical eosinophilia. Br J Radiol 1963;36:889–901.
65. Khoo FY, Danaraj TJ. The roentgenographic appearance of eosinophilic lung (tropical eosinophilia). Am J Roentgenol Radium Ther Nucl Med 1960;83:251–9.
66. Sandhu M, Mukhopadhyay S, Sharma SK. Tropical pulmonary eosinophilia: a comparative evaluation of plain chest radiography and computed tomography. Australas Radiol 1996;40(1):32–7.
67. Ghoshal AG, Sarkar S, Saha K, et al. Hydatid lung disease: an analysis of five years cumulative data from Kolkata. J Assoc Physicians India 2012;60: 12–6.
68. Kantarci M, Bayraktutan U, Karabulut N, et al. Alveolar echinococcosis: spectrum of findings at cross-sectional imaging. Radiographics 2012; 32(7):2053–70.
69. Erdem CZ, Erdem LO. Radiological characteristics of pulmonary hydatid disease in children: less common radiological appearances. Eur J Radiol 2003;45(2):123–8.
70. Boland JM, Vaszar LT, Jones JL, et al. Pleuropulmonary infection by Paragonimus westermani in the United States: a rare cause of Eosinophilic pneumonia after ingestion of live crabs. Am J Surg Pathol 2011;35(5):707–13.
71. Im JG, Whang HY, Kim WS, et al. Pleuropulmonary paragonimiasis: radiologic findings in 71 patients. AJR Am J Roentgenol 1992;159(1):39–43.
72. Kim TS, Han J, Shim SS, et al. Pleuropulmonary paragonimiasis: CT findings in 31 patients. AJR Am J Roentgenol 2005;185(3):616–21.
73. Seon HJ, Kim YI, Lee JH, et al. Differential chest computed tomography findings of pulmonary parasite infestation between the paragonimiasis and nonparagonimiatic parasite infestation. J Comput Assist Tomogr 2015;39(6):956–61.
74. Shim SS, Kim Y, Lee JK, et al. Pleuropulmonary and abdominal paragonimiasis: CT and ultrasound findings. Br J Radiol 2012;85(1012):403–10.
75. Lee KH, Kim TJ, Lee KW. Pulmonary toxocariasis: initial and follow-up CT findings in 63 patients. AJR Am J Roentgenol 2015;204(6):1203–11.
76. Hur JH, Lee IJ, Kim JH, et al. Chest CT findings of toxocariasis: correlation with laboratory results. Clin Radiol 2014;69(6):e285–90.
77. Solomon J, Schwarz M. Drug-, toxin-, and radiation therapy-induced eosinophilic pneumonia. Semin Respir Crit Care Med 2006;27(2):192–7.

78. Baptista JP, Casanova PC, Sousa JP, et al. Acute eosinophilic pneumonia associated with acute respiratory distress syndrome: case report. Rev Port Pneumol 2004;10(4):355–64 [in Portuguese].

79. Kabbara WK, Kordahi MC. Nitrofurantoin-induced pulmonary toxicity: a case report and review of the literature. J Infect Public Health 2015;8(4):309–13.

80. Martins RR, Marchiori E, Viana SL, et al. Chronic eosinophilic pneumonia secondary to long-term use of nitrofurantoin: high-resolution computed tomography findings. J Bras Pneumol 2008;34(3):181–4.

81. Adar T, Tayer-Shifman O, Mizrahi M, et al. Dapsone induced eosinophilic pneumonia. Eur Ann Allergy Clin Immunol 2012;44(3):144–6.

82. Kaur J, Khandpur S, Seith A, et al. Dapsone-induced eosinophilic pneumonitis in a leprosy patient. Indian J Lepr 2005;77(3):267–71.

83. Espeleta VJ, Moore WH, Kane PB, et al. Eosinophilic pneumonia due to duloxetine. Chest 2007;131(3):901–3.

84. Rochford AP, Smith PR, Khan SJ, et al. Perindopril and pulmonary eosinophilic syndrome. J R Soc Med 2005;98(4):163–5.

85. Watanabe K, Nishimura K, Shiode M, et al. Captopril, an angiotensin-converting enzyme inhibitor, induced pulmonary infiltration with eosinophilia. Intern Med 1996;35(2):142–5.

86. Faller M, Quoix E, Popin E, et al. Migratory pulmonary infiltrates in a patient treated with sotalol. Eur Respir J 1997;10(9):2159–62.

87. Gagnadoux F, Roiron C, Carrie E, et al. Eosinophilic lung disease under chemotherapy with oxaliplatin for colorectal cancer. Am J Clin Oncol 2002;25(4):388–90.

88. Richeldi L, Rossi G, Ruggieri MP, et al. Churg-Strauss syndrome in a case of asthma. Allergy 2002;57(7):647–8.

89. Reques FG, Rodriguez JL. Tolerability of leukotriene modifiers in asthma: a review of clinical experience. BioDrugs 1999;11(6):385–94.

90. Soy M, Ozer H, Canataroglu A, et al. Vasculitis induced by zafirlukast therapy. Clin Rheumatol 2002;21(4):328–9.

91. Bonniaud Ph, Baudouin N, Fanton A, et al. The drug-induced respiratory disease website. Dijon (France): Department of Pulmonary Medicine and Intensive Care University Hospital; 2016. Available at. http://www.pneumotox.com/.

92. Souza CA, Muller NL, Johkoh T, et al. Drug-induced eosinophilic pneumonia: high-resolution CT findings in 14 patients. AJR Am J Roentgenol 2006;186(2):368–73.

93. Shintani H, Fujimura M, Yasui M, et al. Acute eosinophilic pneumonia caused by cigarette smoking. Intern Med 2000;39(1):66–8.

94. Uchiyama H, Suda T, Nakamura Y, et al. Alterations in smoking habits are associated with acute eosinophilic pneumonia. Chest 2008;133(5):1174–80.

95. McCormick M, Nelson T. Cocaine-induced fatal acute eosinophilic pneumonia: a case report. WMJ 2007;106(2):92–5.

96. Oh PI, Balter MS. Cocaine induced eosinophilic lung disease. Thorax 1992;47(6):478–9.

97. Strong DH, Westcott JY, Biller JA, et al. Eosinophilic "empyema" associated with crack cocaine use. Thorax 2003;58(9):823–4.

98. Orriols R, Munoz X, Ferrer J, et al. Cocaine-induced Churg-Strauss vasculitis. Eur Respir J 1996;9(1):175–7.

99. Chaaban S, Salloum V. Chronic eosinophilic pneumonia in a breast cancer patient post-radiation therapy: a case report. Respir Care 2014;59(5):e81–3.

100. Cottin V, Frognier R, Monnot H, et al. Chronic eosinophilic pneumonia after radiation therapy for breast cancer. Eur Respir J 2004;23(1):9–13.

Imaging of Small Airways Diseases

Abigail V. Berniker, MD, Travis S. Henry, MD*

KEYWORDS

- Small airways diseases • Bronchiolitis • Centrilobular nodules • Tree-in-bud • Air trapping
- High-resolution computed tomography • Constrictive bronchiolitis

KEY POINTS

- Small airways diseases, or bronchiolitis, refers to bronchiolar inflammation and fibrosis that is caused by numerous entities. Small airways diseases is broadly classified into either cellular or constrictive subtypes.
- High-resolution computed tomography (HRCT) plays an important role in diagnosing small airways diseases and is used in conjunction with clinical data and pathologic findings to solidify a diagnosis. Normal small airways are too small to be visible on HRCT.
- Cellular bronchiolitis is an inflammatory process that usually presents as centrilobular nodules, which is a direct finding of the disease. Centrilobular nodules may vary in size and attenuation.
- Constrictive bronchiolitis is a fibrotic process that usually manifests as mosaic attenuation from air trapping, an indirect finding of airway obstruction. Constrictive bronchiolitis often appears similar, despite etiology, so clinical history is crucial.
- Many mimics of small airways diseases exist. Centrilobular nodules may be a result of arteriolar disease or aerogenous spread of adenocarcinoma. Mosaic attenuation may be secondary to small vessels disease or ground-glass opacity.

INTRODUCTION

Small airways diseases, or bronchiolitis, is a broad term encompassing numerous diseases that cause bronchiolar inflammation or fibrosis. Bronchioles are small airways located at the center of the secondary pulmonary lobule (SPL), which are too small to see on imaging when they are normal, and are therefore usually visible only when abnormal.[1] High-resolution computed tomography (HRCT) plays an important role in detecting small airways diseases and is used in conjunction with clinical data and pathologic findings to solidify a diagnosis. Direct signs of bronchiolitis include centrilobular nodules or opacities, typically reflecting a cellular or inflammatory form of bronchiolitis. Air trapping is an indirect sign and usually represents a constrictive, or obliterative bronchiolitis where the small airways are obstructed. This article reviews the following topics: normal bronchiolar anatomy, HRCT protocols for evaluating small airways diseases, a histologic classification of bronchiolitis, the imaging features of small airways diseases (divided into cellular and constrictive subcategories), and important radiologic mimics.

NORMAL ANATOMY

The SPL refers to the smallest functional anatomic unit of the lungs that is recognizable on imaging. A basic knowledge of the SPL anatomy is critical to recognizing and understanding small airways diseases. SPLs measure 10 mm to 25 mm in size and are bounded by the interlobular septa, which

---

Disclosure: The authors have no relevant disclosures for this article.
Department of Radiology and Biomedical Imaging, University of California, San Francisco, 505 Parnassus Avenue, San Francisco, CA 94143, USA
* Corresponding author.
E-mail address: Travis.Henry@ucsf.edu

Radiol Clin N Am 54 (2016) 1165–1181
http://dx.doi.org/10.1016/j.rcl.2016.05.009
0033-8389/16/$ – see front matter © 2016 Elsevier Inc. All rights reserved.

contain peripheral connective tissue, veins, and lymphatics. At the heart of the SPL are the small airways, arterioles, and additional lymphatics.[2]

The small airways, or bronchioles, are less than 2 mm internal diameter and lack cartilage. Membranous bronchioles are purely air conducting, whereas respiratory bronchioles supply alveoli and provide gas exchange. These airways provide little resistance in the normal lung, but their total cross-sectional area is so large that even mild abnormalities of the small airways can have a profound effect on lung function.[2,3]

Normal bronchioles are below the size threshold for HRCT. As such, visible bronchiolar abnormalities are a clue to underlying small airways inflammation and/or fibrosis. Bronchiolar inflammation typically manifests as centrilobular nodules on HRCT. These nodules may vary in size (as small as 1–2 mm, or large enough to occupy nearly an entire SPL) and attenuation (ranging from faint ground-glass to soft tissue attenuation) but the most important characteristic is that centrilobular nodules should spare the pleural and fissural surfaces, thus distinguishing them from random or perilymphatic nodules (Fig. 1).[2]

Similarly, bronchiolar fibrosis often manifests as mosaic attenuation because of air trapping. This air trapping often has sharply delineated borders where abnormal SPLs interface with normal SPLs. Bronchial wall thickening and bronchiectasis may be present.

Both imaging patterns seen in small airways diseases (nodules and mosaic attenuation) are commonly encountered on CT. However, there are many mimics of small airways diseases that are also frequently encountered, which are also discussed in this article.

IMAGING TECHNIQUE

HRCT is the primary imaging tool for evaluation of small airways diseases. HRCT uses thin sections

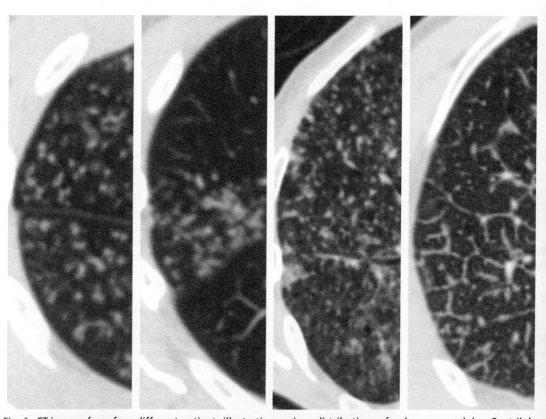

Fig. 1. CT images from four different patients illustrating various distributions of pulmonary nodules. Centrilobular nodules (*far left image*) are distinguishable because they spare the pleural and fissural surfaces (note the 1- to 2-mm gap between the nodules and these surfaces). Many of these nodules have a tree-in-bud pattern, a subset of centrilobular nodules, in this case representing tuberculosis. Perilymphatic (*second from left,* sarcoidosis) and random (*second from right,* miliary tuberculosis) nodules both touch pleural surfaces, thus distinguishing them from centrilobular nodules. *Far right* image shows nodular beading of the interlobular septae from esophageal cancer, nicely outlining the secondary pulmonary lobules.

(0.625–1.5 mm slice thickness) with a high spatial frequency reconstruction algorithm to enhance evaluation of pulmonary parenchyma and small airways.[4]

Basic HRCT protocols include supine inspiratory and expiratory images (**Table 1**). Noncontiguous image acquisition, the so-called step and shoot technique, is a traditional HRCT method and obtains axial images spaced at 10-mm to 20-mm intervals. The benefit of this technique is lower radiation dose. An alternate method uses volumetric acquisition to image the entire lungs. This technique allows for thin-section reconstructions and postprocessing, such as multiplanar reformats and maximum and minimum intensity projections, but at the expense of higher radiation doses.[4] These postprocessing techniques may improve detection and characterization of nodules (**Fig. 2**).[5,6]

Expiratory imaging is a critical component in the evaluation of small airways diseases to detect air trapping, because air trapping may be imperceptible on inspiratory images. Like the variety of inspiratory techniques, expiratory imaging may be acquired using different methods. One common method scans the entire lungs at 10- to 20-mm intervals during end-exhalation (suspended respiration after forced exhalation). A second method (preferred at the authors' institution) acquires a series of dynamic images at three different levels in the thorax. At each level, six to eight images are obtained during forceful exhalation. There are some data that this second technique may accentuate the differences between normal and abnormal lung, but either method should be acceptable if performed appropriately (**Fig. 3**).[7,8] Regardless of technique, expiratory imaging has been shown to increase the accuracy and diagnostic confidence for air trapping.[9]

Prone images may be included to help differentiate posterior lung disease from dependent atelectasis; however, they are not generally as beneficial in the evaluation of small airways diseases as in interstitial lung disease.

CLASSIFICATION OF SMALL AIRWAYS DISEASES

Bronchiolitis is a general term referring to bronchiolar inflammation. Originally, it described peripheral airway inflammation in smokers,[10] but now is applied more broadly as a synonym for small airways diseases. Bronchiolitis may be focal or diffuse, acute or chronic, idiopathic or caused by a known underling mechanism. Clinical, radiologic, and histologic features are complementary in the diagnosis of small airways diseases.

Unfortunately, there is no consensus classification system for small airways diseases, which can lead to confusion among clinicians, radiologists, and pathologists. This lack of consensus is troublesome, because many of these diseases require multidisciplinary input to reach a correct diagnosis. In the most general sense, histologic classification of small airways diseases can be divided into cellular/proliferative and constrictive/obliterative categories (a more detailed pathologic classification scheme is beyond the scope of this

Table 1
HRCT protocol

Patient Position	Respiration	Slice Thickness (mm)	Acquisition	Reconstruction and Reformats
Supine	Inspiratory[a]	0.625–1.5	• Noncontiguous (every 10–20 mm) Or • Volumetric	High spatial frequency +/− MIP, minIP
	Expiratory[b]	0.625–1.5	• Entire lungs at 10- to 20-mm intervals Or • 6–8 dynamic images obtained at three levels	
+/− Prone	Inspiratory	0.625–1.5	• Noncontiguous (every 10–20 mm) Or • Volumetric	High spatial frequency

Abbreviations: minIP, minimum intensity projection; MIP, maximum intensity projection.
[a] Obtained at suspended respiration following deep inspiration.
[b] Obtained at suspended respiration following deep exhalation.

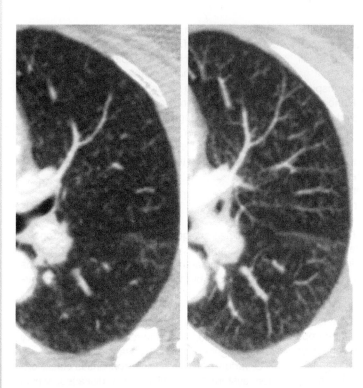

Fig. 2. A 45-year-old woman with hypersensitivity pneumonitis (bird fancier's lung). HRCT image (*left*) shows faint ground-glass nodules. Maximum intensity projection (MIP) (*right*) depicts the extent and centrilobular distribution of the nodules more clearly.

article but is provided by other resources).[3,11] This histologic system loosely correlates with radiologic features and provides a convenient structure for the two major imaging patterns that are encountered: centrilobular nodules (a direct finding of inflammation and proliferative/cellular bronchiolitis) and air trapping (an indirect finding indicative of obliterative bronchiolitis).

CELLULAR BRONCHIOLITIS

Cellular (inflammatory or proliferative) bronchiolitis is characterized by inflammatory cells in the bronchiolar wall and lumen. Although the causes of small airways inflammation are diverse, there are only a limited number of radiologic patterns,[3] and thus the imaging findings overlap. Several entities may cause cellular bronchiolitis (summarized in Table 2):

- Aspiration bronchiolitis
- Infectious bronchiolitis
- Hypersensitivity pneumonitis
- Respiratory bronchiolitis
- Follicular bronchiolitis
- Diffuse panbronchiolitis
- Other exposures

At HRCT, the primary manifestation of cellular bronchiolitis is centrilobular nodules. Centrilobular nodules may range in size and vary in attenuation. Centrilobular nodules result from inflammation in the peribronchiolar alveoli and may be 1- to 2-mm nodules, or coalesce into nodular foci of consolidation or ground-glass opacities that occupy nearly the entire SPL.[12] The attenuation of nodules may be faint ground-glass, or more well defined and solid. The tree-in-bud pattern refers to a specific subset of centrilobular nodules with multiple, branching, soft tissue attenuation opacities originating from a single stalk, so-named because of their resemblance with a budding tree in springtime.[13] Tree-in-bud opacities result from inspissated bronchiolar secretions or bronchiolar wall thickening, sometimes with peribronchiolar granulomas.[14,15]

In general, the different causes of cellular bronchiolitis have overlapping appearances at HRCT, but some findings may help narrow the differential diagnosis (in addition to using clinical information). For example, the presence of tree-in-bud can help narrow the differential diagnosis further because it is most frequently encountered in patients with infectious bronchiolitis or aspiration.[2,16] Conversely, ill-defined ground-glass centrilobular nodules are frequently seen in either hypersensitivity pneumonitis or respiratory bronchiolitis (RB), especially when they are bilateral and symmetric.

Aspiration Bronchiolitis

Aspiration is a common cause of cellular bronchiolitis and may be acute, chronic, or acute on

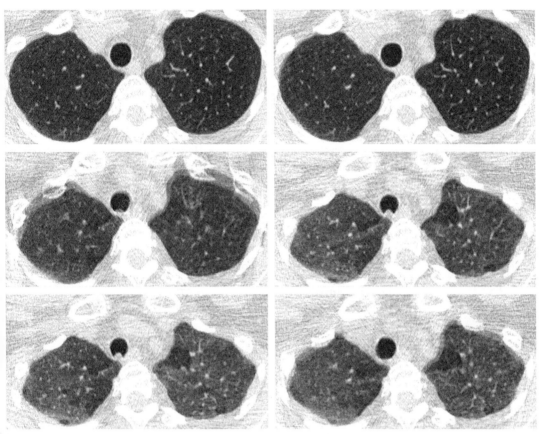

Fig. 3. Air trapping on dynamic expiratory sequence in a 58-year-old woman with chronic hypersensitivity pneumonitis. Six CT images were obtained at the same table position during a forced exhalation maneuver (*top left to bottom right*). The *top left* image (obtained during end-inspiration) shows relatively uniform attenuation of the lung parenchyma. The *bottom left* image (obtained at end-exhalation) shows the greatest degree of air trapping with minimal respiratory motion. Note the bowing of the posterior membrane of the trachea indicative of expiratory physiology.

chronic. Acute aspiration may occur from any number of insults resulting in retained foreign material.[13] Diffuse aspiration bronchiolitis is a specific entity characterized by chronic bronchiolar inflammation resulting from recurrent aspiration. Commonly, patients with diffuse aspiration bronchiolitis are elderly or bedridden with neurologic conditions or dementia predisposing to oropharyngeal dysphagia.[17] Such patients may have bronchorrhea, wheezing, or dyspnea associated with oral food ingestion. Histologically, it is characterized by chronic bronchiolar inflammation and foreign body reaction.[3] At HRCT, acute and chronic aspiration manifest with tree-in-bud opacities with or without bronchocentric consolidation. Acute aspiration tends to be more focal and limited to dependent areas, whereas diffuse aspiration bronchiolitis is more diffuse in distribution as the name implies.[14] Aspiration does not always result from oropharyngeal dysphagia. For example, it

may rarely occur from anatomic abnormalities, such as a tracheoesophageal or bronchopleural fistula in patients with congenital anomalies or postoperative complications (**Fig. 4**).

Infectious Bronchiolitis

Infectious bronchiolitis may result from viral, bacterial, or fungal etiologies. Clinical manifestations are nonspecific and may include dyspnea, productive cough, and wheezing.[18] Acute infectious bronchiolitis most often afflicts infants and children with viral infection, such as from parainfluenza, respiratory syncytial virus, adenovirus, or mycoplasma.[3] When acute infectious bronchiolitis occurs in adults, patients are often immunocompromised; in this specific patient population, fungal infections, such as airway invasive aspergillosis, may occur, in addition to more common viral and bacterial etiologies.[3,13] Chronic infective

Table 2
Cellular bronchiolitis: differential diagnosis

Cause	Imaging	Clinical
Aspiration bronchiolitis	• Tree-in-bud • Often dependent • Focal or multifocal	• Known oropharyngeal dysfunction • Head and neck cancer • Other predisposition to aspiration
Infectious bronchiolitis	• Tree-in-bud • Focal or multifocal • Cavitation → mycobacterium	• Infectious symptoms • May be immunocompromised • Underlying history of bronchiectasis
Hypersensitivity pneumonitis	• Often diffuse, symmetric nodules • +/− Air trapping • +/− Ground-glass opacity	• Usually nonsmoker • History of exposure
Respiratory bronchiolitis	• Bilateral, diffuse, upper-lobe predominant • +/− Other smoking related diseases (emphysema, DIP, LCH)	• Almost always a smoker

Follicular bronchiolitis	• Nodules may be focal/multifocal or diffuse
	• May be seen with other ILD (in context of CTD)
		• Usually develops in context of systemic disorder
		  ○ CTD
		  ○ Common variable immunodeficiency
		  ○ HIV

Diffuse panbronchiolitis	• Nodules and bronchial wall thickening • Progression to bronchiectasis, air trapping and cysts/bullae	• Usually of Asian descent • Chronic sinusitis + cough/dyspnea • Often have *Pseudomonas aeruginosa* or *Haemophilus influenzae* in sputum

Abbreviations: CTD, connective tissue disease; DIP, desquamative interstitial pneumonia; HIV, human immunodeficiency virus; ILD, interstitial lung disease; LCH, Langerhans cell histiocytosis.

bronchiolitis commonly often results from bacterial culprits, such as *Mycobacterium tuberculosis* and nontuberculous mycobacteria.[13]

Histologically, infectious bronchiolitis is characterized by bronchiolar injury with bronchiolar wall epithelial necrosis and inflammation and intraluminal exudates. At HRCT, infectious bronchiolitis shows tree-in-bud opacities and centrilobular nodules corresponding to bronchiolar mural inflammation and associated cellular bronchiolitis (**Fig. 5**).[19] Some clues can help narrow the differential diagnosis. Infectious bronchiolitis is often patchy and asymmetric and certain features may suggest specific agents (eg, tuberculosis should be considered when both tree-in-bud and cavitation are present in the upper lobes or superior segments of lower lobes; nontuberculous mycobacterial infection often involves the middle lobe and lingua with tree-in-bud, bronchiectasis, and volume loss) (**Fig. 6**).[13]

Hypersensitivity Pneumonitis

Hypersensitivity pneumonitis is an allergic lung disease caused by inhalational exposure to numerous offending agents, including organic dust, chemical compounds, and household mold.[18] Unlike RB, hypersensitivity pneumonitis is more common in nonsmokers.[20] Signs and symptoms of hypersensitivity pneumonitis include inspiratory crackles, weight loss, fatigue, identifiable antigen, recurring cough and dyspnea after antigen exposure, and serum antibodies to antigen exposure. Pathologically, hypersensitivity pneumonitis is characterized by inflammation and granulomatous infiltration of the interstitium and bronchioles. Active hypersensitivity pneumonitis manifests with diffuse or lower lobe-predominant, symmetric, poorly defined centrilobular nodules or larger ground-glass opacities that correspond to the granulomatous lesions (**Fig. 7**).[18,21] The presence of air trapping is also a helpful feature that can distinguish hypersensitivity pneumonitis from other entities with diffuse ground-glass centrilobular nodules, and may indicate a component of constrictive bronchiolitis.[20]

Respiratory Bronchiolitis

RB and RB-associated interstitial lung disease almost always occur in smokers and are part of a spectrum with desquamative interstitital pneumonia.[19] Rarely, RB has been described in nonsmokers with secondhand cigarette smoke

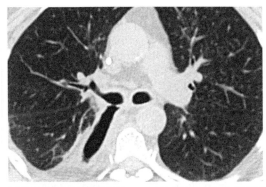

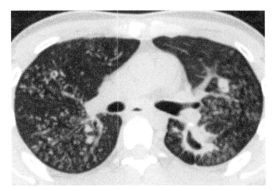

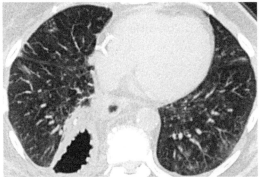

Fig. 6. CT image of a 26-year-old man with infectious bronchiolitis from active tuberculosis. Extensive branching, soft tissue attenuation opacities, so-called tree-in-bud nodules, are present throughout both lungs. Note how these opacities spare the sub-pleural regions and fissures, as expected from a process arising from bronchioles centered in secondary pulmonary lobules. Multiple cavities are also seen, typical of tuberculosis.

Fig. 4. A 66-year-old man who presented with persis-tent cough months after an esophagectomy and gastric pull-through. CT images show basilar-predominant centrilobular nodules (left greater than right; *bottom image*). The dependent distribution was suspicious for aspiration and prompted careful evaluation of the surgical pull-through, which re-vealed a subtle fistula to the posterior wall of the bronchus intermedius (confirmed at bronchoscopy).

exposure, connective tissue disease (CTD), or mineral dust–induced diseases. A distinguishing pathologic feature is brown-pigmented macro-phages filling respiratory bronchiolar lumens

and alveoli.[3,19] RB usually presents with upper lobe–predominant ground-glass nodules, but may overlap with findings of other smoking-related lung diseases, such as emphysema or desquamative interstitital pneumonia (**Fig. 8**). Most patients are asymptomatic with incidental imaging and histologic findings. The imaging find-ings may improve or completely resolve with smoking cessation, whereas the histologic find-ings can persist even years after smoking cessation.[3]

Follicular Bronchiolitis

Follicular bronchiolitis (FB) represents perib-ronchiolar lymphoid hyperplasia and reactive

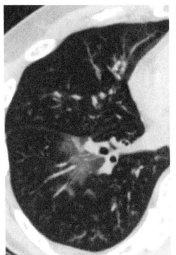 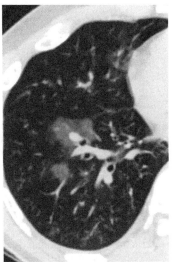

Fig. 5. A 34-year-old man with relapsed multiple myeloma present-ing with fever and cough. Axial thin MIP images through the right lung show subtle centrilobular nodules, ground-glass opacity, and mild bron-chial wall thickening (left lung not involved). The pattern and asym-metric distribution are typical of in-fectious bronchiolitis and cultures were positive for respiratory syncytial virus. Viral bronchiolitis afflicts in-fants and children more commonly, but is seen in adults (especially the immunocompromised).

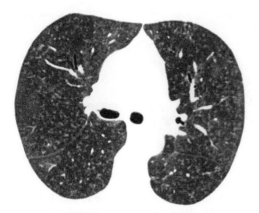

Fig. 7. A 65-year-old woman with active hypersensitivity pneumonitis secondary to bird exposure. HRCT image shows diffuse centrilobular nodules and some areas of more ill-defined ground-glass opacity in the anterior upper lobes. The patient's symptoms coincided with acquiring a pet bird, and symptoms improved after the bird was removed from her household.

germinal centers along the small airways.[3] On imaging, FB manifests as centrilobular nodules, which correspond to obstructed bronchioles and inflammatory cells infiltrating the adjacent alveolar interstitium.[3,19] These nodules range in size and attenuation and can be ground-glass or sometimes tree-in-bud. FB is on the mild end of a spectrum of lymphoproliferative disorders of the lung, which includes lymphoid interstitial pneumonia, and findings may overlap on imaging or pathology.[3,19] FB is most common in middle-aged adults with progressive cough and dyspnea. Typically, it occurs in patients with underlying immunodeficiency, such as from human immunodeficiency virus, or CTD, particularly rheumatoid arthritis (**Fig. 9**).[3,14]

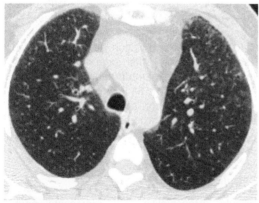

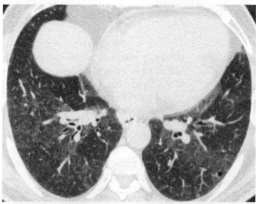

Fig. 8. CT images of a 49-year-old man with a 1.5-pack-per-day smoking history and respiratory bronchiolitis. (*Top*) Diffuse centrilobular ground-glass nodules typical of respiratory bronchiolitis. (*Bottom*) More confluent ground-glass opacity. Also note the presence of a cyst in the left lower lobe, which can be seen in the setting of smoking-related lung disease.

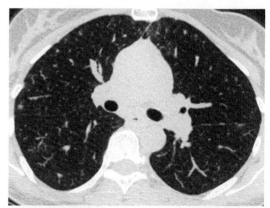

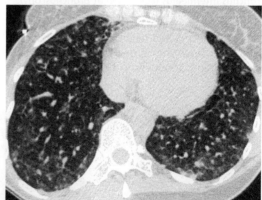

Fig. 9. A 34-year-old woman with follicular bronchiolitis and lymphocytic interstitial pneumonia secondary to underlying common variable immune deficiency. CT images show symmetric mid- and basilar-predominant centrilobular nodules of varying sizes. Because of the history of common variable immune deficiency, follicular bronchiolitis was suspected. Surgical lung biopsy showed polyclonal lymphocytes and germinal centers representing a spectrum of FB and lymphoid interstitial pneumonia, which may overlap.

Diffuse Panbronchiolitis

Diffuse panbronchiolitis is a rare, but progressive inflammatory disease involving the upper and lower respiratory systems, classically occurring in middle-aged men of Asian descent, namely from Japan, although cases have been diagnosed in patients of various races, including white persons.[22] There is no known relationship with smoking.[19] Patients typically report progressive sinusitis, cough, and dyspnea with a subacute course. Histologically, diffuse panbronchiolitis shows peribronchiolar inflammatory cell infiltrates and foamy macrophages in the interstitium and alveolar spaces.[3,22] Early HRCT findings include diffuse or lower-lobe-predominant centrilobular nodules and tree-in-bud opacities, followed in later stages by bronchiolectasis and bronchiectasis, mosaic attenuation, and cystic spaces indicative of evolution to a constrictive bronchiolitis as the airways become further injured (**Fig. 10**).[3] Concomitant *Pseudomonas aeruginosa* superinfection or organizing pneumonia may also be present.[14] Despite maintenance therapy with long-term low-dose macrolide antibiotics, which suppress airway secretions through an immune-modulatory effect, diffuse panbronchiolitis often is progressive and results in respiratory failure. Recurrence following lung transplantation has been reported.[3]

Other Exposures

Various inhalational exposures may cause cellular bronchiolitis and present as centrilobular nodules. These nodules may be the result of inflammatory conditions, such as necrotizing granulomatous inflammation or organizing pneumonia.[2,23,24] Synthetic marijuana is one such inhalational culprit. Synthetic marijuana refers to chemical substances sprayed onto dried plants that are smoked to mimic the appearance and psychoactive effects of natural marijuana. In a series of four young adult men with synthetic marijuana exposure, patients presented with dyspnea, cough, hypoxemia, and respiratory failure.[23] CT scans in all patients were notable for diffuse centrilobular and tree-in-bud nodules, which correlated with organizing pneumonia in the three patients who underwent surgical biopsy (**Fig. 11**).[23] Importantly, standard urine tests for marijuana metabolites can be negative, so the radiologist may be the first to suggest the correct diagnosis. It is always important to think about unusual exposures if there is no clear explanation for centrilobular nodules in the setting of small airways diseases. For example, hookah smoking (hookah lung) is another example of an exposure that can have a similar imaging appearance.[24]

CONSTRICTIVE BRONCHIOLITIS

Constrictive (fibrotic or obliterative) bronchiolitis is characterized by irreversible, concentric submucosal fibrosis resulting in bronchiolar narrowing or occlusion. Fibrosis extends between the epithelium and muscular mucosa of the airway, ultimately leading to airflow obstruction. Causes of cellular bronchiolitis may also have a component of constrictive bronchiolitis (eg, FB, diffuse panbronchiolitis), but there are many diseases where

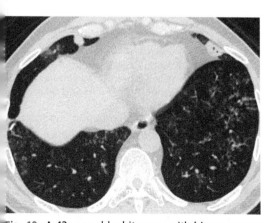

Fig. 10. A 42-year-old white man with biopsy-proven diffuse panbronchiolitis. CT image shows bilateral tree-in-bud nodules and later stage findings including bronchiectasis and bronchiolectasis. A staple line is present in the right lower lobe from the excisional biopsy that proved the diagnosis.

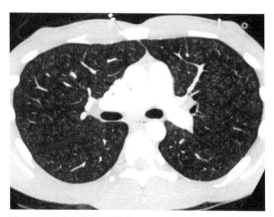

Fig. 11. Axial thin MIP image of a 21-year-old man with diffuse centrilobular and tree-in-bud nodules secondary to smoking synthetic marijuana. The patient presented with respiratory failure and required prolonged intubation. Surgical lung biopsy demonstrated organizing pneumonia as the correlate for the diffuse centrilobular nodules.

constrictive bronchiolitis is the dominant imaging feature (summarized in **Table 3**):

- Childhood infection
- Transplant-related
  - Lung transplant rejection: bronchiolitis obliterans syndrome

- Stem cell transplant: graft-versus-host disease
- Inhalational lung disease
- CTD
- Diffuse idiopathic pulmonary neuroendocrine cell hyperplasia
- Idiopathic

Table 3
Constrictive bronchiolitis: differential diagnosis

Cause	Imaging	Clinical
Childhood infection	• Hyperlucent lobe(s) or lung (may be bilateral) with air trapping, diminished vascularity, bronchiectasis	• Childhood airway infection, most often viral
Lung transplant	• Air trapping	• Sign of chronic allograft rejection (≥3 mo after transplant)
Graft-versus-host disease	• Air trapping	• Hematopoietic stem cell transplant recipient • Other organ involvement (eg, skin, gastrointestinal tract)
Inhalational lung disease	• Air trapping • +/− bronchiectasis	• Exposure to nitrous acid/oxide, popcorn flavoring agent, or fire smoke
CTD	• Air trapping	• Known CTD (usually rheumatoid arthritis) • Progressive dyspnea/cough
Diffuse idiopathic pulmonary neuroendocrine cell hyperplasia	• Air trapping • Nodular bronchial wall thickening • Small parenchymal nodules	• Middle-aged or elderly female
Idiopathic	• Air trapping indistinguishable from other causes	• Rare, diagnosis of exclusion • Often older women • May have rapidly worsening course

Diagnostic Criteria		
Pattern	**Histologic Finding**	**Imaging Appearance**
Centrilobular nodules (direct finding of small airways inflammation)	• Inflammation in walls of airways • Inflammatory exudates/debris in airway lumen	• Nodules at the center of secondary pulmonary lobules that spare the pleural and fissural surfaces • Vary in attenuation and size
Tree-in-bud nodules (subset of centrilobular nodules most often seen with infection or aspiration)	• Peribronchiolar inflammation + lumen impacted with pus, fluid, mucus or debris	• Branching V- or Y-shaped nodules • Spare fissural/pleural surfaces
Air trapping (indirect finding of bronchiolar obstruction)	• Collagen deposition with narrowing and/or obliteration of small airways	• Geographic areas of decreased attenuation • Regions remain more lucent than surrounding lung on expiratory imaging • Bronchial wall thickening/bronchiectasis may also be present

At HRCT, constrictive bronchiolitis manifests with air trapping, which is an indirect sign of small airways diseases. Air trapping refers to heterogeneous parenchyma on inspiratory images, termed mosaic attenuation, and accentuated geometric areas of decreased attenuation on expiratory images. On expiratory images, the lucent areas represent abnormally hypoaerated and hypoperfused portions of lung, whereas the high-attenuation areas are normal.[15] Large airways disease may also be present, with bronchial wall thickening and/or bronchiectasis.

Childhood Infection

Constrictive bronchiolitis may occasionally result from childhood airway infection, primarily viral etiologies, such as adenovirus. Alveoli mature by age 8, so bronchiolitis before this time can disrupt alveoli and associated pulmonary vessel development, leading to an obliterative bronchiolitis with mosaic attenuation and air trapping.[19] Swyer-James (or Swyer-James-MacLeod) syndrome is the most advanced, long-term complication of postinfectious bronchiolitis with involvement of an entire lobe, entire lung, and sometimes even both lungs.[25] Imaging findings include regions of hyperlucent lung (and often decreased volume) with diminished vascularity, bronchiectasis, and air trapping (**Fig. 12**).

Lung Transplant

Bronchiolitis obliterans syndrome, a form of constrictive bronchiolitis, is a known complication of lung transplantation occurring in up to 50% of patients.[19] It is considered a manifestation of chronic allograft rejection, developing at least 3 months after transplantation, and is associated with decreased pulmonary function. Air trapping on expiratory HRCT images is the most sensitive and specific imaging feature of bronchiolitis obliterans syndrome in patients post–lung transplant, although the degree of air trapping does not necessarily correlate with severity of rejection (**Fig. 13**). The presence of bronchiolitis obliterans syndrome portends a poor prognosis in lung transplant recipients with 5-year survival about 30% to 40% after onset of disease.[14]

Graft-Versus-Host Disease

Constrictive bronchiolitis is also a common manifestation of graft-versus-host disease associated with hematopoietic stem cell transplantation, occurring in approximately 10% of recipients. Air trapping is the predominant imaging finding, and is similar in appearance to other causes of constrictive bronchilolitis.[26] The clinical history of

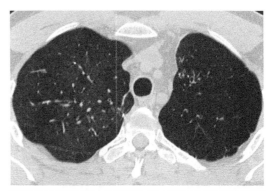

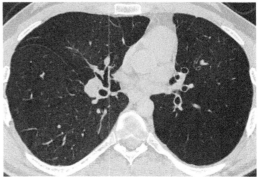

Fig. 12. A 37-year-old man with a history of severe viral illness as a child and resultant Swyer-James syndrome. CT images performed during lung transplant evaluation show a hyperlucent left lung (from severe air trapping) with decreased vascularity and bronchiectasis. Note that there is volume loss in the left lung, with leftward mediastinal shift, but that there are areas of the right lung that are also involved.

graft-versus-host disease, often affecting other organs, such as skin and gastrointestinal tract, helps confirm the diagnosis.[19,27]

Inhalational Lung Disease

Various inhalational exposures have been implicated in constrictive bronchiolitis, including nitrous acid and nitrous oxide chemical compounds, popcorn flavoring agents, and fire smoke. These exposures cause epithelial injury leading to granulation tissue accumulation that ultimately results in airway obliteration, manifesting as air trapping on expiratory HRCT.[1,12] Bronchiectasis may also be seen in cases of inhalation injury (**Fig. 14**).[28]

Connective Tissue Disease

Constrictive bronchiolitis has been described in CTD, most commonly women with advanced rheumatoid arthritis. Such patients may present with dyspnea or cough, typically with a severe and progressive course that is refractory to treatment.[18] Although many cases have occurred in

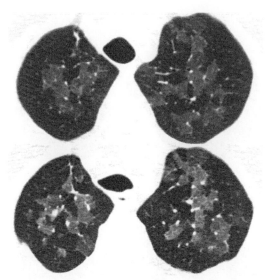

Fig. 13. A 60-year-old man who underwent bilateral lung transplant 7 years earlier with bronchiolitis obliterans syndrome as a manifestation of chronic rejection. Axial images through the upper lobes during inspiration (*top*) shows a striking mosaic attenuation pattern. Without expiratory views it could be difficult to determine which regions of lung are abnormal, but expiratory image (*bottom*) confirms that the mosaic pattern is caused by air trapping because the lucent regions remain lucent.

patients on penicillamine for rheumatoid arthritis, constrictive bronchiolitis may arise independent of such therapy.[14,29] Imaging findings are similar to other causes of constrictive bronchiolitis, and

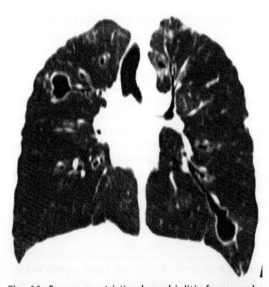

Fig. 14. Severe constrictive bronchiolitis from smoke inhalation in a house fire. This coronal reformatted CT image shows mosaic attenuation from severe air trapping and cystic bronchiectasis, findings that are seen from inhalational injury.

are usually seen independent of CTD-related interstitial lung disease (Fig. 15).

Diffuse Idiopathic Pulmonary Neuroendocrine Cell Hyperplasia

Diffuse idiopathic pulmonary neuroendocrine cell hyperplasia refers to proliferation of neuroendocrine cells confined to bronchial or bronchiolar epithelial basement membranes.[30] Most patients are middle-aged or elderly women, and may be asymptomatic or report chronic cough, dyspnea, or "asthma."[31] Histologically, the proliferation of neuroendocrine cells results in narrowing and obstruction of small airway lumens with progressive fibrosis. The cell proliferation and luminal obstruction corresponds to the HRCT findings of air trapping, nodular bronchial wall thickening, and multiple small parenchymal nodules (Fig. 16).[30,32] Nodules may remain stable for several years or show slow growth. Diffuse idiopathic pulmonary neuroendocrine cell hyperplasia is a mild form of neuroendocrine cell proliferation: the term "tumorlets" refers to tumors less than 5 mm with extension beyond the epithelial basement membrane, and "carcinoids" describe extension greater than 5 mm.[32]

MIMICS

Several entities may present with imaging findings similar to small airways diseases and it is important for radiologists to be aware of these mimics. Mimics of small airways nodules include aerogenous spread of adenocarcinoma, and vascular and lymphatic causes of centrilobular nodules. Small vessel disease or ground-glass opacity may cause a mosaic attenuation pattern and mimic obliterative bronchiolitis.

Aerogenous Spread of Adenocarcinoma

Aerogenous spread of lung adenocarcinoma is thought to represent a mechanism whereby the tumor metastasizes to other parts of the lungs via the airways. In contrast to multiple synchronous primary lung cancers, where each tumor may be of different histologic subtypes, aerogenous spread represents a monoclonal tumor at different sites. Typical imaging findings of aerogenous spread of adenocarcinoma include persistent centrilobular or tree-in-bud nodules that slowly enlarge over serial examinations, especially in the context of a known lung adenocarcinoma. These nodules may cluster and coalesce into areas of ground-glass opacity or consolidation (Fig. 17).[33]

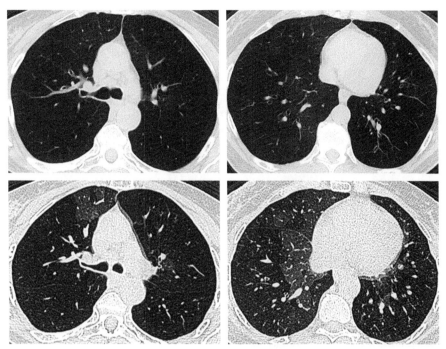

Fig. 15. A 60-year-old woman with scleroderma and worsening dyspnea. Inspiratory HRCT images (*top row*) depict very subtle findings of constrictive bronchiolitis including mosaic attenuation and mild bronchial wall thickening. Expiratory images (*bottom row*), however, reveal severe air trapping with areas of relative high attenuation representing normal lung. The severity of mosaic attenuation would be easy to overlook without the expiratory images.

VASCULAR AND LYMPHATIC CAUSES OF CENTRILOBULAR NODULES

Arterioles and lymphatics course alongside bronchioles at the center of the SPL. As such, arteriolar and lymphatic diseases may mimic the entire spectrum of small airways imaging findings from ill-defined centrilobular nodules to a tree-in-bud pattern.[13] Arteriolar causes of centrilobular nodules include intravascular metastases, excipient lung, and pulmonary arterial hypertension. A history of malignancy or signs of elevated pulmonary pressures (including right heart enlargement/hypertrophy and pulmonary artery dilation) can be helpful clues to the presence of vascular centrilobular nodules or a vascular tree-in-bud pattern.

Malignancy

Malignancy may mimic small airways diseases because tumors may spread through airways, along lymphatics, or within pulmonary arterioles. Intravascular metastases may manifest as centrilobular or tree-in-bud nodules on CT. Any tumors that result in hematogenous spread to the lung can cause this pattern and the visible abnormality usually represents filling of peripheral vessels with tumor cells.[13] In patients with cancer, the presence of growing centrilobular or tree-in-bud nodules (often with a beaded appearance) over multiple restaging scans is a big clue to the presence of intravascular metastases (**Fig. 18**). Tumor

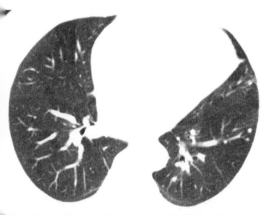

Figs. 16. A 60-year-old woman with diffuse idiopathic pulmonary neuroendocrine cell hyperplasia. CT image through the lung bases shows patchy mosaic attenuation and two small nodules in the periphery of the left lower lobe representing carcinoid tumorlets. Numerous nodules of similar size were present throughout the remainder of the lungs.

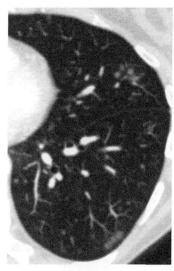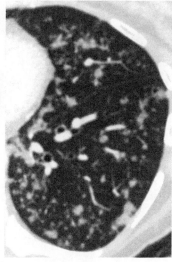

Figs. 17. A 64-year-old woman with endobronchial (aerogenous) spread of mucinous lung adenocarcinoma. Axial thin MIP from baseline CT (*left*) shows clustered centrilobular ground-glass nodules in the left lung, thought to represent an acute infectious bronchiolitis. CT performed 6 months later (*right*) shows enlargement of preexisting nodules and extensive new centrilobular nodules throughout the lung, subsequently confirmed to represent diffuse adenocarcinoma.

thrombotic angiopathy is a rare complication of tumor emboli where diffuse centrilobular or tree-in-bud nodules are the result of widespread fibro-cellular intimal hyperplasia of arterioles.[34] Patients with intravascular metastases may present with worsening dyspnea, hypoxia, and pulmonary hypertension, and tumor thrombotic angiopathy in particular may cause rapid decline.

Excipient Lung Disease

Excipient lung disease, also known as drug abuser's lung, is a foreign body reaction within

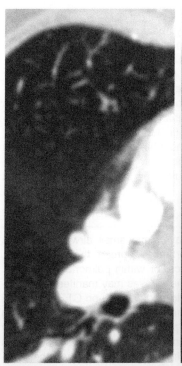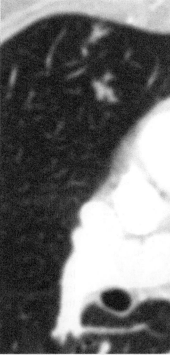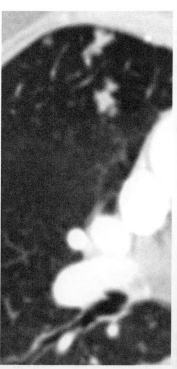

Figs. 18. A 77-year-old woman with metastatic colon adenocarcinoma. On the initial staging CT (*left*) very faint centrilobular nodules are visible in the anterior segment of the right upper lobe. Subsequent CT scans at 3 months (*center*) and 6 months (*right*) show progressive enlargement with a beaded or tree-in-bud appearance consistent with intravascular metastases.

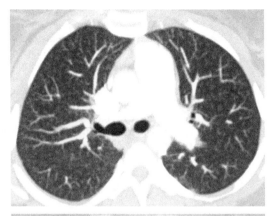

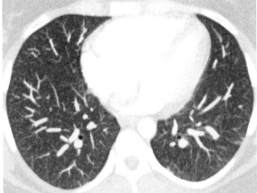

Figs. 19. A 24-year-old woman with excipient lung disease who presented with syncope and dyspnea. Axial MIP images from a pulmonary-embolism protocol CT performed on arrival show diffuse centrilobular nodules involving all lobes. The right ventricle is dilated with leftward bowing of the interventricular septum (*lower image*) from elevated pulmonary arterial pressures. Patient had an indwelling catheter (not shown, but another clue to the possibility of excipient lung disease) through which she admitted injecting crushed hydromorphone hydrochloride tablets.

pulmonary arterioles caused by intravenous injection of crushed oral tablets.[35] Excipients are the various insoluble, inert fillers that are added to a pill during production and, when injected, become lodged in the pulmonary arterioles and capillaries. These particles can incite an angiogranulomatous reaction that causes pulmonary hypertension and potentially death.[35] Imaging findings in excipient lung disease include diffuse centrilobular nodules (nodules may favor the mid lower lung zones presumably caused by increased blood flow) and signs of pulmonary hypertension (**Fig. 19**). Patients often have a history of drug use, chronic pain, and/or an indwelling catheter, and the radiologist may be the first to suggest the diagnosis because excipient lung disease is clinically underrecognized.

AIR TRAPPING MIMICS

The presence of mosaic attenuation does not equate to air trapping in all cases. Vessel disease (eg, chronic pulmonary embolism, pulmonary arterial hypertension) and ground-glass opacity (eg, *Pneumocystis* pneumonia) may be difficult to differentiate on routine inspiratory imaging.[36] Expiratory imaging improves the accuracy of differentiating air trapping from other causes of mosaic attenuation. Whereas air trapping is accentuated with expiratory imaging, lung attenuation becomes more uniform on expiratory imaging in small vessels disease or ground-glass opacity (**Figs. 20** and **21**). In the setting of pulmonary arterial hypertension, mosaic attenuation and ill-defined regions of ground-glass opacities may represent a combination of differential perfusion, plexogenic arterial lesions, and/or cholesterol granulomas.[36]

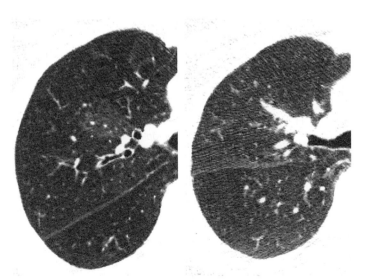

Figs. 20. A 71-year-old woman with mosaic perfusion caused by chronic thromboembolic disease. Axial image at full inspiration (*left*) shows mosaic attenuation with large regions of decreased perfusion associated with small caliber vessels. Expiratory image at a similar level (*right*) shows no air trapping; the entire right lung becomes more uniform with increased attenuation, whereas in air trapping the lucent areas would remain lucent during exhalation.

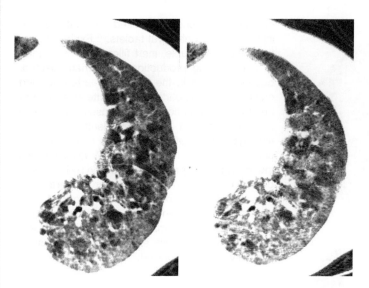

Figs. 21. A 31-year-old woman with dyspnea. Axial HRCT images during inspiration (*left*) and dynamic expiration (*right*) show mosaic attenuation from ground-glass opacity. Although the mosaic pattern persists on expiratory image, all regions of lung increase in attenuation (ie, no air trapping). The patient was subsequently diagnosed with pneumocystis pneumonia.

SUMMARY

Small airways diseases, or bronchiolitis, encompasses an array of conditions that cause inflammation or fibrosis of the small airways within SPL. Centrilobular nodules are a direct sign of a cellular, or inflammatory, bronchiolitis. Air trapping is an indirect sign of a constrictive, or obliterative, bronchiolitis. Combining the imaging patterns with the clinical history and pathologic features can usually narrow the differential or solidify a diagnosis.

REFERENCES

1. Hansell DM. Small airways diseases: detection and insights with computed tomography. Eur Respir J 2001;17(6):1294–313.
2. Webb WR. Thin-section CT of the secondary pulmonary lobule: anatomy and the image–the 2004 Fleischner lecture. Radiology 2006;239(2):322–38.
3. Rice A, Nicholson AG. The pathologist's approach to small airways disease. Histopathology 2009;54(1):117–33.
4. American College of Radiology. ACR–STR practice parameter for the performance of high-resolution computed tomography (HRCT) of the lungs in adults. 2015. Available at: http://www.acr.org/~/media/17AF593BAF2E47AE9A51B10A60BC09D1.pdf. Accessed February 27, 2016.
5. Gruden JF, Ouanounou S, Tigges S, et al. Incremental benefit of maximum-intensity-projection images on observer detection of small pulmonary nodules revealed by multidetector CT. Am J Roentgenol 2002;179(1):149–57.
6. Beigelman-Aubry C, Hill C, Guibal A, et al. Multi-detector row CT and postprocessing techniques in the

assessment of diffuse lung disease. Radiographics 2005;25(6):1639–52.
7. Gotway MB, Freemer MM, King TE Jr. Challenges in pulmonary fibrosis. 1: Use of high resolution CT scanning of the lung for the evaluation of patients with idiopathic interstitial pneumonias. Thorax 2007;62(6):546–53.
8. Gotway MB, Lee ES, Reddy GP, et al. Low-dose, dynamic, expiratory thin-section CT of the lungs using a spiral CT scanner. J Thorac Imaging 2000;15(3):168–72.
9. Arakawa H, Webb WR, McCowin M, et al. Inhomogeneous lung attenuation at thin-section CT: diagnostic value of expiratory scans. Radiology 1998;206(1):89–94.
10. Hogg JC, Macklem PT, Thurlbeck WM. Site and nature of airway obstruction in chronic obstructive lung disease. N Engl J Med 1968;268:1355–60.
11. Visscher DW, Myers JL. Bronchiolitis: the pathologist's perspective. Proc Am Thorac Soc 2006;3(1):41–7.
12. Pipavath SN, Stern EJ. Imaging of small airway disease (SAD). Radiol Clin North Am 2009;47(2):307–16.
13. Rossi SE, Franquet T, Volpacchio M, et al. Tree-in-bud pattern at thin-section CT of the lungs: radiologic-pathologic overview. Radiographics 2005;25(3):789–801.
14. Abbott GF, Rosado-de-Christenson ML, Rossi SE, et al. Imaging of small airways disease. J Thorac Imaging 2009;24(4):285–98.
15. Naidich DP, Webb WR, Müller NL, et al. Computed tomography and magnetic resonance of the thorax. 4th edition. Philadelphia (PA): Lippincott Williams and Wilkins; 2007.
16. Aquino SL, Gamsu G, Webb WR, et al. Tree-in-bud pattern: frequency and significance on thin section CT. J Comput Assist Tomogr 1996;20(4):594–9.

17. Fukuchi Y, Matsuse T, Kida K. Clinico-pathological profile of diffuse aspiration bronchiolitis (DAB). Nihon Kyobu Shikkan Gakkai Zasshi 1989;27:571–7.

18. Burgel PR, Bergeron A, de Blic J, et al. Small airways diseases, excluding asthma and COPD: an overview. Eur Respir Rev 2013;22(128):131–47.

19. Pipavath SJ, Lynch DA, Cool C, et al. Radiologic and pathologic features of bronchiolitis. Am J Roentgenol 2005;185(2):354–63.

20. Elicker BM, Jones KD, Henry TS, et al. Multidisciplinary approach to hypersensitivity pneumonitis. J Thorac Imaging 2016;31(2):92–103.

21. Franks TJ, Galvin JR. Hypersensitivity pneumonitis: essential radiologic and pathologic findings. Surg Pathol Clin 2010;3(1):187–98.

22. Poletti V, Casoni G, Chilosi M, et al. Diffuse panbronchiolitis. Eur Respir J 2006;28(4):862–71.

23. Berkowitz EA, Henry TS, Veeraraghavan S, et al. Pulmonary effects of synthetic marijuana: chest radiography and CT findings. AJR Am J Roentgenol 2015; 204(4):750–7.

24. De Dios JA, Javaid AA, Mesologites T, et al. 20-year-old man with fever, chest pain, and lung nodules. Chest 2011;140(5):1378–81.

25. Lucaya J, Gartner S, García-Peña P. Spectrum of manifestations of Swyer-James-MacLeod syndrome. J Comput Assist Tomogr 1998;22(4):592–7.

26. Coy DL, Ormazabal A, Godwin JD, et al. Imaging evaluation of pulmonary and abdominal complications following hematopoietic stem cell transplantation. Radiographics 2005;25(2):305–17 [discussion: 318].

27. Gunn MLD, Godwin JD, Kanne JP, et al. High-resolution CT findings of bronchiolitis obliterans syndrome after hematopoietic stem cell transplantation. J Thorac Imaging 2008;23(4):244–50.

28. Tasaka S, Kanazawa M, Mori M, et al. Long-term course of bronchiectasis and bronchiolitis obliterans as late complication of smoke inhalation. Respiration 1995;62(1):40–2.

29. Penny WJ, Knight RK, Rees AM, et al. Obliterative bronchiolitis in rheumatoid arthritis. Ann Rheum Dis 1982;41(5):469–72.

30. Koo CW, Baliff JP, Torigian DA, et al. Spectrum of pulmonary neuroendocrine cell proliferation: diffuse idiopathic pulmonary neuroendocrine cell hyperplasia, tumorlet, and carcinoids. AJR Am J Roentgenol 2010;195(3):661–8.

31. Aguayo SM, Miller YE, Waldron JA, et al. Brief report - idiopathic diffuse hyperplasia of pulmonary neuroendocrine cells and airways disease. N Engl J Med 1992;327(18):1285–8.

32. Davies SJ, Gosney JR, Hansell DM, et al. Diffuse idiopathic pulmonary neuroendocrine cell hyperplasia: an under-recognized spectrum of disease. Thorax 2007;62:248–52.

33. Gaikwad A, Souza CA, Inacio JR, et al. Aerogenous metastases: a potential game changer in the diagnosis and management of primary lung adenocarcinoma. AJR Am J Roentgenol 2014;203(6):W570–82.

34. Franquet T. Imaging of pneumonia: trends and algorithms. Eur Respir J 2001;18(1):196–208.

35. Nguyen VT, Chan ES, Chou SH, et al. Pulmonary effects of i.v. injection of crushed oral tablets: "excipient lung disease". AJR Am J Roentgenol 2014; 203(5):W506–15.

36. Kligerman SJ, Henry T, Lin CT, et al. Mosaic attenuation: etiology, methods of differentiation, and pitfalls. Radiographics 2015;35(5):1360–80.

Imaging of Diseases of the Large Airways

Brent P. Little, MD*, Phuong-Anh T. Duong, MD

KEYWORDS

- Imaging of large airways • CT of airways • Bronchiectasis • Tracheal imaging

KEY POINTS

- A variety of congenital and acquired disorders of the trachea and bronchi can be characterized at noninvasive chest imaging.
- Although many large airway diseases are suspected at radiography, computed tomography offers detailed characterization of airway abnormalities with reformatting techniques and dynamic expiratory protocols.
- The morphology and pattern of involvement can point to an accurate differential diagnosis of large airway diseases.

INTRODUCTION

Imaging of the large airways is key to the diagnosis and management of a wide variety of congenital, infectious, malignant, and inflammatory diseases. Involvement can be focal, regional, or diffuse, and abnormalities can take the form of masses, thickening, narrowing, enlargement, or a combination of patterns. Recognition of the typical morphologies, locations, and distributions of large airways disease is central to an accurate imaging differential diagnosis.

NORMAL ANATOMY AND IMAGING TECHNIQUES

The large airways include the trachea and bronchi, a set of branching structures that serve as the interface between the lungs and the environment. As part of the conducting system, the large airways do not participate in gas exchange. However, the trachea and bronchi are more than simple tubes for entry and exit of gases of respiration. Cilia within the pseudostratified columnar epithelium of the mucosal layer of both the trachea and bronchi help clear inhaled toxins, organisms, and debris. A submucosal layer contains secretory glands producing secretions that assist clearance and serve a protective role. The large airways, unlike the small airways—the bronchioles—have a cartilaginous component, with cartilaginous rings in the trachea and more amorphous sheets in the bronchi. Additional components of the large airways include other glandular tissue, including neuroendocrine and mucosal-associated lymphoid tissue.[1]

The trachea is typically 6 to 9 cm in length; multiple rings of cartilage comprise the anterior and lateral portions of the trachea, whereas the posterior tracheal wall—the "membranous trachea"—is noncartilagenous and composed of a thinner muscular layer and connective tissue layer. The bronchioles have a more uniform composition of sheetlike layers of cartilage and other constituents.[1]

Chest radiography plays a limited but important role in the examination of the large airways. The trachea, mainstem bronchi, and lobar bronchi are readily identified on chest radiography (Fig. 1). Focal tracheal narrowing or filling defects can suggest stenoses or masses, and tracheomegaly or diffuse thickening or narrowing of the trachea can

Disclosure Statement: The authors have nothing to disclose.
Department of Radiology and Imaging Sciences, Emory University Hospital, Emory University School of Medicine, Clinic Building A, 1365 Clifton Road Northeast, Atlanta, GA 30322, USA
* Corresponding author.
E-mail address: brent.p.little@emory.edu

Radiol Clin N Am 54 (2016) 1183–1203
http://dx.doi.org/10.1016/j.rcl.2016.05.014

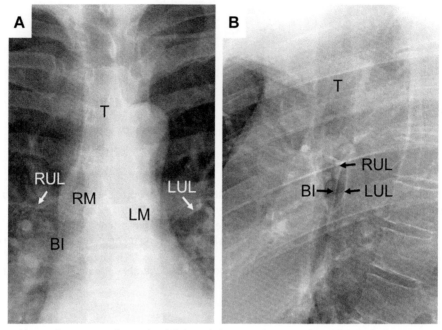

Fig. 1. Normal large airways at radiography. (*A*) Coned-down posteroanterior radiograph shows normal large airways; the mainstem and lobar bronchi are visible as tubular air-filled structures with smooth, thin walls. (*B*) Coned-down lateral radiograph of the normal large airways; the trachea (T) is a long air-filled column. The left upper lobe bronchus (LUL) and right upper lobe bronchus (RUL) are seen on end as circular lucencies. The posterior wall of bronchus intermedius (BI) is seen as a line bisecting the LUL bronchial lucency. BI, bronchus intermedius; LM, left main bronchus; LUL, left upper lobe bronchus; RM, right main bronchus; RUL, right upper lobe bronchus.

at times be identified. However, many tracheal or bronchial masses can be relatively inconspicuous at radiography, and computed tomography (CT) is central to examination of any suspected large airway narrowing or thickening. In addition, although radiographs can often be used in the detection and preliminary characterization of diffuse diseases of the airways such as bronchiectasis and bronchial wall thickening, thin slice CT of the chest is more sensitive in detecting these abnormalities and more helpful in characterizing their severity, distribution, and morphology.

COMPUTED TOMOGRAPHY IMAGING PROTOCOLS
Acquisition of Images

Multidetector CT has become an essential tool for noninvasive assessment of the airways for both neoplastic and nonneoplastic causes of airway narrowing and thickening. Not only does CT provide diagnostic information to determine the cause of airways disease, but 3-dimensional (3D) rendered images allow detailed visualization of these lesions and the surrounding structures for preoperative planning. Volumetric, spiral acquisition with thin collimation (3 mm) and thin slice

reconstructions (1-2 mm) in the axial plane are preferred, allowing for the detection and evaluation of airway thickening, nodularity, masses, or other abnormalities; coronal and sagittal reformatted series should be reconstructed as part of a standard examination (**Fig. 2**). An expiratory series can be obtained during maximum forced expiration to maximize sensitivity for air trapping, and to allow for assessment of expiratory airway collapse that can be seen in tracheobronchomalacia; imaging obtained during forced expiration rather than at end expiration is preferred for detection of airway collapse.[2] Dynamic 4-dimensional imaging of the trachea and bronchi during inspiration and expiration has also been used in detection and planning of therapy for abnormalities of the large airways, especially in children.[3]

Although CT is the mainstay in airway evaluation, fluorine-18-fluoro(2)deoxyglucose (FDG) PET may be also helpful to distinguish malignant disease and evaluate posttreatment response.[4,5]

Postprocessing of Images

Several methods of reformatting volumetric CT data sets can be used to evaluate the large airways. 3D multiplanar reformatted images in the

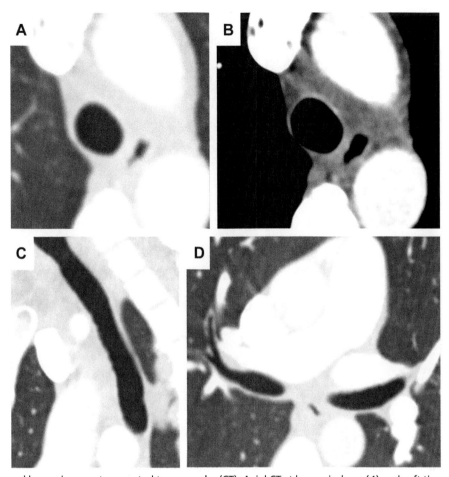

Fig. 2. Normal large airways at computed tomography (CT). Axial CT at lung windows (*A*) and soft tissue windows (*B*) showing a normal intrathoracic trachea at inspiration. The normal trachea has a smooth, soft tissue attenuation wall and is typically circular or ovoid shape. (*C*) Sagittal reformatted CT through the trachea at lung windows shows a normal tubular appearance with a smooth contour. (*D*) Axial CT at lung windows shows normal mainstem bronchi and right upper lobe segmental bronchi. Normal bronchi have smooth, thin walls and taper in diameter as they ramify.

coronal, sagittal, and other planes are helpful for detection and characterization of both focal and diffuse abnormalities. Maximum intensity projection reformatted images are often obtained in the axial and often other planes, and can provide an overview of the anatomic relationships between the airways and adjacent vessels, lymph nodes, and other constituents of the mediastinum. 3D volume-rendered images can also be helpful for assessing relationships between the airways and adjacent structures, and can assist planning a surgical approach to a focal large airway abnormality. A 3D dataset can also be processed specifically to simulate bronchoscopic endolumenal views, called "virtual bronchoscopy" (**Fig. 3**). Newer 3D CT reformatting techniques have been found to be of high sensitivity similar to bronchoscopy for detection of lesions of the large airways such as

tracheal stenosis.[6] Minimum intensity projection images can be helpful in assessing the overall distribution and morphology of airway abnormalities such as bronchiectasis (**Fig. 4**).

More recently, there has been much excitement over the use of 3D printing using detailed CT data—early applications have included printing of airway models for hands-on surgical planning and anesthesia airway management.[7–9] CT has also has advantages compared with bronchoscopy when there is a stenotic segment that cannot be traversed or there is a risk of injury from inflammation, trauma, or infection.[4]

Review of Images

Airways should be evaluated at both standard lung windows and soft tissue windows. Lung windows

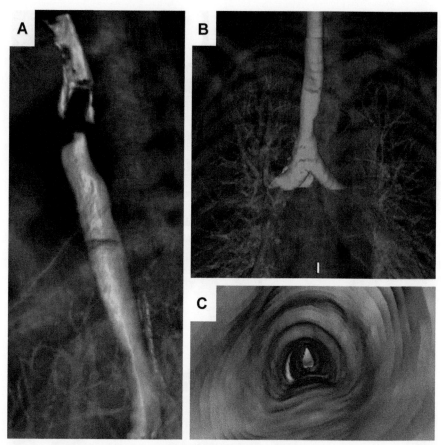

Fig. 3. Three-dimensional reformatting techniques. (*A*) Three-dimensional volume rendering with segmentation and shading of the trachea, highlighting the 3-dimensional structure of the airway. (*B*) Three-dimensional volume rendering of the trachea and bronchi, segmented to demonstrate the overall structure of the tracheobronchial tree. (*C*) "Virtual bronchoscopy" 3-dimensional reformatted image shows the trachea from an endoluminal perspective.

are superior for assessing the diameter and thickness of the airways, as well as for the presence of filling defects or stenoses. Soft tissue windows can be used to assess components of any masses, stenoses, or wall thickening, highlighting the presence and morphology of soft tissue or calcification.[10] Review usually begins with the axial series, with sagittal, coronal, and other 3D reformatted series available for further characterization of abnormalities. Advanced postprocessing is usually reserved for cases in which an abnormality is detected or is known before the examination acquisition.

Manual and semiautomated techniques have been developed for scoring diffuse large airway abnormalities such bronchial wall thickening. Computer algorithms can be used to segment and analyze the diameter and thickness of the tracheobronchial tree at multiple levels, and have been used to correlate bronchial wall thickness with degree of airway obstruction in smokers.[11,12]

NORMAL AND ABNORMAL APPEARANCES OF THE LARGE AIRWAYS
Normal Appearances

At radiography, the normal trachea is seen as an air-filled tubular structure on both frontal and lateral views extending from above the thoracic inlet to the carina (see **Fig. 1**). The tracheal wall should be thin and smooth. The main and lobar bronchi are readily seen, and often many of the segmental bronchi can be identified. Bronchial walls, similar to the trachea, should be smooth and thin at radiography, and the normal bronchial diameter should be similar to the adjacent artery. Tracheal and bronchial calcification can be seen, especially in older age and in the setting of chronic use of some medications such as warfarin.

At CT, the normal trachea at inspiration has a circular or ovoid shape with smooth walls measuring 1 to 3 mm; the posterior membranous trachea is normally thinner than the cartilaginous anterior and lateral portions of the trachea (see

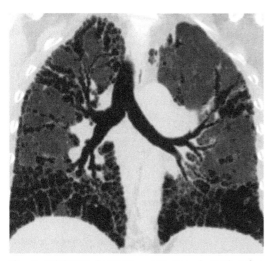

Fig. 4. Minimum intensity projection (minIP) reformatted image. The minIP of an axial computed tomography viewed at lung windows of a patient with sarcoidosis highlights upper lobe traction bronchiectasis and central retraction. The image also shows a complex combination of severe traction bronchiectasis and architectural distortion at the lung bases in a pattern distinctive from that seen in usual interstitial pneumonitis (UIP).

Fig. 2).[13] Although the large airway cartilage can calcify often quite dramatically with age, this calcification should follow the normal distribution of cartilage, with an incomplete ringlike appearance in the trachea and a more diffuse appearance in the bronchi. The upper limit of normal transverse and anteroposterior tracheal diameters are 21 and 23 mm in women and 25 and 27 mm in men.[2]

Similarly, bronchial walls should be smooth and thin at CT. Bronchi should smoothly taper in diameter as they branch from center to the periphery of the lung, and usually have diameters less than or equal to the adjacent pulmonary artery. Although the average bronchial-to-arterial ratio (measured from outer to outer diameter) has been described as approximately 1:1, a range of ratios have been noted in healthy adults, ranging from 0.53 to 1.39.[14] With age, bronchi can increase in thickness and diameter, even in patients without known respiratory disease; 1 study noted a bronchoarterial ratio greater than 1 in 41% of subjects over 65 years of age.[15]

Abnormal Appearances

Abnormal appearances of the airways include a variety of types of airway thickening, airway narrowing, or airway enlargement. Thickening and narrowing can be characterized as diffuse, regional, or focal. Airway thickening can be smooth or irregular/nodular, and can show soft tissue attenuation or calcification. At CT, thickening and nodularity can be circumferential or can spare the posterior noncartilagenous trachea, a clue to etiology. Tracheal enlargement can be readily detected at radiography and CT, and the latter can be used to measure tracheal diameters and areas. Bronchial dilation can be suspected when the bronchus is larger than the adjacent artery, or when bronchi do not show normal peripheral tapering.

DIFFUSE LARGE AIRWAY NARROWING: TRACHEOBRONCHOMALACIA AND SABER SHEATH TRACHEA
Tracheobronchomalacia

The normal trachea usually has an ovoid or circular appearance at inspiration. At expiration, the posterior membranous trachea can flatten or can bow anteriorly, a common finding at routine CT owing to difficulty in breath holding during the examination. However, patients with tracheobronchomalacia show excessive collapse of the trachea and bronchi at expiration, often leading to symptoms such as chronic cough, wheezing, and stridor.[16] Congenital tracheobronchomalacia is the most common congenital large airway disease and is caused by a deficiency in the cartilaginous walls of the trachea and central bronchi, leading to a lack of airway support during expiration.[17] Tracheomalacia and bronchomalacia can also be acquired as part of prolonged intubation with mechanical ventilation, or as part of a number of other diseases that involve the large airways, such as chronic obstructive pulmonary disease (COPD).[16] Focal or diffuse malacia of the large airways was found at expiratory CT in 72% patients with relapsing polychondritis in 1 study.[18] Bronchomalacia has been detected in up to 61% of patients with sarcoidosis.[19]

In severe cases, the trachea and mainstem bronchial lumens can be nearly completely obliterated at expiration, causing what is known as the "frown sign" (**Fig. 5**).[20] However, the degree of collapse at which one should suggest tracheomalacia has been revised over the past few years. CT and MR imaging studies have shown that the tracheas of normal volunteers can collapse significantly at forced expiration, with 1 study noting a decrease in cross-sectional area of more than 50% in 78% of healthy volunteers (mean age 50).[21] In men, the degree of collapse is age dependent, with a tendency toward greater percentage collapse in older patients.[22] The main bronchi can also narrow significantly with expiration; 1

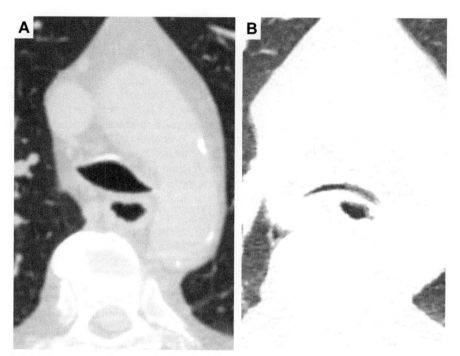

Fig. 5. Lunate trachea and tracheomalacia. (*A*) Coned-down axial computed tomography (CT) image at inspiration shows a "lunate" shape of the trachea, with an elongated posterior wall and a flattened appearance. (*B*) Axial CT at same level shows near complete collapse of the trachea, in keeping with tracheomalacia.

study showed an average of 70% collapse of the right main bronchus and 61% of the left main bronchus.[23] A threshold of 70% tracheal luminal collapse at expiration may be more suggestive of tracheobronchomalacia than the 50% threshold originally proposed. At inspiration, a "lunate" configuration of the trachea with an elongated transverse diameter can be noted in a subset of patients, and is highly associated with tracheomalacia (see **Fig. 5**).[20]

Dedicated protocols for tracheomalacia typically include both a helically acquired CT of the chest at maximum inspiration and a series obtained at forced expiration, usually performed helically at lower kV or mAs. Postprocessing with multiplanar reformatting in the sagittal and coronal planes is routinely performed, and 3D volume-rendered images are often also obtained, demonstrating the overall geometry of the tracheal and bronchial collapse.

Saber Sheath Trachea

Although tracheomalacia is a cause of narrowing of the trachea in the anterior/posterior dimension, narrowing of the intrathoracic trachea in the coronal plane is often seen in patients with COPD, and has been termed a "saber sheath" appearance (**Fig. 6**). The saber sheath trachea was originally

defined as a trachea with an internal transverse diameter less than or equal to two-thirds that of the anteroposterior dimension; clinical evidence of COPD was found in 95% of patients with this tracheal configuration.[24] This smooth narrowing of the trachea begins just below the thoracic inlet and often involves most or all of the intrathoracic trachea, and may be owing to chronically increased intrathoracic pressures in COPD. For unknown reasons, the saber sheath trachea appearance has a strong male predominance with a female instance, reported in only 1 of 200 patients originally described with the morphology.[24] Recognition of a saber sheath appearance can avoid confusion with strictures or extrinsic tracheal compression, and can suggest the presence of COPD in cases in which other findings of the disease are not obvious.

TRACHEOMEGALY AND BRONCHOMEGALY

A variety of diseases can cause dilation of the trachea, with tracheal dimensions measuring over the normal upper limit of 21 and 23 mm for women and 25 and 27 mm for men in transverse and anteroposterior diameters. In moderate to severe cases, an abnormal, irregular, "corrugated" contour of the trachea can often be observed. Dilation of the central bronchi is often also present.

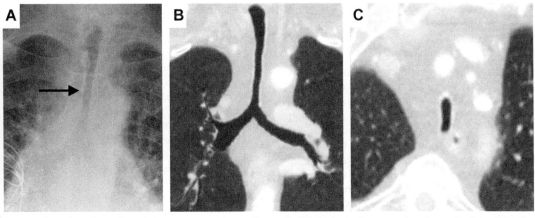

Fig. 6. Saber-Sheath trachea. (*A*) Posteroanterior radiograph shows smooth narrowing (*arrow*) of the intrathoracic trachea. (*B*) Coronal reformatted computed tomography (CT) image shows narrowing of the trachea in the coronal plane. (*C*) Axial CT image shows the "Saber-sheath" shape of the involved trachea, with a transverse diameter substantially smaller than anteroposterior diameter.

Acquired Tracheomegaly and Bronchomegaly

Acquired tracheomegaly and bronchomegaly can occur as a result of airway damage and remodeling from a variety of causes, including prolonged ventilation, radiation therapy, infection, and pulmonary fibrosis, and should be entertained as causes before a congenital source of tracheobronchomegaly is considered.[25]

Mounier–Kuhn Syndrome

Mounier–Kuhn syndrome is an uncommon congenital condition that causes both tracheomegaly and central bronchiectasis (**Fig. 7**). The condition can present in a wide range of ages, from 18 months of age to the elderly, with a mean age of approximately 54 years.[26] The disease is owing to a deficiency of the elastic fibers and thinning of muscular mucosa of the trachea and central bronchi, producing a dilated, irregular, "corrugated" appearance of the trachea and central bronchi.[25] Patients typically have a history of chronic infections that in turn result in worsening airway damage and progressive tracheal and bronchial enlargement; chronic cough and obstructive physiology is often present. In addition to supportive therapy such as mucolytics and physical therapy, surgical measures such as

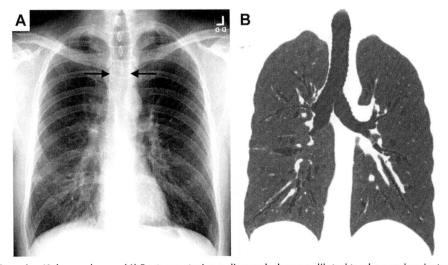

Fig. 7. Mournier–Kuhn syndrome. (*A*) Posteroanterior radiograph shows a dilated trachea and mainstem bronchi, with a suggestion of mild central bronchial wall thickening and bronchiectasis (*arrows*). (*B*) Coronal reformatted minimum intensity projection computed tomography image shows a dilated trachea and mainstem bronchi, with cystic and varicoid bronchiectasis involving the segmental and proximal subsegmental bronchi. An irregular "corrugated" appearance of the trachea is noted, in keeping with deficiency of elastic and muscular fibers.

tracheobronchoplasty and silicone airway stents have shown promise.[25]

Williams–Campbell Syndrome

Williams–Campbell syndrome is a rare cartilage deficiency of the midorder bronchi that causes bronchiectasis at the fifth- or sixth-order subsegmental level, often with a cystic morphology (**Fig. 8**). Unlike Mounier–Kuhn syndrome, Williams–Campbell syndrome spares the trachea and central bronchi.[27] Similar to the former condition, patients usually have a history of recurrent infections, obstructive pulmonary function tests, cough, and wheezing. Although a congenital cartilage deficiency is widely considered the cause of most cases, acquired causes of midorder bronchiectasis include infections such as adenoviral pneumonia.[28]

BRONCHIECTASIS

Bronchiectasis—irreversible dilation of bronchi—can occur in a large variety of airway diseases. Many cases of airway dilation are caused by direct damage to the airway mucosa that occurs in infection, aspiration, and other diseases, resulting in a deleterious cascade of cytokine release, immune cell attraction and activation, and release of enzymes and free radicals. The resulting damage to

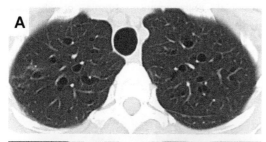

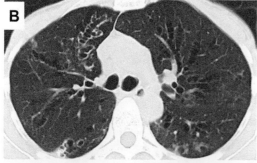

Fig. 8. Williams–Campbell syndrome. (*A, B*) Axial computed tomography images show varicoid and mildly cystic bronchiectasis affecting the midorder bronchi; the central bronchi and trachea are not involved primarily. Note the smooth contour of the trachea and central bronchi, contrasting with the corrugated appearance in Mounier–Kuhn syndrome.

cartilage and other connective tissue causes airway remodeling and enlargement, compounded by elevated intraluminal pressures in the setting of repeated coughing. Impairment of airway defenses increases the frequency and severity of additional airway infections, causing a "vicious cycle" of airway damage. A second major mechanism of airway dilation is "traction bronchiectasis" caused by parenchymal fibrosis, with resulting distortion, dilation, and tethering of bronchi, findings seen in many interstitial lung diseases, such as idiopathic pulmonary fibrosis, connective tissue diseases, and sarcoidosis.

Detection

At radiography, moderate to severe bronchiectasis can often be detected as parallel branching lines representing dilated bronchi radiating from the hila, known as the "tram track" appearance. Bronchial wall thickening and nodular or tubular opacities representing mucous impaction are frequent accompanying findings in many large airways diseases. CT has a high sensitivity for detection of bronchiectasis, and can reveal bronchiectasis in cases in which chest radiography is inconclusive. At CT, bronchial diameters exceed those of adjacent pulmonary arteries, and bronchi show a lack of tapering. CT accurately characterizes the severity, morphology, and distribution of bronchiectasis, which is helpful in formulating a differential diagnosis.[29]

Morphology

Morphologies of bronchiectasis are typically characterized as either cylindrical (smooth and tubular), cystic (saccular), or varicoid (irregular or undulating). Although at times a dominant morphology can suggest a particular cause, 2 or more morphologies are frequently seen in the same patient.[30] Cylindrical bronchiectasis is a very common morphology, and is usually present to some degree in most cases of bronchiectasis. Cystic bronchiectasis is often present in cystic fibrosis, but is neither present in all cases nor specific to this disease, also occurring in many other causes of moderate to severe bronchiectasis in which bronchial wall injury and remodeling occur. Varicoid bronchiectasis suggests the presence of external bronchial traction, and is common in diseases such as sarcoidosis, pneumoconioses, and usual interstitial pneumonitis or fibrotic nonspecific interstitial pneumonitis patterns of pulmonary fibrosis.

Distribution of Bronchiectasis

At CT, the distribution of bronchiectasis is often paramount in determining a differential diagnosis.

Although the craniocaudal and anteroposterior distributions are often the most helpful clues to an etiology, a central or peripheral predominance, symmetric or asymmetric distribution are also helpful to note[30] (**Box 1**).

Lower lung predominant

- Aspiration and prior infection are important causes of lower lobe–predominant bronchiectasis (**Fig. 9**). Chronic aspiration can occur in the bedridden and neurologically impaired, or in patients with chronic gastroesophageal reflux; direct damage to the airways occurs from acidic gastric contents, and a foreign body reaction can occur owing to aspirated food.[31] A relatively symmetric, basilar distribution of bronchiectasis can be a clue to aspiration, but some cases can be asymmetric, presumably owing to favoring of 1 decubitus position over another.

- Congenital immunodeficiencies cause frequent pneumonias from a young age, leading to direct damage to the airways and resulting cartilage loss, remodeling, and bronchiectasis. Congenital immunodeficiencies such as common variable immunodeficiency and agammaglobulinemia often cause a pronounced cystic and cylindrical bronchiectasis that is readily detected at both radiography and CT, most frequently present in the right middle lobe and lower lobes.[32] Fluid levels and mucoid impaction are often noted within dilated bronchi, and chronic bronchial wall thickening, tree-in-bud nodules and air trapping are common.

- Pulmonary fibrosis often causes traction bronchiectasis that is lower lobe predominant. Usual interstitial pneumonitis in diseases such as idiopathic pulmonary fibrosis and rheumatoid lung disease can cause a moderate amount of varicoid lower lobe traction bronchiectasis. However, fibrotic forms of nonspecific interstitial pneumonitis in connective tissue diseases such as scleroderma can cause much more striking lower lobe central traction bronchiectasis accompanied by adjacent bronchocentric ground glass opacities.[33]

- Alpha-1 antitrypsin deficiency often causes a panlobular pattern of lower lobe emphysema that can often be severe. However, clinically significant bronchiectasis (confirmed at CT, with history of abnormal sputum production) is a finding in a substantial percentage of cases (27% in one study),[34] and can appear in the lower lobes before emphysema is noticeable.[35]

Box 1
Selected etiologies of bronchiectasis by distribution

Central or midorder bronchi

- Mounier–Kuhn syndrome (trachea and bronchi)
- Williams–Campbell (midorder bronchi)

Lower Lung Predominant

- Aspiration
- Prior infection
- Congenital immunodeficiency
- Pulmonary fibrosis
- Bronchiolitis obliterans
- Alpha-1 antitrypsin deficiency

Mid to Upper Lung Predominant

- Cystic fibrosis
- Sarcoidosis
- Pneumoconiosis
- Tuberculosis
- Allergic bronchopulmonary aspergillosis

Anterior/Middle Lobe and Lingula Predominant

- Chronic *mycobacterium avium-intracellulare* infection
- Primary ciliary dyskinesia
- Acute respiratory distress syndrome fibrosis

Asymmetric or Focal

- Airway tumors and foreign bodies
- Swyer–James syndrome

Diffuse

- Bronchiolitis obliterans

Anterior, often middle lobe and lingula predominance

- Chronic mycobacterium avium intracellulare infection can cause an anterior predominant bronchiectasis that preferentially affects the right middle lobe and lingula (**Fig. 10**). *Mycobacterium avium-intracellulare* is the most common chronic atypical mycobacterial infection, and is seen predominantly in elderly females or in men with predisposing conditions such as COPD. Radiographs may suggest the diagnosis, with volume loss, bronchiectasis, and clustered nodules in the middle lobes and lingula. CT can confirm these features, and is also revealing in cases

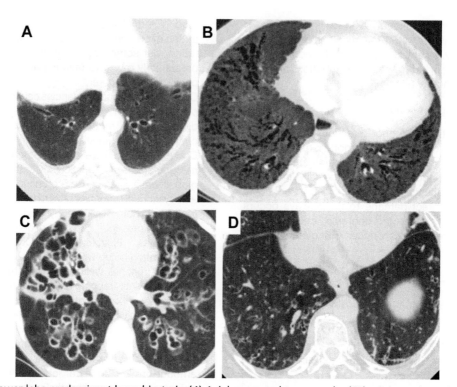

Fig. 9. Lower lobe-predominant bronchiectasis. (*A*) Axial computed tomography (CT) minimum intensity projection (minIP) reformatted image shows lower lobe bronchiectasis and mild bronchial wall thickening in a patient with reflux and symptoms of chronic aspiration. (*B*) Axial minIP reformatted CT image shows varicoid bronchiectasis within the lower lungs with adjacent ground glass opacity in a patient with scleroderma and a nonspecific interstitial pneumonitis pattern of interstitial lung disease; note the dilated distal esophagus. (*C*) Axial CT image of a patient with common variable immunodeficiency shows cystic and varicoid bronchiectasis with a lower zone distribution involving the lower lobes, middle lobe and lingua. (*D*) Axial CT image of a patient with alpha-1 antitrypsin deficiency shows lower lobe cylindrical bronchiectasis and bronchial wall thickening.

in which radiographic findings are subtle or confusing. Typical CT findings include bronchiectasis with clustered centrilobular nodules in the right middle lobe and lingula, often with a tree-in-bud pattern representing small airways mucoid impaction. These findings are often also seen in the anterior portions of the upper lobes, and to a lesser extent within the lower lobes. One study found that severity of bronchiectasis decreased with favorable sputum conversion (clearing of infection) under successful antimycobacterial drug therapy.[36]

- Primary ciliary dyskinesia is an autosomal-recessive congenital defect in any of a diverse set of mucosal ciliary proteins; patients develop repeated infections from a young age, leading to airway damage and bronchiectasis. The distribution tends to be right middle lobe and lingula predominant, a distribution seen in 100% of adult patients with the disorder and in 56% of pediatric patients in 1 series.[37] Substantial additional

involvement of the lower lobes is often noted. A subset of patients with primary cilia dyskinesia have Kartagener's syndrome, a triad of situs inversus, bronchiectasis, and chronic sinusitis.

- Acute respiratory distress syndrome fibrosis is a cause of chronic bronchiectasis and volume loss in the anterior lungs, usually with a middle lobe and lingula distribution. Damage to the airways is caused by prolonged mechanical ventilation, compounded by traction on the airways from parenchymal fibrosis of acute respiratory distress syndrome.[38] The characteristically gravitationally dependent consolidation in acute respiratory distress syndrome is thought to confer relative protection of the posterior lungs from ventilatory barotrauma, explaining the anterior predominance of bronchiectasis and fibrosis. Unlike cases of chronic *Mycobacterium avium* intracellulare infection, tree-in-bud nodules and mucoid impaction are usually not prominent features.

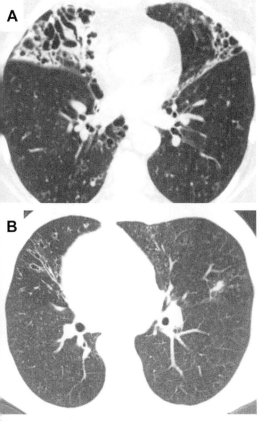

Fig. 10. Middle lobe and lingular predominant bronchiectasis. (A) Axial computed tomography (CT) image show right middle lobe and lingual predominant cystic and varicoid bronchiectasis in a patient with chronic *Mycobacterium avium* intracellulare infection. (B) Axial CT image shows right middle lobe predominant cylindrical bronchiectasis, scattered tree-in-bud nodules and dextrocardia/situs inversus in a patient with primary ciliary dyskinesia and Kartagener syndrome.

Mid to upper lung predominant

- Cystic fibrosis is a major cause of morbidity and mortality in children and young adults, with an average life expectancy of just over 40 years in 2013 (Fig. 11). Cystic fibrosis is caused by an autosomal-recessive defect in a key cell membrane chloride transporter that causes abnormally thick airway secretions, inhibiting normal ciliary clearance and causing chronic airway infection, leading to airway damage and bronchiectasis.[39] A classic tram track appearance of upper lobe predominant bronchiectasis can usually be noted on chest radiographs; nodular opacities along bronchial courses represent mucous plugging. Chest CT shows upper lobe predominant airway thickening, bronchiectasis,

and mucous plugging.[29] These findings can worsen to involve the remainder of the lungs and cause extensive architectural distortion as the disease progresses.

- Sarcoidosis, silicosis, and tuberculosis are granulomatous diseases that can cause traction bronchiectasis with a typically upper lung distribution; these diseases incite granuloma formation and subsequent fibrosis with traction on adjacent bronchi. Sarcoidosis can cause varicoid bronchiectasis, upper lobe volume loss, and bronchocentric architectural distortion,[40] with a "clumped" appearance of the centrally retracted bronchi.[30] In the fibrotic stages of sarcoidosis and silicosis, perilymphatic nodules can coalesce into large central upper lobe masses, termed "progressive massive fibrosis." Tuberculosis can cause architectural distortion in the upper lobes, with traction bronchiectasis that is frequently more asymmetric than that caused by sarcoidosis or pneumoconioses.[41] In 1 study, bronchiectasis was identified 71% of postprimary latent/inactive tuberculosis infections, and in 56% of cases of active infection, whereas tree-in-bud nodularity, consolidation, or cavities were more often found in active tuberculosis infection.[42]

- Allergic bronchopulmonary aspergillosis is a chronic airways disease caused by immune reaction to aspergillus colonization in the airways (Fig. 12). Patients typically have a history of asthma, chronic cough with thick secretions, and expectoration of often large mucous plugs, and have elevated immunoglobulin E antibodies. Radiographs can show branchial tubular opacities representing mucoid impaction of bronchi, the "finger-in-glove sign." Allergic bronchopulmonary aspergillosis cases typically show upper lobe predominance, central bronchiectasis, bronchial wall thickening, and at times pronounced mucoid impaction; high attenuation of mucous within bronchi is seen in approximately 30% of patients.[43]

Asymmetric or focal distribution

- Focal airway tumors and foreign bodies can cause bronchiectasis through a ball–valve mechanism of intermittent obstruction that results in elevated luminal pressures and often impaction of bronchi distal to the lesion. Endobronchial carcinoid tumors and other malignant and benign tumors can cause focal bronchiectasis, as can chronically impacted foreign bodies in the airways.[33]

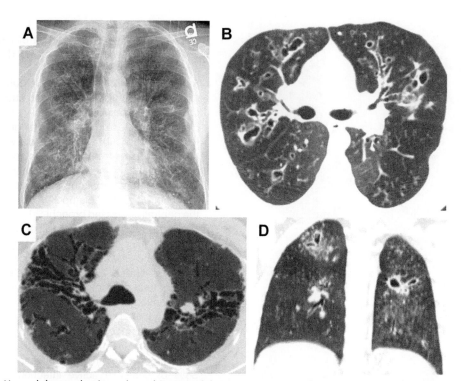

Fig. 11. Upper lobe-predominant bronchiectasis. (*A*) Posteroanterior radiograph of a young patient with cystic fibrosis shows extensive bilateral bronchial wall thickening and bronchiectasis, with an upper lobe predominance. Parallel branching tubular opacities have been called a "tram-track" appearance. (*B*) Axial computed tomography (CT) of the same patient shows bilateral symmetric cystic and cylindrical bronchiectasis and bronchial wall thickening; regional areas of parenchymal lucency represent air trapping. (*C*) Axial reformatted minimum intensity projection (minIP) image of a patient with sarcoidosis shows bilateral, symmetric, upper lobe varicoid bronchiectasis and bronchial retraction, a perilymphatic pattern of bronchiectasis. (*D*) Coronal reformatted minIP CT image of a patient with active tuberculosis shows upper lobe cystic bronchiectasis and bronchial wall thickening with upper lobe volume loss and upper lobe cavitation. Numerous tree-in-bud nodules represent endobronchial spread of infection.

- Swyer–James syndrome is an asymmetric bronchiolitis obliterans primarily affecting 1 lung, usually owing to a severe pneumonia in early life. The lung with primary involvement is usually smaller and more lucent than the contralateral lung, and shows a diffuse bronchiectasis that ranges from mild to severe (**Fig. 13**). In 1 study, all patients had cylindrical bronchiectasis in the lung primarily affected, and a subset had cystic and/or varicoid bronchiectasis.[44] A lesser degree of involvement of the contralateral lung is common.

Diffuse distribution

Bronchiolitis obliterans is the histology of chronic rejection in lung transplantation, with more than 60% of patients affected 3 years posttransplantation, and is the most common cause of death in the chronic setting.[45] Bronchiolitis obliterans can also be seen less frequently after other solid organ and bone marrow transplants, infections, exposures, and systemic inflammatory conditions. Although air trapping with mosaic attenuation is the most common finding at CT, bronchial wall thickening and bronchiectasis are also common findings (**Fig. 14**), especially in severe cases, with bronchiectasis present in 36% of lung transplant patients with confirmed bronchiolitis obliterans in 1 study.[46] When present, bronchiectasis is usually smooth and cylindrical, and often has a diffuse distribution. In severe cases, diffuse but uniform hyperlucency of the lungs at CT may be mistaken for normal lungs; the presence of even mild bronchiectasis and bronchial wall thickening can be a clue to the diagnosis in these cases.

AIRWAY NARROWING AND THICKENING: NEOPLASTIC CAUSES

Most tumors involving the central airways are caused by direct invasion by an adjacent tumor arising from the thyroid, lung, or esophagus.[47]

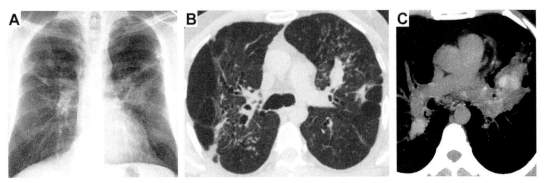

Fig. 12. Allergic bronchopulmonary aspergillosis. (*A*) Frontal chest radiograph shows central mid to upper lung branching opacities representing bronchiectasis and mucoid impaction, called the "finger-in-glove" sign. (*B*) Axial computed tomography (CT) image shows central bronchiectasis with the upper lobes with mucoid impaction. (*C*) Same CT viewed with lung windows shows high attenuation mucoid impaction within the bronchi owing to the iron and manganese content of mucous plugs in this condition.

Primary airway neoplasms are rare, comprising 1% to 2% of all respiratory tract tumors, and arise from the respiratory endothelium, salivary glands or mesenchymal tissue.[48] Benign neoplasms of the airway are more common in children (70%–80%) and uncommon in adults (10%). The vast majority of airways neoplasms are seen adults. Breast, colorectal, renal, lung, ovarian, thyroid, uterine, testicular, melanoma, and sarcomas all have the potential to metastasize to the airway but are extremely rare.[49]

Benign Neoplasms

- Hamartomas are the most common benign endobronchial neoplasms in adults.[50] Lesions are well-circumscribed, may contain fat or calcifications, and are usually solitary.[50] Endobronchial lesions are more likely to contain fat than parenchymal lesions. Most are not FDG avid, but atypical hamartomas may have increased FDG activity, mimicking malignant neoplasm.[5] Because these lesions are slow growing, they may be asymptomatic but they can cause airway obstruction resulting in cough, hemoptysis, dyspnea, or obstructive pneumonia.

- Papillomas are another common benign neoplasm of the trachea and larynx. The pathogenesis of laryngotracheal papillomatosis, also called recurrent respiratory papillomatosis, is through vertical transmission of the human papilloma viruses 6 and 11 during birth. These lesions may undergo malignant transformation to squamous cell carcinoma in 10% of cases.[50] Papillomas arise from the endothelium and may seem to be polypoid, sessile, or pedunculated (**Fig. 15**). Multiple lesions protruding into the trachea are common. Cavitary and polypoid lesions in the lung

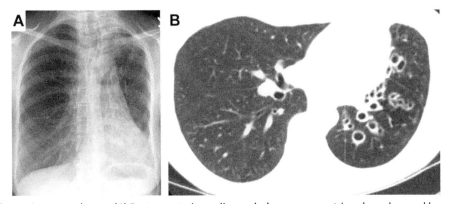

Fig. 13. Swyer–James syndrome. (*A*) Posteroanterior radiograph shows asymmetric volume loss and lucency of the left lung, with tubular branching structures along the central left lung in keeping with bronchiectasis. (*B*) Axial computed tomography image shows a small volume left lung with cylindrical bronchiectasis and bronchial wall thickening; the right lung is grossly normal in appearance.

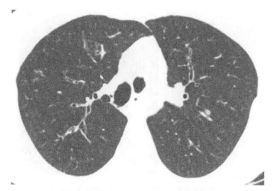

Fig. 14. Bronchiolitis obliterans (BO). A patient with BO several years after undergoing lung transplantation shows mild, bilateral, diffuse bronchiectasis and bronchial wall thickening.

parenchyma with irregular borders are a less common associated finding, occurring in less than 1% of patients.[50,51] Squamous cell papilloma is a rare, solitary type of human papillomavirus–associated papillomatosis in adults, most commonly presenting in men age 50 to 70 years of age. Malignant

transformation to invasive carcinoma is strongly associated with tobacco use.[52]

- Lipomas, chondromas, schwannomas, and leiomyomas are other rare benign endobronchial and endotracheal neoplasms.[49,50] Arising from interstitial adipose tissue, lipomas also grow slowly and seem to be pedunculated.[49] Chondromas are rare polypoid cartilaginous tumors that may have focal calcification. Schwannomas and leiomyomata are smooth, ovoid lesions. Schwannomas homogeneously and strongly enhance with intravenous contrast, whereas leiomyomata enhance only slightly. Leiomyomata may also have a large extraluminal component (iceberg tumor).[49]

Malignant Neoplasms

Malignant tumors of the tracheobronchial tree account for less than 1% of all thoracic malignancies.[53] Two-thirds of primary tumors arise from the surface endothelium (squamous cell carcinoma) or salivary glands (adenoid cystic carcinoma).[5,52] Other primary malignancies that occur

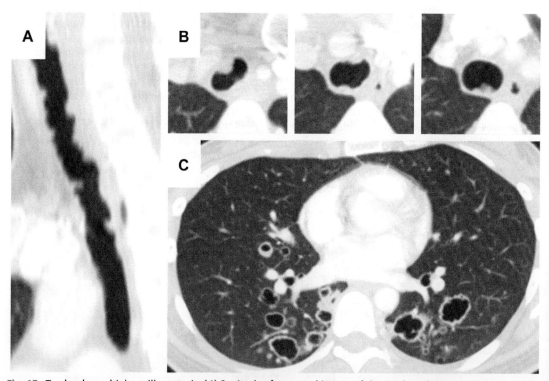

Fig. 15. Tracheobronchial papillomatosis. (*A*) Sagittal reformatted image of the trachea shows numerous nodules arising from the inner tracheal wall, representing multiple papillomata. (*B*) Sequential axial images show the polypoid nodules in multiple locations along the inner margin of the trachea. (*C*) Axial computed tomography at lung windows of the same patient shows multiple cavitary nodules with walls of varying thicknesses in the dependent lungs, a distribution common for parenchymal involvement in this disease. Squamous cell carcinoma can arise in the lungs or trachea in this condition.

n the tracheobronchial tree include mucoepidermoid carcinoma, carcinoid tumor, lymphoma, plasmacytoma, sarcoma, and adenocarcinoma.[5,48,49]

- Squamous cell carcinoma is related strongly to smoking and is most often seen in men in their sixth and seventh decades. These tumors typically arise from the posterior wall in the distal two-thirds of the trachea, and one-third of patients present with mediastinal or pulmonary metastases.[48] On CT, these tumors have a range of appearances—they may be polypoid and exophytic, focal and sessile, eccentric narrowing, or circumferential thickening (**Fig. 16**). These lesions seem to be irregular as they arise from the endothelium. On PET imaging, the majority are FDG avid.[5]
- Adenoid cystic carcinoma occurs with equal frequency in men and women, and typically presents in the fourth and fifth decades.[48] These slow-growing salivary gland neoplasms often extend circumferentially in the submucosal tissue and tend to have a smooth

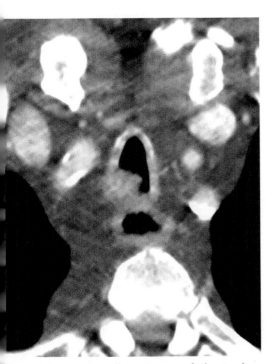

Fig. 16. Squamous cell carcinoma of the trachea. Coned-down axial computed tomography with soft tissue windows shows an irregular soft tissue mass arising from the right lateral wall of the upper trachea, with mild tracheal narrowing. The remainder of the cartilaginous trachea is mildly thickened and calcified, which can be a normal finding in older patients.

contour with intact epithelium, but can be invasive (**Fig. 17**).[5] Perineural extension is common and resection margins are often positive, but metastasis is uncommon.[48,54] Because of their slow growth and submucosal extension, patients with adenoid cystic carcinoma commonly presents with wheezing and stridor owing airway stenosis rather than hemoptysis, as typically seen in squamous cell carcinoma.[48]

- Mucoepidermoid carcinoma also arises from the salivary glands and is very rare (0.1%–0.2% of pulmonary malignancies).[5] It has been reported in patients as young as 4 and old as 78, but most are under the age of 30. The CT appearance is similar to carcinoid tumors: smoothly oval or lobulated mass with mild contrast enhancement and sometimes punctate calcification.[49] These tumors typically occur in the lobar or segmental bronchi, extend within the airways, and have variable FDG avidity.[5]
- Airway carcinoid tumors most often occur in the main, lobar, and segmental bronchi. These tumors may appear as small nodules within the airway, or may have a relatively small airway component with a large extraluminal lesion.[5] Similar to other neuroendocrine tumors, they are often highly vascular in nature, demonstrating intense contrast enhancement on CT, which helps to distinguish this lesion from a mucus plug.[5,49,55] Calcification is present in 25% of cases.[49] Typically, these tumors demonstrate low FDG activity, so PET imaging may not be helpful in assessing these lesions.[55]
- Primary malignant lymphoma is extremely rare and usually related to the mucosa-associated lymphoid tissue. On CT, these lesions can manifest as a solitary mass resulting in focal narrowing, or polypoid thickening of the airway wall owing to diffuse infiltration of the submucosa.[49]

AIRWAY NARROWING AND THICKENING: NONNEOPLASTIC CAUSES

Focal, multifocal, or diffuse airway narrowing may be congenital, traumatic/iatrogenic, infectious, or inflammatory in nature. It is important to characterize the location, length, and distribution of stenosis as well as the presence and distribution of airway wall thickening. The distribution of disease can be very helpful in determining the etiology; for example, disorders of the tracheal cartilage, which spares the posterior membranous wall of the trachea, may be diagnosed by imaging alone.[2]

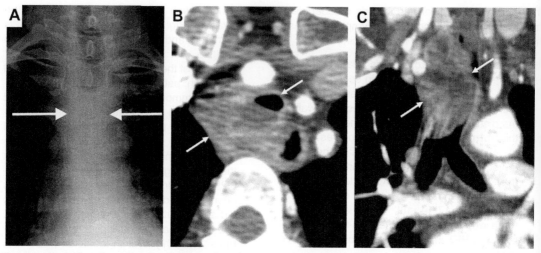

Fig. 17. Adenoid cystic carcinoma of the trachea. (A) Coned-down posteroanterior radiograph shows a mass (arrows) effacing the normal air column of the midtrachea. (B) Axial computed tomography (CT) image shows a large enhancing mass (arrows) with a central area of fluid attenuation; the mass narrows the trachea and displaces the esophagus. (C) Coronal reformatted CT image shows an infiltrative appearance of the mass (arrows), which extends over a long segment of the trachea and extends outside the tracheal wall.

- Congenital tracheal stenosis is caused by complete tracheal cartilaginous rings and absent or deficient posterior membranes. This rare entity may cause short or long segment stenosis and typically presents in the first year of life. Adults rarely presentation is rare but more common with short segment stenosis.[2] The trachea has an O-shaped lumen with complete rings but without wall thickening. Surgical resection is typically necessary.[2]
- Postintubation or tracheostomy stenosis is the most frequent reason for tracheal surgery,

and CT can accurately assess the stenosis for preoperative planning.[56] The stenosis—typically 1.5 to 2.5 cm in length—commonly occurs at the level of the tube balloon or at the tracheostomy stoma. Acute stenosis is characterized by eccentric or concentric edema or granulation tissue internal to normal-appearing tracheal cartilage whereas in chronic stenosis, the cartilage or posterior membrane is deformed and there is an "hourglass" configuration of the stenosis[2,13] (Fig. 18). Another iatrogenic cause of stenosis

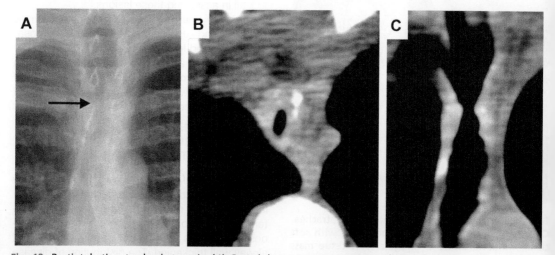

Fig. 18. Postintubation tracheal stenosis. (A) Coned-down posteroanterior radiograph shows a short segment narrowing of the intrathoracic trachea in a patient several months after prolonged intubation (arrow). (B, C) Axial and coronal computed tomography images at soft tissue windows show severe narrowing of the intrathoracic trachea several centimeters below the thoracic inlet; circumferential soft tissue represents granulation tissue, and a small amount of calcification is present.

is posttransplant stricture at the bronchial anastomosis, seen in approximately 10% of cases and typically occurring 2 to 4 weeks after transplantation.[57] External beam radiation to the lung is also a cause of bronchial stenosis, particularly in doses of greater than 70 Gy.[58]

- Tuberculosis is the most common infectious cause of airway stenosis. Airway stenosis in patients with tuberculosis may be caused by granulomatous involvement of the trachea or by extrinsic compression from enlarged lymph nodes. The left mainstem bronchus is most frequently involved. Irregular luminal narrowing with enhancement and wall thickening are seen in the acute stage, whereas in the fibrotic stage there is concentric thickening and uniform narrowing involving a long segment.[41]

- Relapsing polychondritis affects the tracheal cartilage and spares the posterior membrane of the trachea. Relapsing polychondritis is an autoimmune disorder that affects the cartilage of the peripheral joints, nose, ear, and airway. Airway involvement is seen in 50% of affected patients and may be focal or diffuse with smooth wall thickening of the anterior and lateral tracheal walls[18,59] (Fig. 19). Patients may be more symptomatic and have poorer prognosis owing to associated tracheomalacia, so it is important to assess for malacia

with dynamic expiratory CT.[2,18] Air trapping is another common feature.

- Tracheobronchopathia osteochondroplastica (TBO) is an idiopathic disease of the large airways that also spares the posterior membrane. Characterized by multiple submucosal osteocartilagenous nodules that may be focal or diffuse, TBO affects the distal two-thirds of the trachea and proximal mainstem bronchi. On CT, there is wavy thickening of the cartilage, calcified nodules sparing the posterior membrane, and long segment stenosis[59] (Fig. 20). In some cases, narrowing may be so severe that it is difficult to tell if there is involvement of the posterior membrane.[60]

- Granulomatosis with polyangitis (or Wegener's granulomatosis) is a systemic necrotizing granulomatous vasculitis that involves the upper airways (sinusitis, nasal mucosal ulcers, bone deformities and subglottic stenosis), lung, and kidneys. Thoracic involvement in granulomatosis with polyangitis most commonly presents as nodules or masses in the lung, but can affect the trachea in 14% and the main bronchi in 22% of patients[61] (Fig. 21). Focal disease is most common, usually affecting a 2- to 4-cm segment of airway, most commonly the subglottic trachea; however, involvement may also be multifocal. Nodular or smooth circumferential wall thickening distinguishes this entity from TBO and

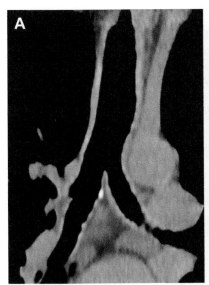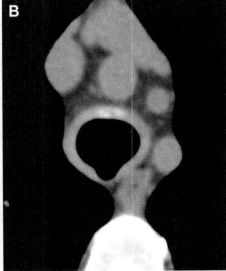

Fig. 19. Relapsing polychondritis. (A) Coronal reformatted image at soft tissue windows shows diffuse thickening of the tracheal wall, with a small amount of calcification. (B) Axial computed tomography image shows smooth thickening and mild calcification of the cartilaginous trachea with relative sparing of the posterior membranous trachea.

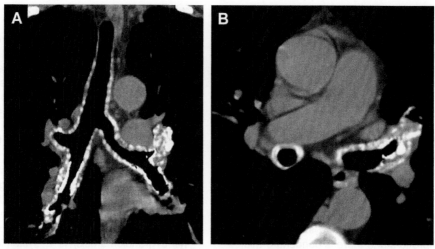

Fig. 20. Tracheobronchopathia osteochondroplastica. (*A*) Coronal reformatted computed tomography (CT) image at soft tissue windows shows extensive thickening and nodularity of the trachea and central bronchi, with a large amount of nodular calcification along the courses of the tracheal and bronchial cartilage. (*B*) Axial CT image shows these findings within the central bronchi.

relapsing polychondritis, which spare the posterior membrane. Airway stenosis is observed in 18% of patients, which may necessitate stenting or surgery.[62] In addition to the imaging findings, the diagnosis is confirmed by increased circulating antineutrophil cytoplasmic antibodies against proteinase 3.

- Amyloidosis may manifest as pulmonary nodules, alveolar and septal parenchymal disease, or airway involvement. Usually, submucosal plaques are found diffusely in the tracheobronchial tree. However, occasionally these plaques are solitary and may mimic an endobronchial neoplasm.[63] On CT, the airway wall may be high in attenuation from either ossification or calcification but, unlike TBO, the posterior membrane may be involved. The combination of long segmental stenosis and high attenuation wall is highly suggestive of amyloidosis[63] (**Fig. 22**).

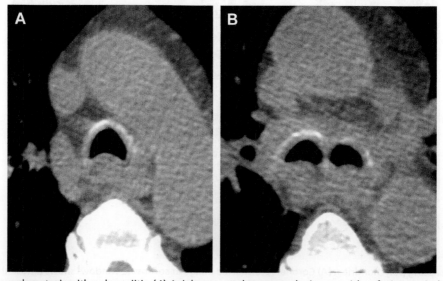

Fig. 21. Granulomatosis with polyangiitis. (*A*) Axial computed tomography image with soft tissue windows shows circumferential soft tissue thickening of the lower trachea with linear calcification. The posterior membranous trachea is not spared. (*B*) Image at the level of the carina shows similar findings involving the mainstem bronchi.

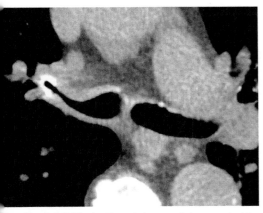

Fig. 22. Amyloidosis. Coned-down axial computed tomography image with soft tissue windows shows smooth thickening of the right mainstem and proximal right upper lobe bronchus, with calcification of the thickened airway. The left mainstem bronchus is involved to a minor extent.

SUMMARY

A wide variety of congenital and acquired conditions can affect the large airways. Although many large airway diseases are often first suspected at radiography, CT offers detailed characterization of airway abnormalities with a variety of reformatting techniques and dynamic expiratory protocols. Knowledge of the typical morphologies, distributions, and clinical backgrounds of large airway diseases is central to accurate diagnosis.

REFERENCES

1. Ross MH, Pawlina W. Histology: a text and atlas: with correlated cell and molecular biology. 5th edition. Baltimore (MD): Lippincott Williams & Wilkins; 2006.
2. Boiselle PM. Imaging of the large airways. Clin Chest Med 2008;29(1):181–93, vii.
3. Lee EY, Zucker EJ, Restrepo R, et al. Advanced large airway CT imaging in children: evolution from axial to 4-D assessment. Pediatr Radiol 2013;43(3): 285–97.
4. Kligerman S, Sharma A. Radiologic evaluation of the trachea. Semin Thorac Cardiovasc Surg 2009;21(3): 246–54.
5. Park CM, Goo JM, Lee HJ, et al. Tumors in the tracheobronchial tree: CT and FDG PET features. Radiographics 2009;29(1):55–71.
6. Koletsis EN, Kalogeropoulou C, Prodromaki E, et al. Tumoral and non-tumoral trachea stenoses: evaluation with three-dimensional CT and virtual bronchoscopy. J Cardiothorac Surg 2007;2:18.
7. Miyazaki T, Yamasaki N, Tsuchiya T, et al. Airway stent insertion simulated with a three-dimensional printed airway model. Ann Thorac Surg 2015;99(1): e21–3.
8. Wilson CA, Arthurs OJ, Black AE, et al. Printed three-dimensional airway model assists planning of single-lung ventilation in a small child. Br J Anaesth 2015;115(4):616–20.
9. Tam MD, Laycock SD, Brown JR, et al. 3D printing of an aortic aneurysm to facilitate decision making and device selection for endovascular aneurysm repair in complex neck anatomy. J Endovasc Ther 2013; 20(6):863–7.
10. Little BP. Approach to chest computed tomography. Clin Chest Med 2015;36(2):127–45, vii.
11. Washko GR, Diaz AA, Kim V, et al. Computed tomographic measures of airway morphology in smokers and never-smoking normals. J Appl Physiol (1985) 2014;116(6):668–73.
12. Hackx M, Gyssels E, Garcia TS, et al. Chronic obstructive pulmonary disease: CT quantification of airway dimensions, numbers of airways to measure, and effect of bronchodilation. Radiology 2015; 277(3):853–62.
13. Webb EM, Elicker BM, Webb WR. Using CT to diagnose nonneoplastic tracheal abnormalities: appearance of the tracheal wall. AJR Am J Roentgenol 2000;174(5):1315–21.
14. Kim SJ, Im JG, Kim IO, et al. Normal bronchial and pulmonary arterial diameters measured by thin section CT. J Comput Assist Tomogr 1995;19(3):365–9.
15. Matsuoka S, Uchiyama K, Shima H, et al. Bronchoarterial ratio and bronchial wall thickness on high-resolution CT in asymptomatic subjects: correlation with age and smoking. AJR Am J Roentgenol 2003;180(2):513–8.
16. Ridge CA, O'Donnell CR, Lee EY, et al. Tracheobronchomalacia: current concepts and controversies. J Thorac Imaging 2011;26(4):278–89.
17. Lee EY, Boiselle PM. Tracheobronchomalacia in infants and children: multidetector CT evaluation. Radiology 2009;252(1):7–22.
18. Lee KS, Ernst A, Trentham DE, et al. Relapsing polychondritis: prevalence of expiratory CT airway abnormalities. Radiology 2006;240(2):565–73.
19. Nishino M, Kuroki M, Roberts DH, et al. Bronchomalacia in sarcoidosis: evaluation on volumetric expiratory high-resolution CT of the lung. Acad Radiol 2005;12(5):596–601.
20. Boiselle PM, Ernst A. Tracheal morphology in patients with tracheomalacia: prevalence of inspiratory lunate and expiratory "frown" shapes. J Thorac Imaging 2006;21(3):190–6.
21. Boiselle PM, O'Donnell CR, Bankier AA, et al. Tracheal collapsibility in healthy volunteers during forced expiration: assessment with multidetector CT. Radiology 2009;252(1):255–62.
22. O'Donnell CR, Litmanovich D, Loring SH, et al. Age and sex dependence of forced expiratory central

airway collapse in healthy volunteers. Chest 2012; 142(1):168–74.

23. Litmanovich D, O'Donnell CR, Bankier AA, et al. Bronchial collapsibility at forced expiration in healthy volunteers: assessment with multidetector CT. Radiology 2010;257(2):560–7.

24. Greene R. "Saber-sheath" trachea: relation to chronic obstructive pulmonary disease. AJR Am J Roentgenol 1978;130(3):441–5.

25. Krustins E, Kravale Z, Buls A. Mounier-Kuhn syndrome or congenital tracheobronchomegaly: a literature review. Respir Med 2013;107(12):1822–8.

26. Krustins E. Mounier-Kuhn syndrome: a systematic analysis of 128 cases published within last 25 years. Clin Respir J 2016;10(1):3–10.

27. Noriega Aldave AP, William Saliski D. The clinical manifestations, diagnosis and management of Williams-Campbell syndrome. N Am J Med Sci 2014;6(9):429–32.

28. Manzke H. [Irreversible generalized pulmonary emphysema resulting from destructive bronchitis and bronchiolitis following adenovirus infection]. Klin Padiatr 1982;194(6):387–92.

29. Cartier Y, Kavanagh PV, Johkoh T, et al. Bronchiectasis: accuracy of high-resolution CT in the differentiation of specific diseases. AJR Am J Roentgenol 1999;173(1):47–52.

30. Milliron B, Henry TS, Veeraraghavan S, et al. Bronchiectasis: mechanisms and imaging clues of associated common and uncommon diseases. Radiographics 2015;35(4):1011–30.

31. Matsuse T, Oka T, Kida K, et al. Importance of diffuse aspiration bronchiolitis caused by chronic occult aspiration in the elderly. Chest 1996;110(5): 1289–93.

32. Touw CM, van de Ven AA, de Jong PA, et al. Detection of pulmonary complications in common variable immunodeficiency. Pediatr Allergy Immunol 2010; 21(5):793–805.

33. Javidan-Nejad C, Bhalla S. Bronchiectasis. Radiol Clin North Am 2009;47(2):289–306.

34. Parr DG, Guest PG, Reynolds JH, et al. Prevalence and impact of bronchiectasis in alpha1-antitrypsin deficiency. Am J Respir Crit Care Med 2007; 176(12):1215–21.

35. Shin MS, Ho KJ. Bronchiectasis in patients with alpha 1-antitrypsin deficiency. A rare occurrence? Chest 1993;104(5):1384–6.

36. Kuroishi S, Nakamura Y, Hayakawa H, et al. Mycobacterium avium complex disease: prognostic implication of high-resolution computed tomography findings. Eur Respir J 2008;32(1):147–52.

37. Kennedy MP, Noone PG, Leigh MW, et al. High-resolution CT of patients with primary ciliary dyskinesia. AJR Am J Roentgenol 2007;188(5):1232–8.

38. Treggiari MM, Romand JA, Martin JB, et al. Air cysts and bronchiectasis prevail in nondependent areas in severe acute respiratory distress syndrome: a computed tomographic study of ventilator-associated changes. Crit Care Med 2002;30(8):1747–52.

39. Spoonhower KA, Davis PB. Epidemiology of cystic fibrosis. Clin Chest Med 2016;37(1):1–8.

40. Nunes H, Uzunhan Y, Gille T, et al. Imaging of sarcoidosis of the airways and lung parenchyma and correlation with lung function. Eur Respir J 2012;40(3):750–65.

41. Kim HY, Song KS, Goo JM, et al. Thoracic sequelae and complications of tuberculosis. Radiographics 2001;21(4):839–58 [discussion: 859–60].

42. Hatipoglu ON, Osma E, Manisali M, et al. High resolution computed tomographic findings in pulmonary tuberculosis. Thorax 1996;51(4):397–402.

43. Jeong YJ, Kim KI, Seo IJ, et al. Eosinophilic lung diseases: a clinical, radiologic, and pathologic overview. Radiographics 2007;27(3):617–37 [discussion: 637–9].

44. Marti-Bonmati L, Ruiz Perales F, Catala F, et al. CT findings in Swyer-James syndrome. Radiology 1989;172(2):477–80.

45. Choi YW, Rossi SE, Palmer SM, et al. Bronchiolitis obliterans syndrome in lung transplant recipients: correlation of computed tomography findings with bronchiolitis obliterans syndrome stage. J Thorac Imaging 2003;18(2):72–9.

46. Leung AN, Fisher K, Valentine V, et al. Bronchiolitis obliterans after lung transplantation: detection using expiratory HRCT. Chest 1998;113(2):365–70.

47. Gamsu G, Webb WR. Computed-tomography of the trachea - normal and abnormal. Am J Roentgenol 1982;139(2):321–6.

48. Macchiarini P. Primary tracheal tumours. Lancet Oncol 2006;7(1):83–91.

49. Ferretti GR, Bithigoffer C, Righini CA, et al. Imaging of tumors of the trachea and central bronchi. Thorac Surg Clin 2010;20(1):31–45, xiii.

50. Wilson RW, Kirejczyk W. Pathological and radiological correlation of endobronchial neoplasms: Part I, Benign tumors. Ann Diagn Pathol 1997;1(1):31–46.

51. Marchiori E, Araujo Neto C, Meirelles GS, et al. Laryngotracheobronchial papillomatosis: findings on computed tomography scans of the chest. J Bras Pneumol 2008;34(12):1084–9.

52. Jamjoom L, Obusez EC, Kirsch J, et al. Computed tomography correlation of airway disease with bronchoscopy–part II: tracheal neoplasms. Curr Probl Diagn Radiol 2014;43(5):278–84.

53. Gaissert HA, Grillo HC, Shadmehr MB, et al. Long-term survival after resection of primary adenoid cystic and squamous cell carcinoma of the trachea and carina. Ann Thorac Surg 2004;78(6):1889–96 [discussion: 1896–7].

54. Shadmehr MB, Farzanegan R, Graili P, et al. Primary major airway tumors: management and results. Eur J Cardiothorac Surg 2011;39(5):749–54.

55. Chong S, Lee KS, Kim BT, et al. Integrated PET/CT of pulmonary neuroendocrine tumors: diagnostic and prognostic implications. AJR Am J Roentgenol 2007;188(5):1223–31.

56. Taha MS, Mostafa BE, Fahmy M, et al. Spiral CT virtual bronchoscopy with multiplanar reformatting in the evaluation of post-intubation tracheal stenosis: comparison between endoscopic, radiological and surgical findings. Eur Arch Otorhinolaryngol 2009; 266(6):863–6.

57. Ng YL, Paul N, Patsios D, et al. Imaging of lung transplantation: review. AJR Am J Roentgenol 2009;192(3 Suppl):S1–13 [quiz: S14–9].

58. Miller KL, Shafman TD, Anscher MS, et al. Bronchial stenosis: an underreported complication of high-dose external beam radiotherapy for lung cancer? Int J Radiat Oncol Biol Phys 2005;61(1):64–9.

59. Obusez EC, Jamjoom L, Kirsch J, et al. Computed tomography correlation of airway disease with bronchoscopy: part I–nonneoplastic large airway diseases. Curr Probl Diagn Radiol 2014;43(5): 268–77.

60. Restrepo S, Pandit M, Villamil MA, et al. Tracheo-bronchopathia osteochondroplastica: helical CT findings in 4 cases. J Thorac Imaging 2004;19(2): 112–6.

61. Lohrmann C, Uhl M, Kotter E, et al. Pulmonary manifestations of Wegener granulomatosis: CT findings in 57 patients and a review of the literature. Eur J Radiol 2005;53(3):471–7.

62. Martinez F, Chung JH, Digumarthy SR, et al. Common and uncommon manifestations of Wegener granulomatosis at chest CT: radiologic-pathologic correlation. Radiographics 2012;32(1): 51–69.

63. Czeyda-Pommersheim F, Hwang M, Chen SS, et al. Amyloidosis: modern cross-sectional imaging. Radiographics 2015;35(5):1381–92.

Index

Note: Page numbers of article titles are in **boldface** type.

Radiol Clin N Am 54 (2016) 1205–1212
http://dx.doi.org/10.1016/S0033-8389(16)30130-0
0033-8389/16/$ – see front matter

Statement of Ownership, Management, and Circulation
(All Periodicals Publications Except Requester Publications)

1. Publication Title	2. Publication Number	3. Filing Date
RADIOLOGIC CLINICS OF NORTH AMERICA	596 – 510	9/18/2016

4. Issue Frequency	5. Number of Issues Published Annually	6. Annual Subscription Price
JAN, MAR, MAY, JUL, SEP, NOV	6	$466.00

7. Complete Mailing Address of Known Office of Publication (Not printer) (Street, city, county, state, and ZIP+4®)

ELSEVIER INC.
360 PARK AVENUE SOUTH
NEW YORK, NY 10010-1710

Contact Person
STEPHEN R. BUSHING

Telephone (Include area code)
215-239-3688

8. Complete Mailing Address of Headquarters or General Business Office of Publisher (Not printer)

ELSEVIER INC.
360 PARK AVENUE SOUTH
NEW YORK, NY 10010-1710

9. Full Names and Complete Mailing Addresses of Publisher, Editor, and Managing Editor (Do not leave blank)

Publisher (Name and complete mailing address)

ADRIANNE BRIGIDO, ELSEVIER INC.
1600 JOHN F KENNEDY BLVD. SUITE 1800
PHILADELPHIA, PA 19103-2899

Editor (Name and complete mailing address)

JOHN VASSALLO, ELSEVIER INC.
1600 JOHN F KENNEDY BLVD. SUITE 1800
PHILADELPHIA, PA 19103-2899

Managing Editor (Name and complete mailing address)

PATRICK MANLEY, ELSEVIER INC.
1600 JOHN F KENNEDY BLVD. SUITE 1800
PHILADELPHIA, PA 19103-2899

10. Owner (Do not leave blank. If the publication is owned by a corporation, give the name and address of the corporation immediately followed by the names and addresses of all stockholders owning or holding 1 percent or more of the total amount of stock. If not owned by a corporation, give the names and addresses of the individual owners. If owned by a partnership or other unincorporated firm, give its name and address as well as those of each individual owner. If the publication is published by a nonprofit organization, give its name and address.)

Full Name	Complete Mailing Address
WHOLLY OWNED SUBSIDIARY OF REED/ELSEVIER US HOLDINGS	1600 JOHN F KENNEDY BLVD. SUITE 1800 PHILADELPHIA, PA 19103-2899

11. Known Bondholders, Mortgagees, and Other Security Holders Owning or Holding 1 Percent or More of Total Amount of Bonds, Mortgages, or Other Securities. If none, check box ► ☐ None

Full Name	Complete Mailing Address
N/A	

12. Tax Status (For completion by nonprofit organizations authorized to mail at nonprofit rates) (Check one)
The purpose, function, and nonprofit status of this organization and the exempt status for federal income tax purposes:
☐ Has Not Changed During Preceding 12 Months
☐ Has Changed During Preceding 12 Months (Publisher must submit explanation of change with this statement)

13. Publication Title	14. Issue Date for Circulation Data Below
RADIOLOGIC CLINICS OF NORTH AMERICA	JULY 2016

15. Extent and Nature of Circulation		Average No. Copies Each Issue During Preceding 12 Months	No. Copies of Single Issue Published Nearest to Filing Date
a. Total Number of Copies (Net press run)		1517	1597
b. Paid Circulation (By Mail and Outside the Mail)	(1) Mailed Outside-County Paid Subscriptions Stated on PS Form 3541 (Include paid distribution above nominal rate, advertiser's proof copies, and exchange copies)	774	914
	(2) Mailed In-County Paid Subscriptions Stated on PS Form 3541 (Include paid distribution above nominal rate, advertiser's proof copies, and exchange copies)	0	0
	(3) Paid Distribution Outside the Mails Including Sales Through Dealers and Carriers, Street Vendors, Counter Sales, and Other Paid Distribution Outside USPS®	316	392
	(4) Paid Distribution by Other Classes of Mail Through the USPS (e.g., First-Class Mail®)	0	0
c. Total Paid Distribution (Sum of 15b (1), (2), (3), and (4))		1090	1306
d. Free or Nominal Rate Distribution (By Mail and Outside the Mail)	(1) Free or Nominal Rate Outside-County Copies included on PS Form 3541	43	101
	(2) Free or Nominal Rate In-County Copies Included on PS Form 3541	0	0
	(3) Free or Nominal Rate Copies Mailed at Other Classes Through the USPS (e.g., First-Class Mail)	0	0
	(4) Free or Nominal Rate Distribution Outside the Mail (Carriers or other means)	0	0
e. Total Free or Nominal Rate Distribution (Sum of 15d (1), (2), (3) and (4))		43	101
f. Total Distribution (Sum of 15c and 15e)		1133	1407
g. Copies not Distributed (See Instructions to Publishers #4 (page 83))		384	190
h. Total (Sum of 15f and g)		1517	1597
i. Percent Paid (15c divided by 15f times 100)		96%	93%

* If you are claiming electronic copies, go to line 16 on page 3. If you are not claiming electronic copies, skip to line 17 on page 3.

16. Electronic Copy Circulation	Average No. Copies Each Issue During Preceding 12 Months	No. Copies of Single Issue Published Nearest to Filing Date
a. Paid Electronic Copies ►	0	0
b. Total Paid Print Copies (Line 15c) + Paid Electronic Copies (Line 16a) ►	1090	1306
c. Total Print Distribution (Line 15f) + Paid Electronic Copies (Line 16a) ►	1133	1407
d. Percent Paid (Both Print & Electronic Copies) (16b divided by 16c × 100) ►	96%	93%

☒ I certify that 50% of all my distributed copies (electronic and print) are paid above a nominal price.

17. Publication of Statement of Ownership

☒ If the publication is a general publication, publication of this statement is required. Will be printed in the NOVEMBER 2016 issue of this publication. ☐ Publication not required.

18. Signature and Title of Editor, Publisher, Business Manager, or Owner

STEPHEN R. BUSHING - INVENTORY DISTRIBUTION CONTROL MANAGER

Date 9/18/2016

I certify that all information furnished on this form is true and complete. I understand that anyone who furnishes false or misleading information on this form or who omits material or information requested on the form may be subject to criminal sanctions (including fines and imprisonment) and/or civil sanctions (including civil penalties).

Moving?

Make sure your subscription moves with you!

To notify us of your new address, find your **Clinics Account Number** (located on your mailing label above your name), and contact customer service at:

Email: journalscustomerservice-usa@elsevier.com

800-654-2452 (subscribers in the U.S. & Canada)
314-447-8871 (subscribers outside of the U.S. & Canada)

Fax number: 314-447-8029

Elsevier Health Sciences Division
Subscription Customer Service
3251 Riverport Lane
Maryland Heights, MO 63043

*To ensure uninterrupted delivery of your subscription, please notify us at least 4 weeks in advance of move.

Printed and bound by CPI Group (UK) Ltd, Croydon, CR0 4YY

08/05/2025

U1864693-0002